D1030235

TEXTBOOK OF MEN'S MENTAL HEALTH

TEXTBOOK OF MEN'S MENTAL HEALTH

Edited by

JON E. GRANT, M.D., M.P.H., J.D.

MARC N. POTENZA, M.D., PH.D.

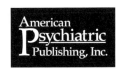

Washington, DC
London, England

Note: The authors have worked to ensure that all information in this book is accurate at the time of publication and consistent with general psychiatric and medical standards, and that information concerning drug dosages, schedules, and routes of administration is accurate at the time of publication and consistent with standards set by the U.S. Food and Drug Administration and the general medical community. As medical research and practice continue to advance, however, therapeutic standards may change. Moreover, specific situations may require a specific therapeutic response not included in this book. For these reasons and because human and mechanical errors sometimes occur, we recommend that readers follow the advice of physicians directly involved in their care or the care of a member of their family.

Books published by American Psychiatric Publishing, Inc., represent the views and opinions of the individual authors and do not necessarily represent the policies and opinions of APPI or the American Psychiatric Association.

All patient names in this book are fictional. To protect confidentiality, these cases are composites of several people's stories, and case details have been changed to protect patients.

Copyright © 2007 American Psychiatric Publishing, Inc.
ALL RIGHTS RESERVED

Manufactured in the United States of America on acid-free paper
10   09   08   07   06   5   4   3   2   1
First Edition

**WA
305
T3558
2007**

Typeset in Palatino and Futura Condensed.

American Psychiatric Publishing, Inc.
1000 Wilson Boulevard
Arlington, VA 22209–3901
www.appi.org

Library of Congress Cataloging-in-Publication Data
Textbook of men's mental health / edited by Jon E. Grant, Marc N. Potenza.—
    1st ed.
        p. ; cm.
    Includes bibliographical references and index.
    ISBN 1-58562-215-X (hardcover : alk. paper)
    1. Men—Mental health. 2. Men—Psychology.   I. Grant, Jon E.
II. Potenza, Marc N., 1965–   . III. Title: Men's mental health.
    [DNLM: 1. Men—psychology. 2. Mental Health. 3. Mental Disorders.
    4. Sex Factors.   WA 305 T3558 2006]
    RC451.4.M45T49 2006
    616.89'0081—dc22

                                                                    2006014699

British Library Cataloguing in Publication Data
A CIP record is available from the British Library.

CONTENTS

I

Boys and Men at Different Life Stages

II

Psychiatric Disorders in Men: Assessment and Treatment

III

Sociocultural Issues for Men

CONTRIBUTORS

DECLAN T. BARRY, PH.D.
Associate Research Scientist, Yale University School of Medicine, New Haven, Connecticut

DONALD W. BLACK, M.D.
Professor of Psychiatry, Department of Psychiatry, The University of Iowa Roy J. and Lucille A. Carver College of Medicine, Iowa City, Iowa

CARLOS BLANCO, M.D., PH.D.
Assistant Clinical Professor of Psychiatry, New York State Psychiatric Institute at Columbia University Medical Center, New York, New York

R. ANDREW CHAMBERS, M.D.
Director, Laboratory for Translational Neuroscience of Dual Diagnosis Disorders, Institute of Psychiatric Research, Department of Psychiatry, Indiana University School of Medicine, Indianapolis, Indiana

RANI DESAI, PH.D.
Associate Professor of Psychiatry and Epidemiology and Public Health, Yale University School of Medicine, West Haven, Connecticut

CAROLINE J. EASTON, PH.D.
Assistant Professor of Psychiatry, Director of Forensic Drug Diversion, and Director of Substance Abuse and Domestic Violence Services, Division of Substance Abuse, Department of Psychiatry, Yale University School of Medicine, New Haven, Connecticut

CRAIG A. ERICKSON, M.D.
Chief Resident in Psychiatry and Fellow in Child Psychiatry, Department of Psychiatry, Indiana University School of Medicine, Indianapolis, Indiana

JON E. GRANT, M.D., M.P.H., J.D.
Associate Professor of Psychiatry, University of Minnesota Medical Center, Minneapolis, Minnesota

SCOTT HALTZMAN, M.D.
Clinical Assistant Professor of Psychiatry and Human Behavior, Brown Medical School, Providence, Rhode Island

DAVID C. HODGINS, PH.D.
Professor of Psychology, Department of Psychology, University of Calgary, Alberta, Canada

NED HOLSTEIN, M.D., M.S.
Clinical Assistant Professor, Department of Community and Environmental Medicine, Mount Sinai School of Medicine, New York, New York

MICHAEL KING, M.D., PH.D., F.R.C.P., F.R.C.G.P., F.R.C.PSYCH.
Professor of Primary Care Psychiatry, Department of Mental Health Sciences, Royal Free and University College Medical School, London, England

ANN M. LAGGES, PH.D.
Assistant Professor of Clinical Psychology in Clinical Psychiatry, Co-chief, Mood Disorders Clinic, Riley Child and Adolescent Psychiatry Clinic, Riley Hospital for Children, Indiana University School of Medicine, Indianapolis, Indiana

YAEL LEVIN, B.A.
Research Assistant, Yale Depression Research Program and Department of Psychiatry, Yale University School of Medicine, New Haven, Connecticut

ORIANA VESGA LÓPEZ, M.D.
Assistant Clinical Professor of Psychiatry, New York State Psychiatric Institute at Columbia University Medical Center, New York, New York

DOLORES L. MANDEL, L.C.S.W.
Program Coordinator of Drug Diversion, Forensic Drug Diversion, and Director of Substance Abuse and Domestic Violence Services, Division of Substance Abuse, Department of Psychiatry, Yale University School of Medicine, New Haven, Connecticut

LAUREN N. MANNING, B.A.
Research Assistant, Northeast Program Evaluation Center, West Haven
Veterans Affairs Medical Center and Department of Psychiatry, Yale
University School of Medicine, New Haven, Connecticut

THOMAS J. MCMAHON, PH.D.
Associate Professor, Yale University School of Medicine, Department of
Psychiatry and Child Study Center, West Haven Mental Health Clinic,
West Haven, Connecticut

SHERRY B. MOSS, M.A.
Lecturer in Psychiatry, Harvard Medical School, Boston, Massachusetts

TARA M. NEAVINS, PH.D.
National Institute on Drug Abuse Postdoctoral Fellow, Forensic Drug Diversion, and Substance Abuse and Domestic Violence Services, Division
of Substance Abuse, Department of Psychiatry, Yale University School of
Medicine, New Haven, Connecticut

ROBERTO OLIVARDIA, PH.D.
Clinical Instructor of Psychology, Department of Psychiatry, Harvard
Medical School, Belmont, Massachusetts

DEBORAH A. PERLICK, PH.D.
Associate Professor of Psychiatry, Mount Sinai School of Medicine, New
York, New York

MARC N. POTENZA, M.D., PH.D.
Associate Professor of Psychiatry, Yale University School of Medicine,
New Haven, Connecticut

DAVID L. ROWLAND, PH.D.
Professor, Department of Psychology, Valparaiso University, Valparaiso,
Indiana

GERARD SANACORA, M.D., PH.D.
Director, Yale Depression Research Program and Associate Professor of
Psychiatry, Yale University School of Medicine, New Haven, Connecticut

ERIC L. SCOTT, PH.D.
Assistant Professor of Clinical Psychology in Clinical Psychiatry, Co-chief, OCD/Tic/Anxiety Disorders Clinic, Riley Child and Adolescent Psychiatry Clinic, Riley Hospital for Children, Indiana University School of Medicine, Indianapolis, Indiana

N. WILL SHEAD, M.SC.
Doctoral Student, Department of Psychology, University of Calgary, Alberta, Canada

STEVEN SOUTHWICK, M.D.
Professor of Psychiatry, Department of Psychiatry, Yale University School of Medicine, New Haven, Connecticut

AARON Z. SPECTOR, M.S.N., A.P.N.
Graduate Student, Yale University School of Nursing, Psychiatric and Mental Health Nursing Specialty Program, New Haven, Connecticut

DOLORES VOJVODA, M.D.
Assistant Professor of Psychiatry, Department of Psychiatry, Yale University School of Medicine, New Haven, Connecticut

INTRODUCTION

Since the late 1990s, the volume of research on gender issues in mental health has grown significantly. One important point that the gender literature has demonstrated, in addition to clarifying how women's health differs from that of men's, is how little we actually know about men's mental health concerns. Although the great body of research in mental health has historically been based on men, until recently the research has largely failed to address how male gender integrally influences the clinical presentation and treatment of various disorders. Thus this volume reflects an exciting moment in the history of men's mental health. Research on women's health has highlighted the important premise that diagnosis, etiology, prevention, and treatment efforts should carefully consider how men and women differ as well as how they are similar. This volume builds on this premise by presenting the latest research on what mental health care professionals should know about men's psychiatric issues.

Although many clinicians encounter men with mental health issues, many have never considered the unique issues faced by men at various stages in life or how men present differently with certain disorders. In addition, clinicians may be relatively unaware of how treatment responses in men differ from those in women. Thus, a primary aim of this book is to document salient aspects of men's mental health throughout the life span, the clinical presentation and treatment of various psychiatric disorders frequently observed in men, and sociocultural topics of particular relevance to men.

The first part of this text highlights three important stages in men's lives. Scott and Lagges (Chapter 1, "Childhood: Normal Development and Psychopathology") and Erickson and Chambers (Chapter 2, "Adolescence: Neurodevelopment and Behavioral Impulsivity") provide comprehensive descriptions of normal childhood and adolescent development, respectively, and highlight the major developmental issues encountered by boys and how boys differ from girls in their developmental trajectories. At the other end of the age spectrum, Desai (Chapter 3, "Older Men") describes the biopsychosocial changes that occur as men age.

A primary aim of this book is to provide clinicians with information on how men differ from and are similar to women with respect to clinical presentation and treatment of psychiatric disorders. As such, the second part of this text addresses areas of clinical care in which men present unique clinical issues. Disorders that are more prevalent in men are examined by Shead and Hodgins in Chapter 6, "Substance Use Disorders," and by Black in Chapter 7, "Antisocial Personality Disorder, Conduct Disorder, and Psychopathy." These chapters provide a comprehensive understanding of these various disorders as well as treatment approaches. Although the treatment of men's sexual functioning has made tremendous advances since 2000, few mental health clinicians address this important topic. To enhance the overall care of male patients, Rowland has provided an invaluable chapter on male sexual functioning (Chapter 8, "Sexual Health and Problems: Erectile Dysfunction, Premature Ejaculation, and Male Orgasmic Disorder").

Certain psychiatric disorders are seen less frequently in men. Therefore, when men present with these disorders, clinicians often assume that the presentation and treatment will be similar to what is seen and used in women. Disorders less commonly seen in men but with important clinical and treatment differences are explored by Blanco and López in Chapter 4, "Anxiety Disorders," by Levin and Sanacora in Chapter 5, "Depression," and by Vojvoda and Southwick in Chapter 10, "Posttraumatic Stress Disorder." Finally, in Chapter 9, "Impulse Control Disorders," we address certain disorders that are seen more frequently in men (pathological gambling, compulsive sexual behavior) and other disorders that are less commonly encountered (trichotillomania, kleptomania, compulsive buying).

The last section of the book, Part III, focuses on several sociocultural issues of particular salience to men. McMahon and Spector discuss the influence of fathers on the family and the impact of fathering on children's mental health in Chapter 11, "Fathering and the Mental Health of Men." Haltzman and colleagues examine how men think about and behave in intimate relationships in Chapter 12, "Men, Marriage, and Divorce." Body image, a problem long associated with women, has become a serious and underrecognized health issue for many men. Olivardia discusses the clinical presentation of and treatment options for male eating disorders, muscle dysmorphia, and steroid abuse in Chapter 13, "Body Image and Muscularity." Easton and colleagues address the complex issues underlying male aggression and violence and how various interventions offer hope for this public health problem in Chapter 14, "Aggression, Violence, and Domestic Abuse." Mental health issues appear to be intrinsically linked to issues of culture and ethnicity in men. In Chapter 15,

"Culture, Ethnicity, Race, and Men's Mental Health," Barry provides insight into how these factors may influence men's willingness to seek treatment and the effectiveness of the services offered. Because of the high rates of psychiatric disorders among gay men and gay men's reluctance to access mental health care, King has provided a thorough look at issues particular to gay men and how clinicians may better understand and address these concerns in Chapter 16, "Mental Health of Gay Men." Finally, an important clinical issue involves the reluctance of many men to access mental health treatment. In Chapter 17, "Overcoming Stigma and Barriers to Mental Health Treatment," Perlick and Manning examine the issues men face as they consider seeking help for their mental health problems and what clinicians may do to address these concerns.

In summary, men's mental health represents an important yet largely neglected area of clinical care. As the chapters of this volume eloquently attest, extraordinary progress has been made regarding how men with various psychiatric disorders present differently from women and how treatment interventions may need to be modified based on gender issues. This volume presents a multidisciplinary perspective on men's mental health issues by addressing developmental issues, incorporating psychosocial issues unique to men, and presenting treatment options for a wide array of psychiatric disorders. We hope that clinicians who wish to better understand how they can make wise decisions regarding the care and well-being of men with mental health issues will find this text valuable.

Jon E. Grant, M.D., M.P.H., J.D.
Marc N. Potenza, M.D., Ph.D.

PART I

BOYS AND MEN AT
DIFFERENT LIFE STAGES

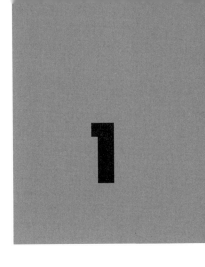

CHILDHOOD

Normal Development and Psychopathology

ERIC L. SCOTT, PH.D.

ANN M. LAGGES, PH.D.

Boys and girls differ during childhood in patterns of normal development and in the psychiatric disorders most frequently encountered. In this chapter, we focus on major developmental issues encountered by boys and girls and highlight how boys and girls differ in their developmental trajectories. For example, boys tend to acquire language more slowly and experience childhood psychiatric disorders like attention-deficit/hyperactivity disorder (ADHD) and autistic disorder more frequently than do girls. Additionally, we highlight areas in which male gender may be a protective factor that enhances the way children can cope with challenges along their developmental paths.

Case Vignette

Mrs. Smith brought her 12-year-old son, Tony, in for an evaluation at the local mental health clinic, believing he had significant mental health problems manifesting as behavioral outbursts, irritability, and a poor attention span. She saw some increased irritability at home, and his teachers complained that he was performing poorly in school, had been uncooperative and refused to do his work, had been fighting more with his peers, and appeared to be having staring spells. His appetite had waned lately, and he had always been a poor sleeper.

Upon his interview with the mental health professional, Tony was irritable and resentful of his mother for making the appointment, choosing to look at the floor of the office rather than make good eye contact. His minimal answers to questions usually ended with "I don't know." He vehemently denied feeling depressed but endorsed sleep and appetite problems, poor concentration, and irritability. He was somewhat hopeful about the future but expressed many comments such as "what difference does it make?" and "who cares?" He had dropped many contacts with his friends and was staying in his room more often than usual. His mother chalked up his behavior as a combination of the cold winter weather and changes in his interests in friends, particularly the drinking that she knew some of his friends were doing. The most bothersome portion for her was the decline in his school performance. She feared the educational implications that would accrue if this downward slide continued into high school.

Considerations in the diagnostic process for Tony would include any history of early attachment problems between Tony and his mother as well as recent stressors such as divorce or fights at school that could indicate a significant adjustment problem. Although the school personnel may consider Tony a prime candidate for ADHD, many of his problems are highly consistent with a major depressive disorder or a learning disability. In a thorough workup for each of these disorders, it may be helpful to observe Tony for several sessions alone, without his parents, and also to speak with the school personnel directly to rule out any learning difficulties. Finding out more about his family's history of depression or other affective problems may also offer a clue about both his genetic and his environmental loading for depression.

TYPICAL EMOTIONAL DEVELOPMENT AND MOOD DISORDERS

Infants are capable of expressing a range of emotions soon after birth. Being able to display feelings such as contentment, distress, and fear allows the infant to communicate on a basic level and therefore have basic needs met long before language develops. Smiling encourages adults to continue interaction, and cries of distress motivate caregivers to try to ascertain and remedy the source of the distress. Interestingly, a spontaneous neonatal smile, a startle response, distress, and disgust are all present at birth. A social smile appears at 4–6 weeks. Anger, surprise, and sadness can be expressed by 3–4 months. Fear and shame or shyness are observable at approximately ages 5–8 months, and contempt and guilt appear in the second year of life (Santrock 1990).

Early studies of gender differences suggested that girls and boys show few, if any, differences in emotional development before age 1 year (Maccoby and Jacklin 1974). However, findings emerged in the decades that followed and suggested that some gender differences in emotional functioning are apparent as early as birth. For example, during the neonatal period, male infants tend to smile less, be more irritable and difficult to soothe, and show greater emotional lability than female infants (Feldman et al. 1980).

Many of these gender differences appear to persist into the first year of life. Weinberg et al. (1999) explored these differences, using Tronick's face-to-face still-face paradigm. This interaction involves 2 minutes of the mother and infant playing, then 2 minutes of the mother looking at the infant, but not smiling, talking, or touching the infant, and finally, 2 minutes of the mother and infant playing (Tronick et al. 1978). The second segment of this procedure, the still-face portion, is theoretically the most difficult for the infants because they must regulate their own emotional state without any cues from their mother. Male infants displayed more difficulty than female infants in regulating their emotional states when faced with these abrupt shifts in interaction with their mothers (Weinberg et al. 1999). As a group, the boys displayed more negative emotion than did the girls during all three portions of the procedure, not just the still-face portion. One possible explanation for this finding is that male infants may rely more on emotional cues from and interaction with others to help regulate emotional states; girls may be more able to self-regulate at an earlier age. It is important to note, however, that individual differences were present; some girls in the study displayed high levels of negative emotion and some boys displayed relatively low levels of negative emotion during the exercise (Weinberg et al. 1999).

Studies have also shown that during the early childhood years, boys tend to show greater emotional effects from parental conflict and stress in caregivers (Kerig 1999; Laumakis et al. 1998). One possible explanation for this finding, given the previously discussed research involving younger children, is that during these early years boys may still be looking to their primary caregivers for assistance in emotional regulation. Highly stressed parents are unlikely to be able to provide calming cues for their young boys.

For many years, it was believed that boys were more vulnerable to parental conflict and environmental stressors throughout development. More recent research has suggested, however, that as girls and boys grow older, girls tend to be more vulnerable than boys to parental conflict; specifically, parental conflict during the adolescent years has been found to be more associated with depressive symptoms in girls than in boys (Davies and Lindsay 2004). One partial explanation for this difference may involve the social expectations for boys to become more independent and self-sufficient as they grow older, whereas girls are expected to become more connected with others on an emotional level as they enter adolescence.

These findings may in part explain why, during the prepubertal years, boys display a slightly higher rate of depressive disorders than do girls; after puberty, rates of depressive disorders in adolescents mirror the gender split of adults, with depressive disorders occurring about twice as frequently in girls than in boys (Hankin et al. 1998). A review of the literature exploring possible reasons for this gender by age interaction in rates of depression suggests that a number of factors are involved, including social (Davies and Lindsay 2004) and biological (Cyranowski et al. 2000) factors. Regarding biological factors, hormonal differences that appear in adolescence (Angold et al. 1998) as well as genetic factors (Merikangas et al. 1985) have been implicated in this gender by age interaction. Differences in gender-based socialization, such as the previously described expectation for girls to be more emotionally connected to others, are also likely to play a role (Wichstrom 1999). Kessler et al. (2001) suggested that cross-cultural studies are likely to be helpful in further separating biological and social influences on adolescent depression.

In considering a diagnosis of a depressive disorder in a boy, either major depression or dysthymic disorder, it is important to remember that in children, mood may be irritable rather than depressed or sad. Depressed boys often express their irritability by throwing tantrums or showing an increase in aggressive or destructive behavior. It is also important to remember that concentration problems can be a symptom of a depressive disorder rather than always indicating ADHD. Grades often drop due to these concentration problems, feelings of worthlessness, and the lack of motivation to do well in school associated with a broader experience of anhedonia; getting good grades is no longer pleasurable. When a boy presents with general "behavior problems," dropping grades, and concerns from parents and teachers regarding poor attention, the child should be screened for depressive disorders as well as the more commonly diagnosed ADHD.

Studies consistently indicate that the majority of both boys and girls diagnosed with depression also carry at least one comorbid diagnosis. Patterns of comorbidity differ with gender; girls are more likely to present with comorbid anxiety disorders, whereas boys are more likely to present with comorbid substance use disorders. Both girls and boys frequently present with comorbid conduct disorder (Kessler et al. 2001; Ruchkin and Schwab-Stone 2003).

Although gender by age differences in rates of depression have been well documented, no comparable differences have been found in rates of new-onset manic symptoms (Kessler 2000). In addition, no gender differences have been found regarding the frequency of cycling between manic and depressive episodes; suicidality; rates of specific manic symptoms such as elated mood, grandiosity, or racing thoughts; psychotic symptoms; or rates of comorbid oppositional defiant disorder (ODD; Geller et al. 2000). Boys diagnosed with bipolar disorder are, however, more likely than girls to carry a comorbid diagnosis of ADHD (Geller et al. 2000).

Suicide is the most serious possible outcome of depression or any other psychiatric disorder. Although it has been well documented that adolescent girls attempt suicide more often than adolescent boys, adolescent boys complete suicide at a higher rate (Salkind 2002). The most frequently cited explanation for the greater completion rate of suicide attempts by adolescent boys is that they tend to choose more violent, lethal methods such as firearms or hanging, whereas adolescent girls are more likely to use methods such as drug overdose that are more frequently less lethal (Salkind 2002). These findings suggest that the intersection between depression and impaired impulse control (see Chapter 9, "Impulse Control Disorders") may be particularly lethal for boys and men.

SOCIAL DEVELOPMENT

The first social task infants face involves forming an attachment to the caregiver. *Attachment* refers to the bond between a caregiver and the child that leads the child to feel safe, secure, and trusting that his or her needs will be met by the caregiver. Insecurely attached infants may be indifferent toward the caregiver or may simultaneously cling to and push away from the caregiver and appear inconsolable.

Although it is commonly believed that females are "more social" than males, research suggests that this supposition may not be the case for infants. Male infants were found to be more likely than female infants to look at, smile at, fuss for, reach to be picked up by, and vocalize to their mothers during a structured interaction (Weinberg et al. 1999). These authors suggest that this higher level of both positive and negative social behavior may serve to assist the infant boys in obtaining more assistance from their mothers in regulating their emotional states, such as when their mother smiles in response to their smile to confirm a happy mood or their mother soothing them in response to their distress. These types of interaction help assure the infant that his mother will help keep him comfortable emotionally and can further facilitate attachment.

Social demands and types of social interaction change as children grow older. The child's social world expands beyond the family, and peer relationships become increasingly important beginning in the preschool years. By middle childhood, friendships and group activities tend to play major roles in a child's life. Although individual differences are always present, boys as a group tend to form friendships based on common activities rather than the emotional intimacy more often cited by girls. Boys are also more likely than girls to select competitive over cooperative forms of play. Both boys and girls display aggression in their social relationships, but boys tend to display more overt forms of aggression, such as physical or verbal aggression, whereas girls tend to rely on more covert forms of aggression, such as social isolation (Salkind 2002).

LANGUAGE DEVELOPMENT AND DISORDERS

Infants typically begin to babble at about ages 3–6 months and usually speak their first words between 10 and 13 months. By ages 18–24 months, children are typically using two-word phrases. Between 27 and 34 months, children normally begin using three-word phrases and are able to use some basic grammatical principles such as plurals and past tense. At this age, they are also able to ask the ever-popular toddler "who, what, where, and why?" questions (Santrock 1990).

There has been some suggestion that expressive language delays are more common in boys (19.2%) than in girls (7.9%) up to approximately age 18 months (Horwitz et al. 2003). Because this difference seems to become nonsignificant in the age groups above 18 months, and because behavior problems first become significantly associated with language delay around age 30 months (Horwitz et al. 2003), it is unclear whether there are any clinically meaningful implications of this difference in the very young age group. It may simply be that boys are more likely than girls to show some initial delay in expressive language but that this delay may not be indicative of later pathology. Therefore, parents who note that their baby boy is not speaking quite as early as his sister did may not have cause for alarm.

COMMUNICATION DISORDERS AND PERVASIVE DEVELOPMENTAL DISORDERS

If an apparent delay persists beyond approximately 18 months, a thorough evaluation is warranted. Communication disorders listed in DSM-IV-TR (American Psychiatric Association 2000) include phonological disorder, expressive language disorder, mixed receptive-expressive language disorder, and stuttering, and all of these disorders are more common in males than in females.

If a language disturbance is accompanied by marked deficits in social functioning and the presence of difficulties such as stereotyped behavior or restricted interests, parents may wish to pursue an evaluation for autistic disorder or other pervasive developmental disorders. Autistic disorder is about four times more common in boys than in girls. Boys as a group, however, tend to have milder symptoms with less severe cognitive impairment (Fombonne 1998). Asperger's disorder, which is characterized by impairment in social interaction and restricted or stereotyped interests or behaviors, is also believed to be more common in boys than in girls (American Psychiatric Association 2000).

NORMAL FEAR AND ANXIETY DISORDERS

Most children experience mild to moderate fears during normal development (Ollendick 1983). Researchers have identified common themes of worry throughout the developmental trajectory, starting with fear of loud noises and strangers from ages 0 to 9 months. At age 1 year, children often begin having some fear of separation from caregivers and heightened alert around strangers. Continuing throughout the early years of development, children's fears are often of concrete objects, people, or stimuli. However, for children around ages 8–9 years, these fears become more abstract, corresponding to the more complex cognitive abilities of children of this age. This feature was illustrated by Kashani and Orvaschel (1990), who demonstrated that most adolescents feared social interactions and ridicule secondary to embarrassing social blunders. Younger children in this study showed much more fear of separation from caretakers and of strangers.

In the early years, attachment is an important element to consider when determining whether fears are developmentally appropriate or problematic. Attachment, as found by Ainsworth et al. (1978) in the Strange Situation Task, can categorize children into three types: securely attached (approximately 65% of children are in this category), avoidant (approximately 25%), and anxious/avoidant (10%). As mentioned earlier, attachment style can significantly influence the experience of normal childhood fears. Children with secure attachments show less fear of strangers and are more easily comforted by caretakers upon reunion during the Strange Situation Task. Attachment styles can have both immediate and more far-reaching implications for children. For example, Fagot and Kavanagh (1993) showed that boys with anxious and avoidant attachment styles were treated differently by their parents (i.e., these boys received less direction and guidance) than girls with the same attachment styles. As compared with insecurely attached girls, insecurely attached boys tended to show more aggression, attention-seeking behavior, and manipulation of peers (Turner 1991). Additionally, anxious and avoidant attachment styles in childhood have been highly predictive of later psychopathology (West et al. 1993). Unfortunately, little has been documented in terms of gender differences in childhood attachment styles. However, Williams and Blunk (2003) in their study of 52 mother–infant dyads found that the majority of boys (76%) but not girls (39%) were securely attached. In their study examining attachment as a protective factor against attention and behavior problems, Fearon and Belsky (2004) categorized more boys than girls into the avoidant attachment style (60% vs. 40%). No gender differences were found among the other attachment styles. Despite good attachment style in both males and females, attachment style did not protect against high levels of social risk for attention problems as reported by mothers—namely, poverty, poor educational opportunities, and poor maternal IQ. However, the study found that boys with avoidant attachment showed less inattention than did girls with avoidant attachment styles.

Gender Differences

In general, in both clinical and nonclinical samples boys show less anxiety and fear than girls (Albano et al. 1996; Ollendick 1983). Unlike the presentation of affective disorders, anxiety manifestation does not appear to have a significant gender by developmental age interaction. Following is a review of some of these gender differences.

Developmentally, one of the first anxiety disorders to present is separation anxiety disorder, with a typical onset between ages 7 and 9 years (Last et al. 1992). It is characterized by intense fear, sadness, emotional distress, and worry upon separation from a parent, caretaker, or guardian. Children fear permanent separation and harm befalling the parent in the child's absence (American Psychiatric Association 2000). Community samples of children show prevalence rates of separation anxiety disorder between 2% and 12% (Bowen et al. 1990; Kashani and Orvaschel 1990). However, children referred for psychiatric treatment have much higher rates, ranging from 29% to 45% (Last et al. 1992, 1996). Separation anxiety disorder follows a developmental course, with a peak between ages 6 and 12 years and declining prevalence thereafter (Weiss and Last 2001).

Two separate findings regarding separation anxiety disorder should be noted. First, the preponderance of children diagnosed with the disorder are female. Kashani and Orvaschel (1990) found that 21% of females compared with 4.8% of males in a community sample of children ages 8–17 years met the diagnosis of separation anxiety disorder. Other studies have found odds ratios between males and females to be between 0.4 (Anderson et al. 1987) and 0.56 (McGee et al. 1990). Second, most children (92% in one sample of children 5–18 years old) recovered from the disorder, but one-quarter subsequently developed other forms of pathology, most often a depressive disorder (Last et al. 1996). Male gender seems protective against anxiety disorder and may prevent an individual from later development of an affective disorder.

Male gender also appears protective against overanxious disorder, now called generalized anxiety disorder (GAD; American Psychiatric Association 2000). GAD is characterized by multiple fears causing clinically significant distress, including headaches, fatigue, stomachaches, and muscle tension. Age at onset within child and adolescent samples indicates GAD begins between ages 9 and 12 years but can be seen in younger children (Last et al. 1992). Children under age 12 generally show fewer symptoms of GAD than do their adolescent counterparts (Cohen et al. 1993; Kashani and Orvaschel 1990). Some studies show equivalent rates of the diagnosis between the genders during early childhood, when the diagnosis is less common, but later in life the prevalence estimates for GAD decrease for males and increase slightly for females over the course of adolescence into adulthood (Strauss et al. 1988; Werry 1991). The most common comorbidity among individuals with GAD during early childhood is ADHD or separation anxiety disorder, whereas in adolescence major depression and simple phobia are more frequently comorbid.

Although social phobia is a relatively rare anxiety disorder in the general population (<1%; Anderson et al. 1987), social phobia is more common among clinically referred samples of individuals, with estimates ranging from 27% to 30% (Last et al. 1992, 1996). Like panic disorder, typical age at onset for social phobia is later than that of separation anxiety disorder, occurring between ages 11 and 15 years (Last et al.

1992) and lasting well into adulthood, with a waxing and waning course (American Psychiatric Association 2000). More females than males are affected (Anderson et al. 1987; Francis et al. 1992; Last et al. 1992), with an odds ratio of 5 between females and males. Specific phobias show largely the same pattern as other anxiety disorders regarding gender distribution, but with a stronger preponderance of females.

Obsessive-compulsive disorder (OCD) does not follow the gender-based pattern for anxiety disorder with respect to prevalence estimates (Last and Strauss 1989; Last et al. 1992). Most studies show that slightly more boys than girls are affected by OCD, with some studies showing that 60% of referred males have the disorder.

Anxiety Summary

The developmental pathway of anxiety in children often follows their cognitive development. For example, younger children are more prone to fear the dark, separations, monsters, and strangers. As children's cognitive and abstract abilities develop, they become more sophisticated and complex in their fears. They start to fear social situations and evaluations by others along with developing a burgeoning sense of social importance. Others' perceptions of them mean more in adolescence than in elementary school. Male gender protects against fears, worries, and anxiety disorders. Whereas female rates of anxiety disorders begin to rise steadily throughout adolescence, male rates tend to remain fixed.

One recent theory for the explanation of the differences between males and females comes from Ginsburg and Silverman (2000). In a sample of 66 boys and girls between 6 and 11 years old, the investigators found that boys and girls scoring higher on self-reported masculine role orientation on the Children's Sex Role Inventory endorsed more statements of assertiveness, leadership, and confidence and had a lower number, frequency, and intensity of fears. Therapists often work to instill this kind of attitude and behavioral style in children of both genders during cognitive-behavioral therapy (e.g., Kendall's Coping Cat manual [Kendall 2000]). However, this assertiveness and confidence is often coupled with oppositional behavior and aggression, behaviors that often lead to more problems for boys, as is described in the following section.

ATTENTION AND BEHAVIOR

Ruff and Rothbart (1996) highlighted two attention systems that are important for the maintenance of attention in youngsters. The first system is *behavioral inhibition*, commonly thought of as "a specific class of behaviors of withdrawal, seeking comfort from a familiar person, and suppression of ongoing behavior, when confronted with unfamiliar people or novelty, as opposed to vocalizing, smiling, and interacting with the unfamiliar object or setting" (Craske 1997, p. A11). With increasing age, an infant or young child will continually develop increasing ability to attend to important stimuli while ignoring other distractions. Although this system has stability over time and across situations, a second system, labeled *attention*, is thought to be more important for sustaining vigilance during structured activities like the school setting. Attention to tasks is evident during infancy but, according to Ruff and Rothbart (1996), becomes increasingly important during the second year of life, continuing into adulthood. It is during this period that most gender differences in attention arise. ADHD, involving impairments in sustained attention and behavioral inhibition (Barkley 1998), is arguably most problematic for boys in school and other structured settings. Attention problems in males are often coupled with oppositional behavior and are more likely to initiate a referral to a mental health clinic. "The considerably higher rate of males among clinic samples of children compared to the community surveys seems to be due to referral bias in that males are more likely than females to be aggressive and antisocial and such behavior is more likely to get a child referred to a psychiatric clinic. Hence, more males than females with ADHD will get referred to such centers" (Barkley 1998, p. 85). Supporting this conclusion is the evidence that males are often more aggressive than females within community samples of children with ADHD but not among clinic samples (Gaub and Carlson 1997).

DSM-IV-TR states that between 3% and 5% of children manifest ADHD in one of its three forms. Symptoms include inattention, poor organizational skills, impulsivity, losing things, excessive fidgeting, frequently leaving one's seat in the classroom, and being easily distracted. The symptoms reach their peak during early childhood, after age 5, with hyperactivity declining throughout adolescence and into adulthood. Symptoms of inattention and poor organizational skills are likely to linger into adulthood. Importantly, males have the disorder more often than females, with reported male-to-female gender differences in ADHD ranging from 2:1 to 9:1.

In a meta-analysis examining the gender differences in boys and girls with and without ADHD, Gaub and Carlson (1997) found that impairments in several domains were not significantly different for boys and girls. These domains included impulsivity; math, reading, and spelling grades; social/peer functioning; and fine motor skills. Boys with ADHD, however, showed higher levels of inattention, more internalizing disorders, and more peer aggression. Boys with ADHD referred for treatment showed no greater risk for internalizing disorders than those not referred for treatment; this finding is in contrast to referred girls with ADHD, who showed substantially higher rates of anxiety than nonreferred girls with ADHD. Boys and girls with ADHD both show higher rates of aggression compared with non-ADHD peers, but among those with ADHD, boys show the highest rate of comorbid aggression. Finally, ADHD children of both genders who are being treated psychiatrically show high rates of impairment compared with their nontreated peers with ADHD.

In a study of aggression and violence in youth, males tended to view "walking away" and nonviolent resolution of problems as less masculine. Boys also tended to select active coping strategies as a way to prevent violence, such as learning to get along with others, compared with girls, who tended to want to avoid problematic situations (Reese et al. 2001). Boys tended not to focus as much on schoolwork or education compared with girls (Reese et al. 2001). Indeed, ODD as defined by DSM-IV-TR includes behaviors that are negativistic, hostile, and defiant toward authority figures and is more prevalent in males than females. Additionally, conduct disorder, a more severe form of ODD, is more prevalent in males, is usually seen in older children, and often leads to adult antisocial and criminal activity (Romano et al. 2001).

PLAY PROCESSES: ROUGH-AND-TUMBLE PLAY AND AGGRESSION

Play is an essential activity for a child's development (Erikson 1950; Frost et al. 2001; Piaget 1962). Play forms the backbone of children's daily lives; it encompasses children's social interactions, learning, and recreation. Providing an opportunity for children to engage in learning through play is a hallmark of childhood. Plato declared in *The Republic*, "Our children from their earliest years must take part in all the more lawful forms of play, for if they are not surrounded with such an atmosphere they can never grow up to be well conducted and virtuous citizens."

In the context of the earlier discussion of aggression, one particular type of play, termed *rough and tumble* (R&T), warrants specific discussion (Pellegrini and Smith 1998). R&T play is distinct from aggression and a normal part of children's everyday play. Aggression includes hitting with fists, pushing, and frowning, whereas R&T includes wrestling, jumping, hitting at, and laughing (Blurton-Jones 1976). During physically aggressive interactions, the use of demeaning language, insulting, harassing, crying, and grimacing are common, whereas laughter and smiling characterize R&T play bouts (Blurton-Jones 1976). Children's reports are positive after participating or watching R&T play on video clips (Boulton 1993). However, when viewing an aggressive interaction they correctly characterize it as negative and aversive (Smith and Boulton 1990).

The consequences of aggressive interactions and friendly play also differ such that directly after R&T play the children continue playing together either in more roughhousing or in other social games, such as tag, hopscotch, marbles, or jumping rope, but they move away from one another after aggression, with little likelihood of a friendship developing (Blurton-Jones 1976; Humphreys and Smith 1987; Pellegrini 1989). Play bouts rarely draw crowds of observers on a playground, whereas aggressive interactions draw other children's attention (Smith and Boulton 1990). Although the perceived aggression seen in R&T play is a healthy developmental stage for male children, aggression in male adolescence may be associated with a range of behavioral difficulties (see Chapter 2, "Adolescence: Neurodevelopment and Behavioral Impulsivity").

There is considerable debate within the developmental literature regarding gender differences in play (Maccoby 1997). Many researchers have concluded that boys' preferences of play partners, objects, and activities are different from those of girls, especially in mixed-gender social settings (Maccoby 1997; Maccoby and Jacklin 1987). Most researchers used playgrounds and other naturalistic settings where groups of boys and girls were together. Based on such studies, certain investigators have concluded that robust gender differences exist in the R&T play of boys and girls, with boys playing more roughly than girls (Humphreys and Smith 1987; Pellegrini 1989; Pellegrini and Smith 1998). However, others have found only modest gender differences (Blurton-Jones 1972; Boulton 1996; DiPietro 1981; Fry 1987; Maccoby and Jacklin 1987). Animal studies using mixed-gender groups in complex social situations yield large gender effects (Meaney and Stewart 1981), whereas "paired encounters" procedures generally do not (Panksepp and Beatty 1980). Similar observations have been made in studies of children (Scott and Panksepp 2003).

In a study of young (ages 3–6 years) same-gender, same-age play pairs, Scott and Panksepp (2003) found only a few modest differences between boys' and girls' R&T play behaviors. These findings contrast with those of previous studies of older children, in which gender differences were commonly identified (DePietro 1981; Humphreys and Smith 1984, 1987; Pellegrini 1989). Scott found that boys showed only modest increases in physical play solicitations like taps on the chest but no difference in wrestling-type behavior. Female pairs demonstrated more gross motor activities like rolling, walking, and gymnastics. In another review, Pellegrini and Smith (1998) noted a slightly higher rate of play solicitations among boys as compared with girls. Elsewhere, Pellegrini (1989) noted that boys were more likely to engage in physical contact play bouts than were girls and concluded that boys are generally rougher than girls.

Age influences the amount of R&T play. Humphreys and Smith (1984, 1987) reported a developmental curve in which 13% of 7-year-olds' time is spent in R&T play, but this percentage declines to 9% and 5%, respectively, in 9- and 11-year-olds. However, Boulton (1996) found no differences in the relative percentage of time spent in R&T play when he tested children ages 8–11 years. Scott and Panksepp (2003) studied the free play of children ages 3–6 years and performed separate analyses for two age groups (children ages 36–52 months and 52–72 months) and found no reliable and systematic differences in frequency of R&T play in these two age groups. These observations, combined with those of Humphreys and Smith (1987), suggest that R&T play remains constant until age 7, when it starts to decline in frequency.

In summary, when boys and girls play together, there may be a preponderance of male-generated R&T play, but in same-gender play pairs, those differences in frequency tend to diminish. Therefore, the common conception of males being rougher and displaying more aggression may in part reflect play within mixed-gender groups.

CONCLUSION

We have highlighted some of the normal trajectories of childhood development, including the cognitive and social development of children, and some of the important gender differences seen in the most common childhood psychiatric disorders. Much of the anecdotal evidence and many of the clinical impressions we have as clinicians are borne out in the literature. For example, males tend toward more aggressive expression of ADHD and depression, whereas females are less physical. Females have the preponderance of cases of anxiety, with the exception of OCD. We hope that this information will guide a thorough and comprehensive examination of the child, especially in those cases in which it may be easy to overlook some anxiety that overshadows aggressive behavioral outbursts.

Less intuitive differences or lack of differences between the genders is also highlighted in this chapter, including the section on R&T play. Much talk and some controversy exist over the frequency of R&T play among girls. Study results depend on how the act of R&T play is examined. Girls prefer a same-gender play partner without many onlookers, whereas boys will engage in R&T play in mixed-gender settings without regard to spectators' presence. This pattern could also have implications regarding aggression as well. Males consistently show little inhibition in their displays of aggression compared with females.

By highlighting gender differences, especially the unexpected ones, we hope that mental health professionals will be inspired to take a closer look at children of both genders to "expect the unexpected"—for example, aggression or pervasive developmental disorders in girls or anxiety in boys. Parents long for well-informed and compassionate care for their children when bringing them for mental health appointments. Our desire is for clinicians to be well informed in order to make good decisions about differential diagnoses in both boys and girls.

KEY POINTS

- Male gender seems protective against depression and anxiety when compared with rates in females.

- Male gender is a risk factor for attention problems, particularly for co-occurring aggression if ADHD is diagnosed.

- Despite a great deal of cultural perceptions that boys and girls engage in very different styles of play, these differences may largely be an artifact of the setting of the play. When children are in mixed-gender play groups, males tend toward more R&T play, but this difference largely dissolves in paired same-gender play situations.

PRACTICE GUIDELINES

1. The majority of both boys and girls diagnosed with depression also carry at least one comorbid diagnosis. Girls are more likely to present with anxiety disorders, whereas boys present with substance use disorders. However, both girls and boys frequently present with conduct disorder when depressed.

2. Be sure to assess males for anxiety disorders even though rates of anxiety disorders are higher among females. Anxiety can easily be overlooked as male children get closer to adulthood, as the gender gap widens, and rates of male anxiety disorders stay relatively stable as compared with a growing incidence of anxiety in females. The one exception is OCD, which is more commonly diagnosed in males than females across all age groups.

3. In assessments of children with ADHD-like symptoms, boys are more likely to be referred for treatment because of a co-occurring behavioral difficulty related to the behavioral inhibition inherent in the ADHD. Be sure to assess boys for their level of anxiety, aggression, and inattention, because these may be elevated compared with females.

REFERENCES

Ainsworth MS, Blehar MC, Waters E, et al: Patterns of Attachment: A Psychological Study of the Strange Situation. Oxford, England, Erlbaum, 1978

Albano AM, Chorpita BF, Barlow DH: Childhood anxiety disorders, in Child Psychopathology. Edited by Mash EJ, Barkley RA. New York, Guilford, 1996, pp 196–241

American Psychiatric Association: Diagnostic and Statistical Manual of Mental Disorders, 4th Edition, Text Revision. Washington, DC, American Psychiatric Association, 2000

Anderson JC, Williams S, McGee R, et al: DSM-III disorders in preadolescent children: prevalence in a large sample from a general population. Arch Gen Psychiatry 44:69–76, 1987

Angold A, Costello EJ, Worthman CM: Puberty and depression: the roles of age, pubertal status and pubertal timing. Psychol Med 28:51–61, 1998

Barkley R: Attention-Deficit Hyperactivity Disorder. New York, Guilford, 1998

Blurton-Jones N: Categories of child-child interaction, in Ethological Studies of Child Behavior. Edited by Blurton-Jones N. New York, Cambridge University Press, 1972, pp 97–127

Blurton-Jones N: Rough-and-tumble play among nursery school children, in Play: Its Role in Development and Evolution. Edited by Bruner JS, Jolly A, Sylva K. New York, Basic Books, 1976, pp 352–363

Boulton MJ: Children's abilities to distinguish between playful and aggressive fighting: a developmental perspective. British Journal of Developmental Psychology 11:249–263, 1993

Boulton MJ: A comparison of 8- and 11-year-old girls' and boys' participation in specific types of rough-and-tumble play and aggressive fighting: implications for functional hypotheses. Aggress Behav 22:271–287, 1996

Bowen RC, Offord DR, Boyle MH: The prevalence of overanxious disorder and separation anxiety disorder: results from the Ontario Child Health Study. J Am Acad Child Adolesc Psychiatry 29:753–758, 1990

Cohen P, Cohen J, Brook J: An epidemiological study of disorders in late childhood and adolescence, II: persistence of disorders. J Child Psychol Psychiatry 34:869–877, 1993

Craske MG: Fear and anxiety in children and adolescents. Bull Menninger Clin 61(suppl):A4–A36, 1997

Cyranowski JM, Frank E, Young E, et al: Adolescent onset of the gender difference in lifetime rates of major depression: a theoretical model. Arch Gen Psychiatry 57:21–27, 2000

Davies PT, Lindsay LL: Interpersonal conflict and adolescent adjustment: why does gender moderate early adolescent vulnerability? J Fam Psychol 18:160–170, 2004

DiPietro JA: Rough and tumble play: a function of gender. Dev Psychol 17:50–58, 1981

Erikson EH: Childhood and Society. New York, WW Norton,1950

Fagot BI, Kavanagh K: Parenting during the second year: effects of children's age, sex, and attachment classification. Child Dev 64:258–271, 1993

Fearon RMP, Belsky J: Attachment and attention: protection in relation to gender and cumulative social-contextual adversity. Child Dev 75:1677–1693, 2004

Feldman JF, Brody N, Miller SA: Sex differences in nonelicited neonatal behaviors. Merrill Palmer Q 26: 63–73, 1980

Fombonne E: Epidemiology of autism and related conditions, in Autism and Pervasive Developmental Disorders. Edited by Volkmar FR. Cambridge, England, Cambridge University Press, 1998, pp 32–63

Francis G, Last CG, Strauss CC: Avoidant disorder and social phobia in children and adolescents. J Am Acad Child Adolesc Psychiatry 31:1086–1089, 1992

Frost JL, Worthan S, Reifel S: Play and Child Development. Upper Saddle River, NJ, Merrill Prentice Hall, 2001

Fry DP: Difference between play fighting and serious fighting among Zapotec children. Ethol Sociobiol 8:285–306, 1987

Gaub M, Carlson CL: Gender differences in ADHD: a meta-analysis and critical review. J Am Acad Child Adolesc Psychiatry 36:1036–1045, 1997

Geller B, Zimerman B, Williams M, et al: Diagnostic characteristics of 93 cases of a prepubertal and early adolescent bipolar disorder phenotype by gender, puberty and comorbid attention deficit hyperactivity disorder. J Child Adolesc Psychopharmacol 10:157–164, 2000

Ginsburg GS, Silverman WK: Gender role orientation and fearfulness in children with anxiety disorders. J Anxiety Disord 14:57–67, 2000

Hankin BL, Abramson LY, Moffitt TE, et al: Development of depression from preadolescence to young adulthood: emerging gender differences in a 10-year longitudinal study. J Abnorm Psychol 107:128–140, 1998

Horwitz SM, Irwin JR, Briggs-Gowan MJ, et al: Language delay in a community cohort of young children. J Am Acad Child Adolesc Psychiatry 42:932–940, 2003

Humphreys A, Smith P: Rough-and-tumble in preschool and playground, in Play in Animals and Humans. Edited by Smith PK. London, England, Blackwell, 1984, pp 241–270

Humphreys A, Smith P: Rough-and-tumble, friendship, and dominance in schoolchildren: evidence for continuity and change with age. Child Dev 58:201–212, 1987

Kashani JH, Orvaschel H: A community study of anxiety in children and adolescents. Am J Psychiatry 147:313–318, 1990

Kendall P: Cognitive Behavioral Therapy for Anxious Children: Treatment Manual, 2nd Edition. Ardmore, PA, Workbook Publishing, 2000

Kerig PK: Gender issues in the effects of exposure to violence on children. Journal of Emotional Abuse 2:87–105, 1999

Kessler RC: Gender differences in major depression: epidemiologic findings, in Gender and Its Effect on Psychopathology. Edited by Frank E. Washington, DC, American Psychiatric Press, 2000, pp 61–84

Kessler RC, Avenevoli S, Merikangas KR: Mood disorders in children and adolescents: an epidemiologic perspective. Biol Psychiatry 49:1002–1014, 2001

Last CG, Strauss CC: Obsessive-compulsive disorder in childhood. J Anxiety Disord 3:294–302, 1989

Last CG, Perrin S, Hersen M, et al: DSM-III-R anxiety disorders in children: sociodemographic and clinical characteristics. J Am Acad Child Adolesc Psychiatry 31:1070–1076, 1992

Last CG, Perrin S, Hersen M, et al: A prospective study of childhood anxiety disorders. J Am Acad Child Adolesc Psychiatry 35:1502–1510, 1996

Laumakis MA, Margolin G, John RS: The emotional, cognitive, and coping responses of preadolescent children to different dimensions of conflict, in Children Exposed to Marital Violence: Theory, Research, and Applied Issues. Edited by Holden GW, Geffner R, Jouriles EN. Washington, DC, American Psychological Association, 1998, pp 257–288

Maccoby EE: Gender and relationships: a developmental account. Am Psychol 45:513–520, 1997

Maccoby EE, Jacklin C: The Psychology of Sex Differences. Stanford, CA, Stanford University Press, 1974

Maccoby EE, Jacklin CN: Gender segregation in childhood, in Advances in Child Development and Behavior, Vol 20. Edited by Reese HW. New York, Academic Press, 1987, pp 239–288

McGee R, Feehan M, Williams S, et al: DSM-III disorders in a large sample of adolescents. J Am Acad Child Adolesc Psychiatry 29:611–619, 1990

Meaney MJ, Stewart J: Neonatal androgens influence the social play of prepubescent rats. Horm Behav 15:197–213, 1981

Merikangas KR, Weissman MM, Pauls DL: Genetic factors in the sex ratio of major depression. Psychol Med 15:63– 69, 1985

Ollendick TH: Reliability and validity of the revised Fear Survey Schedule for Children (FSSC-R). Behav Res Ther 21:395–399, 1983

Panksepp J, Beatty WW: Social deprivation and play in rats. Behav Neural Biol 30:197–206, 1980

Pellegrini AD: Elementary school children's rough-and-tumble play. Early Child Res Q 4:245–260, 1989

Pellegrini AD, Smith PK: Physical activity play: the nature and function of a neglected aspect of play. Child Dev 69:577–598, 1998

Piaget J: Play, Dreams and Imitation in Childhood. New York, WW Norton, 1962

Reese LE, Vera EM, Thompson K, et al: A qualitative investigation of perceptions of violence risk factors in low-income African American children. J Clin Child Psychol 30:161–171, 2001

Romano E, Tremblay RE, Vitaro F, et al: Prevalence of psychiatric diagnoses and the role of perceived impairment: findings from an adolescent community sample. J Child Psychol Psychiatry 42:451–461, 2001

Ruchkin V, Schwab-Stone M: What can we learn from developmental studies of psychiatric disorders? Lancet 362:1951–1952, 2003

Ruff HA, Rothbart MK: Attention in Early Development. New York, Oxford University Press, 1996

Salkind NJ (ed): Child Development (Macmillan Psychology Reference Series). New York, Macmillan Reference USA, 2002

Santrock JW: Children, 2nd Edition. Dubuque, IA, William C Brown Publishers, 1990

Scott E, Panksepp J: Rough-and-tumble play in human children. Aggress Behav 29:539–551, 2003

Smith P, Boulton M: Rough-and-tumble play, aggression and dominance: perception and behavior in children's encounters. Hum Dev 33:271–282, 1990

Strauss CC, Lease CA, Last CG, et al: Overanxious disorder: an examination of developmental differences. J Abnorm Child Psychol 16:433–443, 1988

Tronick EZ, Als H, Adamson L, et al: The infant's response to entrapment between contradictory messages in face-to-face interaction. J Am Acad Child Psychiatry 17:1–13, 1978

Turner PJ: Relations between attachment, gender, and behavior with peers in preschool. Child Dev 62:1475–1488, 1991

Weinberg MK, Tronick EZ, Cohn JF, et al: Gender differences in emotional expressivity and self-regulation during early infancy. Dev Psychol 35:175–188, 1999

Weiss DD, Last CG: Developmental variations in the prevalence and manifestations of anxiety disorders, in The Developmental Psychopathology of Anxiety. Edited by Vasey MW, Dadds MR. New York, Oxford University Press, 2001

Werry JS: Overanxious disorder: a review of its taxonomic properties. J Am Acad Child Adolesc Psychiatry 30:533–544, 1991

West M, Rose MS, Sheldon A: Anxious attachment as a determinant of adult psychopathology. J Nerv Ment Dis 181:422–427, 1993

Wichstrom L: The emergence of gender difference in depressed mood during adolescence: the role of intensified gender socialization. Dev Psychol 35: 232–245, 1999

Williams SW, Blunk EM: Sex differences in infant–mother attachment. Psychol Rep 92:84–88, 2003

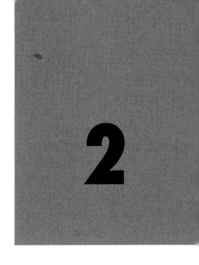

2

ADOLESCENCE

Neurodevelopment and Behavioral Impulsivity

CRAIG A. ERICKSON, M.D.

R. ANDREW CHAMBERS, M.D.

Case Vignette

After 17 years of a troubled marriage marked by frequent absences of the husband due to job requirements, episodes of infidelity, and fighting when both spouses were drinking, Mr. and Ms. Morris decided to divorce. Their two children, Sarah, 13, and Brian, 15, had previously presented as normally adjusted children, active in school and performing better than average academically.

In the 2-year period after Mr. Morris moved out of the house to another city with his girlfriend, both children experienced increasing difficulties. Sarah began to isolate herself more frequently in her bedroom, had frequent crying spells and trouble sleeping, and told her mother that she was becoming scared of her older brother and his friends. Brian began experimenting with marijuana, alcohol, and prescription drugs, including painkillers and sedatives acquired from his peers. On several occasions, he brazenly smoked marijuana in the house and was at other times suspected of being intoxicated on unknown substances. A threatening verbal conflict with his family members resulted in the police being called, and on a separate occasion he was arrested for underage drinking. In one "practical joke" on his mother, Brian filled his mother's clothes drawers and wardrobe with dried cat food. Brian also began staying out at night with a group of his peers who engaged in vandalism, including one incident in which the group rigged a neighbor's mailbox with fireworks and filmed them going off with the home video camera. At school, his grades dropped, and he was recommended for assessment for attention-deficit/hyperactivity disorder (ADHD). A diagnosis of ADHD was made, and Brian was placed on a psychostimulant medication. Soon after this treatment was initiated, Brian was noted to have scored the highest in the school district on yearly academic achievement tests taken just before the ADHD diagnosis. However, new concerns emerged that he was sharing the medication with his friends.

The medication treatment for Brian was stopped. Family and individual psychotherapy for both Sarah and Brian was begun, and Sarah demonstrated remission of her depressive symptoms. Over the next 2 years, Brian stopped experimenting with drugs, acquired a stable dating relationship, and went on to college, which he reported liking much more than high school.

Adolescence is a period of significant change in the brain and body, encompassing alterations in cognitive, emotional, motor, and motivational spheres of functioning. Adolescent neurodevelopment transforms the brain from a childhood design optimized for learning, play, and receiving adult care and resources to a configuration optimized for being a care or resource provider in adult social and occupational roles. In this chapter we describe emerging evidence suggesting that gender differences in brain structure and function interact with adolescent neurodevelopmental events in producing differential vulnerabilities to psychiatric disorders in adulthood. Adolescent neurodevelopment is associated with greater risk-taking, sensation seeking, and impulsive behavior in the exploration of adult roles, especially in boys. Superimposed on a background of a greater tendency toward externalizing disorders, or disorders involving aspects of motor control in young boys, brain changes of adolescence may render males more likely to have a variety of impulse control or motivational disorders in adulthood.

NEUROPSYCHOLOGICAL AND PSYCHIATRIC PROFILES OF MALES IN CHILDHOOD AND ADULTHOOD

Although the existence of and causes behind gender differences in higher-order brain function have long been a topic of debate (Craig et al. 2004), mounting evidence suggests that neuropsychological profiles of males and females do trend differently across ages (Constantino and Todd 2003; Grant et al. 2004). Moreover, differential rates of psychiatric disorders between boys and girls and men and women lend credence to the notion that normative gender differences in brain function instill differential vulnerabilities to psychopathology (Grant et al. 2004; Mash and Dozois 1996).

Neurobehavioral differences between healthy boys and girls have been noted even before and shortly after birth, when male fetuses and babies exhibit increased limb movements (Almli et al. 2001). These differences in psychomotor behavior appear to continue into toddlerhood, as boys tend to show increased rough and tumble play (Pellegrini and Smith 1998) and less symbolic play (Lyytinen et al. 1999) compared with girls (see Chapter 1, "Childhood: Normal Development and Psychopathology"). Still other gender differences encompassing cognitive, sensory processing, emotional, and social behaviors are apparent in early childhood (Braungart-Ricker et al. 1998; Eisenberg et al. 1989; Lundqvist and Sabel 2000; Lundqvist-Person 2001; Malcolm et al. 2002; Weinberg et al. 1999). Toward grade-school ages, these trends continue as the developmental course of boys is marked by increased interest in and displays of externalizing behavior involving physical, nonverbal interactions with the environment or social peers (Mash and Dozois 1996). Boys appear to excel particularly well in visual-spatial skills and mathematics, possibly reflecting some cognitive specialization toward psychomotor interactions with the physical (nonsocial) environment (de Coutern-Myers 1999; Hyde et al. 1990; Silverman and Eals 1992). This propensity in boys contrasts with the internalizing behaviors predominant in girls, which involve emotion-laden perceptions of self and others, increased social aptitude, and verbal communication skills—behaviors that possibly reflect increased specialization toward interactions with the psychosocial milieu (Eisenberg et al. 1995; Thayer and Johnsen 2000). For instance, girls ages 7–15 years show higher social responsiveness and understanding compared with similar-age boys (Constantino and Todd 2003). It remains unclear to what extent these gender trends result from 1) neurogenetic programming responding to evolutionary pressures that favor gender-role dichotomization or 2) the tendency for parenting and culture to instill such gender-biased phenotypes through learning (Hinshaw 2003; Silverman and Eals 1992). Nevertheless, because genes and environmental learning both influence brain form and function, some neurobiological foundation likely supports a tendency toward greater specialization of what might be called cognitive-motivational-motor functioning in boys and cognitive-social-emotional functioning in girls.

Compared with trends in healthy functioning, differentiated forms of psychopathology occurring in boys and girls follow a similar but perhaps more pronounced dichotomization. Preadolescent boys suffer significantly more than girls from the following disorders: pervasive developmental disorders (Klinger et al. 2003), attention-deficit/hyperactivity disorder (ADHD; Barkley 1996), oppositional defiant disorder (Hinshaw and Lee 2003), conduct disorder (Hinshaw and Lee 2003), obsessive-compulsive disorder (Mash and Dozois 1996), and Tourette's syndrome or tic disorders (Giedd 1996). Notably, not only are all of these disorders frequently comorbid in preadolescent boys in various combinations but these disorders also collectively involve core symptoms associated with *dysregulated* behavior within the cognitive-motivational-motor domain, often in association with *deficits* of functionality in the cognitive-social-emotional domain. In contrast, preadolescent girls tend to show greater likelihood for disorders involving the expression of anxiety symptoms (Crick and Zahn-Waxler 2003; Lewinsohn et al. 1998), but without robust behavioral dysregulation. Thus girls may tend to show dysregulated functionality rather than deficits in the cognitive-social-emotional domain while being relatively resistant to dysregulation of behavior within the cognitive-motivational-motor domain.

From an engineering standpoint, evidence for gender trends in healthy mental functioning and psychiatric disorders in childhood suggest that some degree of functional specialization toward cognitive-motivational-motor faculties in boys versus cognitive-social-emotional faculties in girls corresponds to a greater complexity of neurobiological systems that serve each of these gender-biased functional sets. Although such neurobehavioral specialization may protect against deficits within a functional set, increased neurobiological complexity required for such specialization may entail greater vulnerability to dysregulated performance within the functional set, particularly during the complex changes of the brain occurring in adolescence. Thus the prevalence distributions of adult forms of psychopathology show gender trends that appear in many ways to elaborate on or accentuate childhood dichotomizations. For instance, men appear to be particularly vulnerable to disorders of motivation and psychomotor impulse control, showing a 2:1 margin over women in prevalence of alcohol and other substance use disorders, antisocial personality, and completed acts of suicide and homicide (Grant et al. 2004; Kaplan and Sadock 2000). In contrast, women have greater vulnerability, with a greater than 2:1 ratio compared with men, for major depressive and anxiety disorders, borderline personality disorder, and expressions of suicidal ideation rather than completed acts (Grant et al. 2004; Kaplan and Sadock 2000). Even for major psychotic disorders such as schizophrenia and bipolar disorder, in which the prevalence distributions are evenly divided between the genders, there appear to be similar gender-specific subsyn-dromal trends. For instance, males with schizophrenia are particularly vulnerable to developing substance use disorders, have earlier-onset schizophrenia, and appear to have greater deficits within the cognitive-social-emotional sphere of functioning (Lindamer et al. 2003; Opler et al. 2001). In bipolar disorder, some evidence suggests that men may have a higher proportion of manic-impulsive episodes, whereas fe-males may be more prone to the depressive phases of the disorder (Ar-nold 2003; Roy-Byrne et al. 1985).

In sum, both healthy traits and patterns of psychopathology show gender-biased trends through early childhood, adolescence, and adult ages. Characteristics of normative traits and psychopathology commonly emerging during adolescence may relate to the increased complexity and refinement of particular neural systems occurring in adolescent neuro-development (Figure 2–1).

ADOLESCENT BEHAVIOR, IMPULSIVITY, AND PSYCHOPATHOLOGY

Normal adolescence is typified by increased interest in and motivation toward novelty and sensation seeking, associated with a developmen-tally unprecedented desire to explore adult behavior and roles through active participation (Moore and Rosenthal 1992; Yates 1996). Changing cognitive, emotional, motor, and motivational faculties compel or result from adolescent fascination with, and participation in, popular music, fashion, social gatherings, group memberships, sexuality, competition in sports and academia, use of adult tools (e.g., automobile driving), and adult occupational roles (Moore and Rosenthal 1992; Siegel and Shaughnessy 1995).

Yet the interest in and capacity for adult things in adolescence car-ries the risk of inexperience. Despite adolescence being characterized as a time of physical vitality and resilience, overall morbidity and mortal-ity rates increase twofold during this period in association with behav-ior characterized as impulsive, high risk, or the result of poor decision-making (Clayton 1992; Dahl 2004). Disorders that result from or are characterized by impulsive behavior, such as problem gambling, sub-stance use disorders, intermittent explosive disorder, sociopathy, com-pleted suicide, and early-onset schizophrenia, are typified both by periadolescent onset and male predominance (Asarnow and Asarnow 1996; Chambers and Potenza 2003b; Chambers et al. 2003; De Gaston et al. 1996; Kandel et al. 1992; Kohler 1996; Mash and Dozois 1996; Wagner and Anthony 2002). Adolescent male vulnerability to disorders involv-

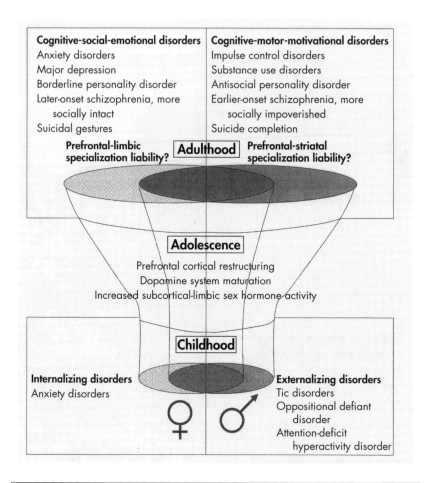

FIGURE 2–1. Conceptual diagram of the developmental trajectories of gender-associated traits and psychopathologies emerging through adolescence.

In males **(right cone),** adolescent neurodevelopmental events may elaborate on and complicate tendencies for specialization in cognitive-motor-motivational domains of mental functioning and produce greater liability for impulse control–related disorders in adulthood. In contrast, a female **(left cone)** tendency for specialization in cognitive-social-emotional domains may interact with adolescent neurodevelopmental events to cause greater liability for anxiety disorders, major depression, and borderline social-emotional defenses in adulthood. Significant areas of overlap between the developmental cones reflect the fact that gender differentiation in vulnerability to psychopathology along a social-emotional versus motor-motivational continuum is only partial, and significant numbers of males and females have disorders on both sides of the continuum.

ing impulsivity as a parameter of dysregulated cognitive-motivational-motor control contrasts with disorders of female preponderance emerging at this developmental stage. Disorders more prevalent in adolescent females include mood and anxiety disorders, borderline defensive structures, and eating disorders (Kaplan and Sadock 2000; Kessler et al. 2001; Mash and Dozois 1996), which involve significant components of dysregulated emotional perceptions of self or others as a dimension of cognitive-social-emotional control.

For both males and females, psychiatric disorders of adult form and gender prevalence distributions begin to emerge in adolescence. Knowing the brain systems involved in impulse control is particularly informative in understanding the neurobiological underpinnings of males' enhanced vulnerability to impulse control disorders.

GENERAL NEUROCIRCUITRY OF IMPULSE CONTROL

A wealth of animal research and human pathophysiological and neuroimaging data indicates that the brain is organized into semisegregated modular systems that 1) collect multimodal sensory data about the internal status of the individual or external environment, 2) process these data according to decision-making computations that optimize the selection and sequencing of behavioral output consistent with survival fitness, and 3) execute specific behavioral programs (see Chambers and Potenza 2003a and 2003b for reviews of corresponding literature). The middle, decision-making stage of this input-output processing is associated with neural substrates localized to the anterior half of the brain (Figure 2–2).

Key components of this primary motivational circuitry include the following: 1) the prefrontal cortex region (encompassing orbitofrontal, anterior cingulate, and dorsolateral sections); 2) the ventral striatum region (nucleus accumbens, shell, and core); and 3) the midbrain source of dopamine to these regions, the ventral tegmental area (VTA). Providing sensory input to primary motivational circuits, the posterior half of the cortex collects and processes primary and multimodal sensory information (e.g., of the five senses) while temporal and midline limbic structures (including the hypothalamus, amygdala, and hippocampus) provide internally generated homeostatic, emotional, and contextual memory information.

Executing behavioral output as directed by primary motivational circuits are the midcoronal motor cortices, the dorsal striatum, and the midbrain source of dopamine to the dorsal striatum, the substantia ni-

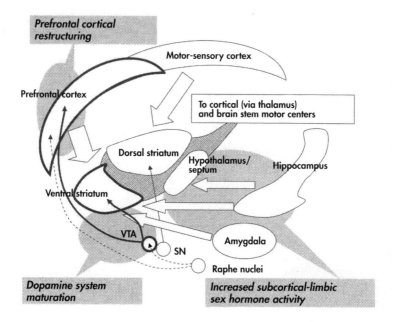

FIGURE 2–2. Major brain systems implicated in adolescent neurodevelopment.

Primary motivational circuits implicated in impulse control (**bold outlined structures**) undergo significant adolescent-age revisions encompassing prefrontal cortical restructuring and functionally robust dopaminergic systems maturation. Subcortical-limbic structures that are important sites of responsivity to sex hormone efflux during adolescence (e.g., hypothalamus/septum, hippocampus, and amygdala) interconnect with primary motivational circuits, possibly mediating neurohormonal influence over impulse control.

Note. Open arrows=major excitatory (glutamatergic) connection pathways; solid arrows=dopamine projections; dotted arrows=serotonin projections; SN=substantia nigra; VTA=ventral tegmental area.

gra. Broadly interconnected with primary motivational circuits at cortical and subcortical levels, this motor output system instantiates the extrapyramidal system, which directly controls the sequencing of concrete motor movements as generated by the classic pyramidal motor system.

Primary motivational circuitry is itself composed of interconnected subsystems that can be viewed as functioning according to how they participate in the promotion or inhibition of motivational programming, so that specific motor routines may be acted on as a result of the decision-making process (Chambers and Potenza 2003b; Chambers et al. 2003). In association with the promotion of motivational programming for behavioral output, dopamine released from neurons in the VTA into the nucleus accumbens (and to a lesser degree into the prefrontal cortex) is associated with responsivity to natural rewards, novelty, stressful or aversive stimuli that require evasive action, and the intake of addictive drugs. In association with the inhibition of motivational programming, the prefrontal cortex sends glutamatergic afferents to the nucleus accumbens. Functional and anatomical abnormalities of the prefrontal cortex have long been associated with disturbances in executive cognitive function, impulsivity, and perseverative behavior—whether occurring in the context of gross neurological disorders or in the broad spectrum of psychiatric disorders associated with poor impulse control. Disruptions of the serotonin system, which projects from midbrain centers (raphe nuclei) into prefrontal cortical, ventral striatal, and VTA stations of primary motivational circuitry, are also implicated in disorders of impulse control in various psychiatric conditions.

Although greatly oversimplified in terms of the countless subsystems, neuronal types, varieties of neurotransmitters, and intracellular and neurocomputational events involved in motivational impulsivity, this depiction of primary motivational circuitry provides a general conceptual platform for understanding disorders of impulse control in which the prefrontal cortex, ventral striatum, and VTA-dopaminergic systems play a central role (Chambers et al. 2003). Generally, pathological or developmental states that in some way represent a compromise of prefrontal cortical function or serotonin functions concomitant with enhanced potency of subcortical dopamine function predispose to traits or clinical phenotypes of psychiatric disorders involving impaired impulse control. Also, because neurocomputational events that subserve healthy versus impaired decision-making are linked with the ventral striatum as a convergence zone of frontal cortical glutamatergic and subcortical dopamine afferents, pathological disturbances or developmental changes in other brain regions (e.g., hippocampus, amygdala) that also project directly into the ventral striatum may also modulate impulse control.

In summary, specific neural substrates located in the anterior portion of the brain, including but not limited to the frontal cortex, ventral striatum, and VTA-dopaminergic system, are key systems involved in motivational programming. Dysregulation in these systems may alter motivational programming to encompass behavioral impulsivity.

ADOLESCENT NEURODEVELOPMENT IN BRAIN AREAS MODULATING IMPULSE CONTROL

Major neurodevelopmental events during adolescence have been characterized as encompassing changes in primary motivational circuitry, predominantly in the prefrontal cortex (Figure 2–2). Additional but more subtle changes may also occur in subcortical components of this circuitry, including the striatum, and with regard to the functionality of monoaminergic transmitter systems (dopamine and serotonin) that innervate primary motivational circuits. Also, subcortical limbic systems such as the hippocampus, amygdala, and hypothalamic nuclei, which are connected with primary motivational circuitry at various points, may change in response to adolescent-age alterations in sex hormone levels.

Because of the relative ease with which the prefrontal cortex can be studied using neuropsychological, histopathological, and neuroimaging approaches, together with the fact that its compromise is arguably the most closely linked with impulsive behavior, most of the available evidence for adolescent brain changes focuses on the prefrontal cortex. Neuropsychological dimensions of prefrontal cortical function such as working memory, complex problem solving, and abstract thinking markedly approach adult levels of performance during adolescence (Feinberg 1983; Woo et al. 1997; Yates 1996). Corresponding to these functional changes are adolescent-age microstructural alterations of the prefrontal cortex that entail the loss of neuronal interconnections, termed *synaptic pruning* (Huttenlocher 1979; Rakic et al. 1994). Aspects of this synaptic pruning may correspond to metabolic and anatomical neuroimaging changes of the prefrontal cortex in adolescence. For instance, metabolic energy usage in the brain globally declines to adult levels during adolescence, with the prefrontal cortex reaching adult levels last (Chugani et al. 1987; Kety 1956). These declines may in part represent decreasing energy requirements associated with decreasing prefrontal cortical synaptic connections pruned in adolescence. Additionally, investigations on the specific patterns of adolescent synaptic pruning indicate that connections between neurons of the prefrontal cortex that are relatively proximal to one another tend to be preferentially pruned (Lewis 1997; Woo et al. 1997). Meanwhile, connections between prefrontal cortical neurons that are relatively distal to one another may be preferentially preserved and strengthened via increases in axonal myelination (Paus et al. 1999; Woo et al. 1997). In sum, these microstructural changes may result in gross changes of frontal cortical gray and white matter observed in adolescence. Possibly as a result of a net reduction of frontal cortical synapses (but not neurons themselves), there is a relative reduction in the volume of cortical gray matter that proceeds in a wavelike fashion from late childhood through early adulthood in a caudal to rostral gradient, where the prefrontal gray shows reductions last (Gogtay et al. 2004; Lewis 1997; Sowell et al. 1999). Conversely, a rostral to caudal pattern of thickening of the corpus callosum up through adolescent ages may correspond to the preservation and myelination-related fortification of prefrontal cortical long-tract connections (Paus et al. 1999; Thompson et al. 2004). Together, these micro- and macrostructural changes may represent adolescent transitioning of the prefrontal cortex to a configuration that increasingly emphasizes broadly distributed, long-range connections over local connectivity; these connections may correlate with enhanced abstract reasoning skills and other adultlike cognitive styles (Gonzalez-Burgos et al. 2000; Woo et al. 1997).

Changes in monoaminergic neurotransmitter systems that project into the primary motivational circuitry are also implicated in adolescent neurodevelopment. In terms of the dopaminergic system, the age-related incidence of several neuropsychiatric illnesses thought to be intrinsically related to dopamine activity appears to reflect a relative functional robustness of dopamine function in late childhood and early adolescence that diminishes later into adulthood. Thus the incidence of tic disorders in late childhood and early adolescence (treated with dopamine receptor antagonists) contrasts with the increasing incidence of Parkinson's syndrome (treated with dopamine agonist drugs) with advanced adult age (Leckman and Cohen 1996; Sano et al. 1996). Moreover, aspects of increased dopaminergic system functionality are associated with both drug addictions and schizophrenia, which in turn most commonly have postadolescent or early adulthood onset (Audrain-McGovern et al. 2004; Chambers et al. 2001, 2003). These clinical observations are paralleled by preclinical studies showing that adolescent rodents are in several measures more sensitive to dopaminergic system stimulation provoked either pharmacologically or by environmental stimuli such as novel contexts (Adriani et al. 1998; Laviola et al. 1995; Spear and Brake 1983).

Cellular protein and neurochemical markers of monoaminergic neurotransmitter function suggest that although dopaminergic system projections to the prefrontal cortex mature up through adolescence, the serotonin system reaches functional maturity much earlier in childhood (Lambe and Krimer 2000; Rosenberg and Lewis 1995; Takeuchi et al. 2000). Notably, although increased functionality of the dopaminergic system may relate to promoting motivations that can be impulsive, several lines of evidence suggest that alterations in serotonin system activity are inversely related to impulsive behavior (Brown and Linnoila 1990; Cherek et al. 2002; Fuller 1996; Nordin and Eklundh 1999). Together, these findings may suggest that impulsive behavior could occur in the context of some increase in the relative ratio of dopamine functionality to serotonin functionality in primary motivational circuitry—a phenomenon that may be maximized during adolescence. Notably, recently emerging evidence for an increased risk of impulsive suicide in adolescents taking selective serotonin reuptake inhibitors would seem to contradict the general notion that upregulation of serotonin activity would inhibit impulsive behavior (Check 2004; Couzin 2004). These data could represent a heretofore unrecognized developmental alteration in serotonin system function specific to adolescence or the capacity of these drugs to adversely affect nonserotonin systems in this developmental stage, such as by increasing dopamine functionality.

Several subcortical brain regions that influence primary motivational circuits are also implicated in adolescent neurodevelopment. Correlating with the process of sexual maturation in adolescence, activation of hypothalamic sources of gonadotropin-releasing hormones causes large increases in somatic and central nervous system levels of sex hormones produced by the testes or ovaries (Romeo et al. 2002). Sexual maturation involves fundamental alterations in motivational repertoires and drives in relation to social and reproductive behavior. Brain regions likely to undergo significant neurodevelopmental changes in adolescence include the hypothalamus, septum, hippocampus, and amygdala; these regions are involved in sexual maturation, are relatively heavily endowed with sex hormone receptors, and maintain connectivity with primary motivational circuitry (Buchanan et al. 1992; Garcia-Segura et al. 1994; Shughrue and Merchenthaler 2000). For example, while sex hormones influence neuroplastic events in the hippocampus (Shughrue and Merchenthaler 2000), the hippocampus regulates responses to dopamine influx in the nucleus accumbens as well as behavioral responses to novelty mediated by the nucleus accumbens (Lipska et al. 1992; McClelland et al. 1995; O'Donnell et al. 1997).

In sum, recent investigations have produced significant inroads in understanding adolescence as a unique period of neurodevelopmental change both in preparation for healthy adult mental life and as a critical period for the development of adult forms of psychopathology. Although contemporary research likely has only scratched the surface of what these changes fully entail and where they occur, a current theme is beginning to emerge: normal adolescence encompasses a brain configuration marked by relative immaturity (and underfunctionality) of the prefrontal cortex, a primary structure of the brain that inhibits motivational programming; at the same time, subcortical dopaminergic systems and sex hormone–responsive brain structures that influence the promotion of motivational programs may operate at particularly robust levels. In combination, these conditions create a state of neuropsychological functioning that may underlie both 1) normative adolescent impulsivity as a transitional trait and 2) increased vulnerability to psychiatric conditions involving disordered impulse control. Investigations of gender differences in adolescent neurodevelopment represent a new frontier toward a greater understanding of this neurodevelopmental phase and how it predisposes to forms of psychopathology frequent in men.

GENDER DIFFERENCES IN ADOLESCENT NEURODEVELOPMENT

As previously described, various lines of evidence suggest that males may generally tend toward greater functional specialization within the cognitive-motivational-motor domain while showing greater vulnerability to disorders characterized by dysregulation of these faculties involving motivational impulsivity. Given that major adolescent neurodevelopmental events appear to occur in brain regions that regulate motivational behavior and impulsivity, boys may undergo adolescent neurodevelopmental changes differently from girls, particularly within primary motivation circuits.

Several studies have examined adolescent-age gender differences related to the frontal cortex. In one study, serial magnetic resonance imaging (MRI) examinations of brain were performed in 164 healthy subjects ages 4–21 years (Giedd et al. 1999). In boys, frontal lobe gray matter peaked at a greater volume and at a later time than in girls (12.1 years vs. 11 years, respectively). Additionally, the normal loss of gray matter volume occurring after this peak and increases in white matter volume, presumably associated with cortical synaptic pruning, were greater in males compared with females. These frontal lobe changes were in contrast to what was observed in the temporal lobe gray matter, where female volumes peaked later than male volumes but decreases showed no gender differences. Similar findings regarding the frontal cortex have emerged in a more recent MRI study, examining 46 healthy subjects ages 6–17 years, in which greater age-associated increases in left inferior frontal gyrus gray and white matter volumes were noted in boys (Blanton et al. 2004). Together, these findings may suggest that adolescent neurodevelopment of the frontal cortex in boys involves greater overall structural revision, which may also entail greater vulnerability to failures associated with the increased complexity of these changes in this brain region. Supporting this idea are findings related to the study of psychiatric disorders in which disturbances in cortical synaptic pruning are implicated. For example, frontal cortical development in early-onset schizophrenia, which is experienced predominantly by boys, follows a course of accelerated gray matter loss as compared with healthy children (Thompson et al. 2001).

Adolescent-age gender differences in subcortical brain regions that are connection targets of the frontal cortex and are involved in motivation and motor behavior have also been characterized. Although serial imaging has shown a general decrease in caudate nucleus (dorsal striatum) volume during the teen years in both genders, boys show lower caudate volumes throughout this period of change (Giedd 2004). Again, this finding is interesting in terms of psychopathological vulnerabilities, given that ADHD and tic disorders, which are more frequent in boys, are also associated with smaller caudate volumes (Giedd 2004).

Few studies have investigated gender-specific neurodevelopmental trends in monoamine neurotransmitter systems that modulate the frontal cortex and striatum. However, a recent investigation has identified a genetic polymorphism on the X chromosome that leads to lower expression of the monoamine oxidase A protein responsible for metabolism of dopamine and serotonin (Huang et al. 2004). This polymorphism occurs in association with early substance abuse and other disorders of impulse control in male adolescents but is not penetrant in females (Huang et al. 2004). This finding may represent an example by which gender-dependent genetic mechanisms that influence monoamine transmitter system activity can become phenotypically expressed in the setting of adolescent neurodevelopmental events.

Several gender differences during childhood and adolescence that are implicated in social-emotional functioning have been identified in brain structures beyond the frontal cortex and striatum. Serial brain MRI examinations of children ages 4–18 years showed increased amygdala volumes in males, whereas girls appeared to have greater increases in hippocampal volumes (Giedd 1996). Additionally, females appear to have more pronounced myelination of subicular regions of the hippocampus from childhood to age 30 compared with males (Benes et al. 1994). In a functional MRI study of children and adolescents ages 9–17 years, gender correlated with different patterns of brain activation associated with exposure to emotion-provoking stimuli (Kilgore et al. 2001). Upon viewing faces expressing fear, girls showed age-related declines in amygdala activation, whereas boys showed age-related decreases in dorsolateral prefrontal cortex activation. Although further research is needed before firm interpretations of the imaging data may be made, it seems clear that structural brain changes throughout adolescence encompass gender differences in structures involved in cognitive-social-emotional functioning as well as primary motivation circuits.

Adolescent-onset gender differences in the function or anatomy of sex hormone–rich limbic regions such as the hypothalamus, amygdala, hippocampus, and nucleus basalis may in part reflect differential activities of sex hormones or neuropeptides in these regions (Fernandez-Guasti et al. 2000; Kruijver and Swaab 2002; Kruijver et al. 2001). In laboratory animals and humans, the onset of male sexual and nonsexual social behavior, including aggression and territorial defensiveness as well as male somatic traits, is mediated by androgenization (Gooren and Kruijver 2002; Romeo et al. 2002). Moreover, testosterone may play a direct role in predisposing males to or protecting males from gender-biased psychiatric disorders. For instance, male-associated externalizing disorders, including oppositional defiant disorder, conduct disorder, and ADHD, have been shown to be associated with specific polymorphisms of the neural androgen receptor gene on the X chromosome (Comings et al. 1999). Conversely, testosterone may protect men against female-typical mood disorder symptoms: whereas testosterone-deficient men show irritability, dysphoria, and fatigue, hormone replacement can ameliorate these symptoms (Rubinow 1996; Wang et al. 1996).

The capacity for sex hormones to mediate certain neurobehavioral or neurodevelopmental effects appears to depend on the particular developmental stage in which the hormones are active. For example, studies of hamsters suggest that some effects of testosterone require the concurrent or past onset of adolescent brain changes. Thus male hamsters given appropriate steroids and social cues do not express a full complement of reproductive behavior before puberty (Meck et al. 1997). Yet, other alterations in sex hormone exposures earlier in development may set the stage for future expression of male versus female traits. For instance, although normal human males may tend to show superior visual-spatial abilities but inferior verbal skills compared with females, males with idiopathic hypogonadatropic hypogonadism may exhibit more female-typical abilities (Hier and Crowley 1982). In a complementary way, females with congenital adrenal hyperplasia have been noted to have male-typical cognitive patterns and increased interest in male-typical toys, activities, or playmates (Hines 2003; Resnick et al. 1986). Additionally, observations that testosterone administration at puberty does not fully alter the course of hypoandrogenized males' cognitive development suggest that androgens very early in development may help establish certain neural pathways that set the stage for further neurodevelopmental effects of testosterone in adolescence (Gooren and Kruijver 2002).

One unexplored area of potential gender difference exists regarding endogenous neurosteroid synthesis in the brain. Although it is known that numerous enzymes exist in the brain that synthesize such steroids, including sex steroids, glucocorticoids, and mineralocorticoids, little is known about potential gender differences in the activity of these enzymes or how they may be influenced by adolescent neurodevelopmental events (Stoffel-Wagner 2003).

To summarize, emerging lines of evidence suggest that adolescent brain maturation involves some degree of differential development based on gender. These gender-biased trends likely represent fairly subtle but identifiable differences in multiple subsystems (neurogenetics, neurotransmitters, neurohormones, local and distributed neural networks, and brain regions). The most compelling current evidence suggests boys show particular vulnerability to adverse developmental alterations in frontal cortical–ventral striatal systems that subserve cognitive-motor-motivational spheres of functioning; these alterations can lead to behavioral impulsivity. Gender differences in temporal-cortical-limbic regions may also be confirmed in future research.

CONCLUSION

This chapter reviewed multiple lines of evidence suggesting that adolescent neurodevelopment in males may proceed along trajectories that differ from females, predisposing men to traits or disorders involving motivational control and impulsivity. Such trends may occur because major neurodevelopmental events of adolescence involve neurobiological revision of primary motivational circuits of brain areas that mediate some degree of male specialization toward cognitive-motor-motivational abilities. The added complexity of neurobiological revision required to achieve such functional specialization may render males more susceptible to motivational system dysregulation manifesting during or after adolescence. Conversely, the relative lack of functional specialization in cognitive-social-emotional abilities in males may protect men from disorders that involve dysregulation of these faculties, as is more characteristic of psychiatric disorders in women.

Further research is required to confirm and further characterize gender dichotomizations of adolescent neurodevelopment as presented here. In particular, future studies are needed to elucidate the extent to which male-female differences in adolescent brain changes and behavior reflect contributions of gender-specific genetic coding as a result of phylogenic evolution versus environmental input during ontological development. Additionally, more sophisticated neurobiological methods should be employed to allow greater resolution in teasing apart the roles of specific neural subcomponents of the major brain systems implicated in adolescent neurodevelopment. For instance, males and females might show differential vulnerabilities to the complexity of adolescent neurodevelopmental events in differing subregions of the prefrontal cortex, depending on whether those regions are subcortical motivational systems (e.g., nucleus accumbens) versus subcortical affective systems (e.g., amygdala), or males and females may differ in the maturational course of monoamine or other specific neurotransmitter systems. A more complete understanding of the neurodevelopmental trajectories of various brain systems in male adolescents holds great promise in discovering more definitive treatments for disorders of impulse control and other psychiatric disorders frequently seen in men.

KEY POINTS

- Adolescence represents a period in which gender trends in adult psychiatric disorders may become manifest, particularly with respect to substance use and other impulsive behavioral syndromes in boys and anxious and depressive behavior in girls.

- Gender differences in cognitive, affective, or motivational spheres of functioning, whether regarded as healthy or pathological and whether of genetic origin or sculpted by sociocultural experiences, likely involve gender-biased trends in the maturation of frontal cortical and temporal-limbic neural systems.

- Further research on gender-biased differences in neural system maturation in adolescence could lead to the development of new treatment modalities that are gender specific or may help interdict or prevent long-term psychiatric morbidity in adulthood.

PRACTICE GUIDELINES

1. Adolescent neurodevelopmental elaboration on vulnerability to dysregulation of cognitive-motor-motivational functions in males, and cognitive-social-emotional functions in females, does not mean that specific diagnoses in childhood (if present) through to adulthood remain diagnostically stable. Use caution in discussing prognosis or long-term symptom course of specific diagnoses evaluated in adolescence.

2. Both genes and environment sculpt the brain. Strive to not alienate parents from treatment by overtly assigning blame to them for their children's difficulty; rather, attempt to refer them to treatment in cases in which their own behaviors or psychiatric difficulties clearly contribute to their adolescent's distress.

3. Maintain healthy scientific skepticism and curiosity about the potential of emerging treatments for childhood and adolescent-age disorders to positively alter the long-term trajectories of adult psychiatric disorders.

REFERENCES

Adriani W, Chiarotti F, Laviola G: Elevated novelty seeking and typical D-amphetamine sensitization in periadolescent compared to adult mice. Behav Neurosci 112:1152–1166, 1998

Almli CR, Ball RH, Wheeler ME: Human fetal and neonatal movement patterns: gender differences and fetal-to-neonatal continuity. Dev Psychobiol 38: 252–273, 2001

Arnold LM: Gender differences in bipolar disorder. Psychiatr Clin North Am 26:595–620, 2003

Asarnow JR, Asarnow RF: Childhood-onset schizophrenia, in Child Psychopathology. Edited by Mash EJ, Barkley RA. New York, Guilford, 1996, pp 455–484

Audrain-McGovern J, Lerman C, Wileyto EP, et al: Interacting effects of genetic predisposition and depression on adolescent smoking progression. Am J Psychiatry 161:1224–1230, 2004

Barkley RA: Attention-deficit/hyperactivity disorder, in Child Psychopathology. Edited by Mash EJ, Barkley RA. New York, Guilford, 1996, pp 75–143

Benes FM, Turtle M, Khan Y, et al: Myelination of a key relay zone in the hippocampal formation occurs in the human brain during childhood, adolescence, and adulthood. Arch Gen Psychiatry 51:477–484, 1994

Blanton RE, Levitt JG, Peterson JR, et al: Gender differences in the left inferior frontal gyrus in normal children. Neuroimage 22:626–636, 2004

Braungart-Ricker J, Garwood MM, Powers BP, et al: Infant affect and affect regulation during the still-face paradigm with mothers and fathers: the role of infant characteristics and parental sensitivity. Dev Psychol 34:1428–1437, 1998

Brown GL, Linnoila MI: CSF serotonin metabolite (5-HIAA) studies in depression, impulsivity, and violence. J Clin Psychiatry 51:31–41, 1990

Buchanan CM, Eccles JS, Becker JB: Are adolescents the victims of raging hormones? evidence for activational effects of hormones on moods and behavior in adolescence. Psychol Bull 111:62–107, 1992

Chambers RA, Potenza MN: Impulse control disorders, in Encyclopedia of the Neurological Sciences. Edited by Aminoff MJ, Daroff RB. San Diego, CA, Academic Press, 2003a, pp 642–646

Chambers RA, Potenza MN: Neurodevelopment, impulsivity, and adolescent gambling. J Gambl Stud 19:53–84, 2003b

Chambers RA, Krystal JH, Self DW: A neurobiological basis for substance abuse comorbidity in schizophrenia. Biol Psychiatry 50:71–83, 2001

Chambers RA, Taylor JR, Potenza MN: Developmental neurocircuitry of motivation in adolescence: a critical period of addiction vulnerability. Am J Psychiatry 160:1041–1052, 2003

Check E: Analysis highlights suicide risk of antidepressants. Nature 430:954, 2004

Cherek DR, Lane SD, Pietras CJ, et al: Effects of chronic paroxetine administration on measures of aggressive and impulsive responses of adult males with a history of conduct disorder. Psychopharmacology (Berl) 159:266–274, 2002

Chugani HR, Phelps ME, Mazziotta JC: Positron emission tomography study of human brain functional development. Ann Neurol 322:487–497, 1987

Clayton R: Transitions in drug use: risk and protective factors, in Vulnerability to Drug Abuse. Edited by Glantz M, Pickens R. Washington, DC, American Psychological Association, 1992, pp 15–52

Comings DE, Chen C, Wu S, et al: Association of the androgen receptor gene (AR) with ADHD and conduct disorder. Neuroreport 10:1589–1592, 1999

Constantino JN, Todd RD: Autistic traits in the general population: a twin study. Arch Gen Psychiatry 60:524–530, 2003

Couzin J: Psychopharmacology. Volatile chemistry: children and antidepressants. Science 305:468–470, 2004

Craig IW, Harper E, Loat CS: The genetic basis for sex differences in human behaviour: role of sex chromosomes. Ann Hum Genet 68:269–284, 2004

Crick NR, Zahn-Waxler C: The development of psychopathology in females and males: current progress and future challenges. Dev Psychopathol 15:719–742, 2003

Dahl RE: Adolescent brain development: a period of vulnerabilities and opportunities (keynote address). Ann N Y Acad Sci 1021:1–22, 2004

de Coutern-Myers GM: The human cerebral cortex: gender differences in structure and function. J Neuropathol Exp Neurol 58:217–226, 1999

De Gaston JF, Weed S, Jensen L: Understanding gender differences in adolescent sexuality. Adolescence 31:217–231, 1996

Eisenberg N, Fabes RA, Schaller M, et al: Sympathy and personal distress: development, gender differences, and interrelations of indexes. New Dir Child Dev 44:107–126, 1989

Eisenberg N, Carlo G, Murphy B, et al: Prosocial development in late adolescence: a longitudinal study. Child Dev 66:1179–1197, 1995

Feinberg I: Schizophrenia: caused by a fault in programmed synaptic elimination during adolescence? J Psychiatr Res 17:319–334, 1983

Fernandez-Guasti A, Kruijver FPM, Fodor M, et al: Sex differences in the distribution of androgen receptors in the human hypothalamus. J Comp Neurol 425:422–435, 2000

Fuller RW: Fluoxetine effects on serotonin function and aggressive behavior. Ann N Y Acad Sci 794:90–97, 1996

Garcia-Segura L, Chowen J, Parducz A, et al: Gonadal hormones as promoters of structural synaptic plasticity: cellular mechanisms. Prog Neurobiol 44:279–307, 1994

Giedd JN: Quantitative MRI of the temporal lobe, amygdala, and hippocampus in normal brain development. J Comp Neurol 223–230, 1996

Giedd JN: Structural magnetic resonance imaging of the adolescent brain. Ann N Y Acad Sci 1021:77–85, 2004

Giedd JN, Blumenthal J, Jeffries NO, et al: Brain development during childhood and adolescence: a longitudinal MRI study. Nat Neurosci 2:861–863, 1999

Gogtay N, Giedd JN, Lusk L, et al: Dynamic mapping of human cortical development during childhood through early adulthood. Proc Natl Acad Sci U S A 101:8174–8179, 2004

Gonzalez-Burgos G, Barrionuevo G, Lewis DA: Horizontal synaptic connections in monkey prefrontal cortex: an in vitro electrophysiological study. Cereb Cortex 10:82–92, 2000

Gooren LJ, Kruijver FP: Androgens and male behavior. Mol Cell Endocrinol 198:31–40, 2002

Grant BF, Hasin DH, Chou SP, et al: Nicotine dependence and psychiatric disorders in the United States. Arch Gen Psychiatry 61:1107–1115, 2004

Hier DB, Crowley WF: Spatial ability in androgen deficient males. N Engl J Med 306:1202–1205, 1982

Hines M: Sex steroids and human behavior: prenatal androgen exposure and sex-typical play behavior in children. Ann N Y Acad Sci 1007:272–282, 2003

Hinshaw SP: Impulsivity, emotion regulation, and developmental psychopathology: specificity versus generality of linkages. Ann N Y Acad Sci 1008: 149–159, 2003

Hinshaw SP, Lee SS: Conduct and oppositional defiant disorders, in Child Psychopathology. Edited by Mash EJ, Barkley RA. New York, Guilford, 2003, pp 144–198

Huang Y, Cate SP, Battistuzzi C, et al: An association between a functional polymorphism in the monoamine oxidase A gene promoter, impulsive traits and early abuse experiences. Neuropsychopharmacology 29:1498–1505, 2004

Huttenlocher PR: Synaptic density in human frontal cortex: developmental changes and effects of aging. Brain Res 163:195–205, 1979

Hyde JS, Fennema E, Lamon SJ: Gender differences in mathematics performance: a meta-analysis. Psychol Bull 107:139–155, 1990

Kandel DB, Yamaguchi K, Chen K: Stages in progression in drug involvement from adolescence to adulthood: further evidence for the gateway theory. J Stud Alcohol 53:447–457, 1992

Kaplan HI, Sadock VA: Kaplan and Sadock's Comprehensive Textbook of Psychiatry. Philadelphia, PA, Lippincott Williams & Wilkins, 2000

Kessler RC, Avenevoli S, Merikangas KR: Mood disorders in children and adolescents: an epidemiologic perspective. Biol Psychiatry 49:1002–1014, 2001

Kety SS: Human cerebral blood flow and oxygen consumption as related to aging. Res Publ Assoc Res Nerv Ment Dis 35:31–45, 1956

Kilgore WD, Oki M, Yurgelun-Todd DA: Sex-specific developmental changes in amygdala responses to affective faces. Neuroreport 12:427–433, 2001

Klinger LG, Dawson G, Renner P: Autistic disorder, in Child Psychopathology. Edited by Mash EJ, Barkley RA. New York, Guilford, 2003, pp 409–454

Kohler MP: Risk-taking behavior: a cognitive approach. Psychol Rep 78:489–490, 1996

Kruijver FP, Swaab DF: Sex hormone receptors are present in the human suprachiasmatic nucleus. Neuroendocrinology 75:296–305, 2002

Kruijver FPM, Fernandez-Guasti A, Fodor M, et al: Sex differences in androgen receptors of the human mammillary bodies are related to endocrine status rather than to sexual orientation or transsexuality. J Clin Metab Endocrinol 86:818–827, 2001

Lambe E, Krimer LS: Differential postnatal development of catecholamine and serotonin inputs to identified neurons in prefrontal cortex of rhesus monkeys. J Neurosci 20:8780–8787, 2000

Laviola G, Wood RG, Kuhn C, et al: Cocaine sensitization in periadolescent and adult rats. J Pharmacol Exp Ther 275:345–357, 1995

Leckman JF, Cohen DJ: Tic disorders, in Child and Adolescent Psychiatry. Edited by Lewis M. Baltimore, MD, Williams & Wilkins, 1996, pp 622–629

Lewinsohn PM, Gotlib IH, Lewinsohn M, et al: Gender differences in anxiety disorders and anxiety symptoms in adolescents. J Abnorm Psychol 107:109–117, 1998

Lewis DA: Development of the prefrontal cortex during adolescence: insight into vulnerable neural circuits in schizophrenia. Neuropsychopharmacology 16:385–398, 1997

Lindamer LA, Bailey A, Hawthorne W, et al: Gender differences in characteristics and service use of public mental health patients with schizophrenia. Psychiatr Serv 54:1407–1409, 2003

Lipska BK, Jaskiw GE, Chrapusta S, et al: Ibotenic acid lesion of the ventral hippocampus differentially affects dopamine and its metabolites in the nucleus accumbens and prefrontal cortex in the rat. Brain Res 585:1–6, 1992

Lundqvist C, Sabel KG: Brief report: the Brazelton Neonatal Behavioral Assessment Scale detects differences among newborn infants of optimal health. J Pediatr Psychol 25:577–582, 2000

Lundqvist-Person C: Correlation between level of self-regulation in the newborn infant and developmental status at two years of age. Acta Paediatr 90:345–350, 2001

Lyytinen P, Laakso ML, Poikkeus AM, et al: The development and predictive relations of play and language across the second year. Scand J Psychol 40:177–186, 1999

Malcolm CA, McCulloch DL, Shepherd AJ: Pattern-reversal visual evoked potentials in infants: gender differences during early visual maturation. Dev Med Child Neurol 44:345–351, 2002

Mash EJ, Dozois DJA: Child psychopathology: a developmental-systems perspective, in Child Psychopathology. Edited by Mash EJ, Barkley RA. New York, Guilford, 1996, pp 3–71

McClelland JL, McNaughton BL, O'Reilly RC: Why are there complementary learning systems in the hippocampus and neocortex? insights from the successes and failures of connectionist models of learning and memory. Psychol Rev 102:419–457, 1995

Meck LR, Romeo RD, Novak CM, et al: Actions of testosterone in prepubertal and postpubertal male hamsters: dissociation of effects on reproductive behavior and brain androgen receptor immunoreactivity. Horm Behav 31:75–88, 1997

Moore SM, Rosenthal DA: Venturesomeness, impulsiveness, and risky behavior among older adolescents. Percept Mot Skills 76:98, 1992

Nordin C, Eklundh T: Altered CSF 5-HIAA disposition in pathologic male gamblers. CNS Spectr 4:25–33, 1999

O'Donnell P, Greene J, Pabello N, et al: Modulation of cell firing in the nucleus accumbens. Ann N Y Acad Sci 877:157–175, 1997

Opler LA, White L, Caton CL, et al: Gender differences in the relationship of homelessness to symptom severity, substance abuse, and neuroleptic noncompliance in schizophrenia. J Nerv Ment Dis 189:449–456, 2001

Paus T, Zijdenbos A, Worsley K, et al: Structural maturation of neural pathways in children and adolescents: in vivo study. Science 283:1908–1911, 1999

Pellegrini AD, Smith PK: Physical activity play: the nature and function of a neglected aspect of playing. Child Dev 69:577–598, 1998

Rakic P, Bourgeois JP, Goldman-Rakic PS: Synaptic development of the cerebral cortex: implications for learning, memory, and mental illness. Prog Brain Res 102:227–243, 1994

Resnick SM, Berenbaum SA, Gottesman II, et al: Early hormone influence of cognitive functioning in congenital adrenal hyperplasia. Dev Psychol 22:191–198, 1986

Romeo RD, Richardson HN, Sisk CL: Puberty and the maturation of the male brain and sexual behavior: recasting a behavioral potential. Neurosci Biobehav Rev 26:381–391, 2002

Rosenberg DR, Lewis DA: Postnatal maturation of the dopaminergic innervation of monkey prefrontal cortices: a tyrosine hydroxylase immunohistochemical analysis. J Comp Neurol 358:383–400, 1995

Roy-Byrne P, Post RM, Uhde TW, et al: The longitudinal course of recurrent affective illness: life chart data from research patients at the NIMH. Acta Psychiatr Scand Suppl 317:1–34, 1985

Rubinow DR: Androgens, brain, and behavior. Am J Psychiatry 153:974–984, 1996

Sano M, Marder K, Dooneief G: Basal ganglia diseases, in Neuropsychiatry. Edited by Fogel BS, Schiffer RB, Rao SM. Baltimore, MD, Williams & Wilkins, 1996, pp 805–834

Shughrue PJ, Merchenthaler I: Estrogen is more than just a "sex hormone": novel sites for estrogen action in the hippocampal lesions. Front Neuroendocrinol 21:95–101, 2000

Siegel J, Shaughnessy MF: There's a first time for everything: understanding adolescence. Adolescence 30:217–221, 1995

Silverman I, Eals M: Sex differences in spatial ability: evolutionary theory and data, in The Adapted Mind: Evolutionary Psychology and the Generation of Culture. Edited by Barkowi JH, Cosmides L, Tooby J. New York, Oxford University Press, 1992, pp 533–549

Sowell ER, Thompson PM, Holmes CJ, et al: In vivo evidence for post-adolescent brain maturation in frontal and striatal regions. Nat Neurosci 2:859–861, 1999

Spear LP, Brake SC: Periadolescence: age-dependent behavior and psychopharmacological responsivity in rats. Dev Psychobiol 16:83–109, 1983

Stoffel-Wagner B: Neurosteroid biosynthesis in the human brain and its clinical implications. Ann N Y Acad Sci 1007:64–78, 2003

Takeuchi Y, Matsushita H, Sakai H, et al: Developmental changes in cerebrospinal fluid concentrations of monoamine-related substances revealed with a Coulochem electrode array system. J Child Neurol 15:267–270, 2000

Thayer JE, Johnsen DH: Sex differences in judgment of facial affect: a multivariate analysis of recognition errors. Scand J Psychol 41:243–246, 2000

Thompson PM, Vidal C, Giedd JN, et al: Mapping adolescent brain change reveals dynamic wave of accelerated gray matter loss in very-early-onset schizophrenia. Proc Natl Acad Sci U S A 98:11650–11655, 2001

Thompson PM, Giedd JN, Woods RP, et al: Growth patterns in the developing brain detected by using continuum mechanical tensor maps. Nature 404:190–193, 2004

Wagner FA, Anthony JC: First drug use to drug dependence: developmental periods of risk for dependence upon marijuana, cocaine, and alcohol. Neuropsychopharmacology 26:479–488, 2002

Wang C, Alexander G, Berman N, et al: Testosterone replacement therapy improves mood in hypogonadal men: a clinical research center study. J Clin Endocrinol Metab 81:3578–3583, 1996

Weinberg MK, Tronick EZ, Cohn JF, et al: Gender differences in emotional expressivity and self-regulation during early infancy. Dev Psychol 35:175–188, 1999

Woo TU, Pucak ML, Kye CH, et al: Peripubertal refinement of the intrinsic and associational circuitry in monkey prefrontal cortex. Neuroscience 80:1149–1158, 1997

Yates T: Theories of cognitive development, in Child and Adolescent Psychiatry. Edited by Lewis M. Baltimore, MD, Williams & Wilkins, 1996, pp 134–155

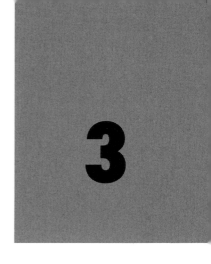

OLDER MEN

RANI DESAI, PH.D.

Case Vignette

Victor was an 80-year-old Polish American World War II combat veteran and a farmer who was placed into a nursing home to recuperate after having a small stroke. He had a lifelong history of alcohol abuse, had had two hip replacements, and experienced difficulty walking and bending. After entering the nursing home, he became withdrawn; he refused to get out of bed, shower, or shave without assistance; and he would not participate in physical or occupational therapy. He also refused to eat and often became combative with staff or family members who tried to feed him. He was informed that he could not go home until he demonstrated that he could get out of bed and take care of himself with minimal assistance, because his elderly wife was frail and physically much smaller. This requirement resulted in a small improvement in his behavior; however, the improvement was short-lived. A consultation was sought from a psychiatrist, who diagnosed major depression and prescribed an antidepressant for Victor. Marked improvement was seen over the next month; Victor regained substantial functional ability and appetite, was less withdrawn, participated more in physical therapy, and interacted more socially with family members who came to visit.

When he was discharged home, it was suggested that Victor receive counseling sessions to monitor his depressive symptoms and prevent further episodes. He refused, saying, "That kind of stuff is for sissies." However, his daughter decided to participate in a Library of Congress program to document the lives of older veterans. He agreed, and as part of the process she interviewed him at length over several weeks about his formative years and experiences during and after the war. She was surprised at his positive reaction to the process as well as by some of the insights and details he offered about his life experiences, many of which he had never previously mentioned.

The U.S. population older than age 65 is rapidly expanding and will continue to grow for the next several decades. By the year 2030, the number of elderly people in the population is projected to be 69.4 million, more than double the 1995 number of 33.5 million (M.M. Desai et al. 1999). Brought about by the aging of the baby boom generation as well as ever-increasing life expectancy rates, this expansion entails large numbers of elderly needing and seeking psychiatric care. Although traditionally women have outnumbered men among the elderly, the gender gap is narrowing as rates of some chronic diseases decline, medical care improves, and changes in lifestyle improve the health of older men.

This chapter focuses on aspects unique to the health of older men that may affect or interact with mental health risk, treatment seeking, assessment, and treatment. First, the most common chronic illnesses among older men, particularly those that are either more prevalent in men than women (e.g., cancer, stroke) or unique to men (e.g., erectile dysfunction, prostate cancer), are reviewed. Next, the mental health effects of changes in social roles (e.g., retirement) and health behaviors, both negative (e.g., smoking, obesity) as well as positive (e.g., social support), that differ either in prevalence or effect between older men and women are described. Third, issues related to help seeking and assessment for psychiatric problems that are unique to the elderly in general and older men specifically are reviewed. Finally, psychiatric treatment issues are described that, although not necessarily unique to men, are important considerations in the treatment of psychiatric disorders or symptoms in this population.

COMMON ILLNESSES

The six most common causes of death among the elderly in the United States mirror the prevalence rates of the most common chronic conditions: heart disease, cancer, stroke, chronic obstructive pulmonary disease, pneumonia/influenza, and diabetes (M.M. Desai et al. 1999). For many of these illnesses, older men have higher rates than older women. For example, cancer mortality rates are considerably higher among older men than older women, as are mortality rates for heart disease, chronic obstructive pulmonary disease, and accidents (M.M. Desai et al. 1999). Older men are more likely to report a history of stroke and heart disease and experience moderate to severe memory impairment (Federal Interagency Forum on Aging-Related Statistics 2000). Hospital discharge rates are higher in older males for diagnoses of malignant neoplasms, stroke, and pneumonia (M.M. Desai et al. 1999). These data imply that, in general, older men are a more medically ill group than are older women and are more likely to experience illnesses that are among the leading causes of death in the country. The higher rates of illness in older men as compared with older women have multiple implications for the assessment and treatment of psychiatric disorders in older men:

1. Identification of psychiatric disorders may be complicated by somatic symptoms of chronic illness, side effects of treatment regimens, or difficulties with communication with a patient (e.g., one who is cognitively impaired). For example, changes in the condition and functioning of the heart can produce many depressive-like symptoms such as lethargy, confusion, and changes in sleep patterns (Burg and Abrams 2004; Lesperance and Frasure-Smith 2000). Similarly, surviving stroke patients can exhibit psychosis-like symptoms such as confusion and violence, and communication difficulties may impede the clinician's ability to detect an underlying psychiatric disorder such as depression (Herrmann et al. 1998; Nys et al. 2005). Depression can also be expressed largely through somatic symptoms, particularly in men (see Chapter 5, "Depression"); and older men are more likely than women to experience co-occurring chronic illness and major depression (Berkman et al. 2003; Borson et al. 1998; Burg and Abrams 2004; Frasure-Smith et al. 1995; Lesperance and Frasure-Smith 2000; Milani and Lavie 1998; Strik et al. 2001). Depressive episodes, although common and associated with poor prognosis, are often not diagnosed or treated in medical settings (Berkman et al. 2003; Lesperance and Frasure-Smith 2000).

2. Primary care physicians often report feeling uncomfortable with psychiatric assessment and difficulty incorporating mental health assessments into a general medical examination (Pincus et al. 2001; Von Korff et al. 2001). They therefore may relegate potential psychiatric symptoms to low priority in the face of competing health care demands for conditions that are more familiar and are perceived to be more serious. They also may prefer to refer patients to psychiatric professionals (Pincus et al. 2001; Von Korff et al. 2001). However, as discussed later, these appointments may be unpalatable to patients, particularly older men, and thus may not be kept.

3. Treatment of psychiatric disorders, if diagnosed, may be complicated by medication regimens for other disorders or by the effects of psychotropic medication on an older medically ill patient (Bartels et al. 2002). Clinical trials for the treatment of psychiatric disorders often exclude participants in poor medical health; thus the efficacies and tolerability of psychotropic medications in physically ill populations are unclear (A.K. Desai 2003). However, even when medications are considered effective, physicians should be aware of potential medication interactions. In addition, coprescribed medications further limit the agents that are appropriate for older patients (Bartels et al. 2002; Hershey and Hales 1984; Olsen et al. 1990).

Aside from the relatively common chronic medical conditions such as heart disease and stroke, there are also prevalent conditions that are unique to the older male. These include diseases of the prostate, erectile dysfunction, and andropause, or "male menopause."

Diseases of the Prostate

Among older men, diseases of the prostate are prevalent, and the risk increases with age. For example, more than 70% of prostate cancer is diagnosed in men over age 65 (American Cancer Society 2003), and the prevalence of benign prostatic hyperplasia is 50% among men age 50 and 80% among men in their 80s (Jakobsson et al. 2004; Yoshimura et al. 2004). Some prostate disease results in only relatively minor inconvenience such as frequent urination; however, other prostate disease results in more debilitating and distressing symptoms such as difficulty urinating or changes in sexual function (Jakobsson et al. 2004; Yoshimura et al. 2004; Zlotta and Schulman 1999). For some patients with benign prostatic hyperplasia or prostate cancer, surgical intervention may be recommended. Diseases of the prostate may influence mental health largely through the disturbing nature of symptoms such as changes in sexual function or through the distress engendered by a surgical procedure and recovery—although the mental health effects of surgery are generally transient.

Erectile Dysfunction

A related condition to diseases of the prostate, erectile dysfunction has also been associated with mental health risks (Shabbir et al. 2004). Erectile dysfunction may result from prostate disease, heart disease, stress, psychiatric symptoms such as alcohol abuse, or normal aging (Shabbir et al.

2004). Erectile dysfunction is reviewed in Chapter 8 ("Sexual Health and Problems: Erectile Dysfunction, Premature Ejaculation, and Male Orgasmic Disorder") and thus will not be covered in detail here. However, the clinician should note that changes in sexual functioning have been associated with depression, anxiety, and increased alcohol consumption (Blanker et al. 2001; Farre et al. 2004; Hedon 2003; Monga and Rajasekaran 2003; Mulhall 2000) and that the prevalence of erectile dysfunction rises substantially with increasing age (Ansong et al. 2000). Consequently, many patients with erectile dysfunction are older men.

Andropause

Controversy exists regarding the concept of andropause, or male menopause. Some clinicians consider andropause to be a syndrome that is treatable with hormone replacement; other clinicians view andropause as a normal part of aging (Asthana et al. 2004; Hafez and Hafez 2004; Hijazi and Cunningham 2005). As men age, testosterone levels decline, and decreased testosterone can influence many aspects of male functioning, including mental health (Morley 2003). Until recently, such symptoms as decreases in lean muscle; loss of bone density; fatigue; increases in fat; anemia; depression; irritability; and mood swings were considered a normal part of aging in older men. Such symptoms are often exacerbated by alcohol consumption, poor diet and exercise, prescription drug use, hypertension, and poor circulation (Hafez and Hafez 2004; Morley and Perry 2003). Recent studies suggest positive effects of hormone replacement therapy (Asthana et al. 2004; Hijazi and Cunningham 2005). However, and possibly more so than many chronic conditions, the symptoms of diminished testosterone both resemble and are influenced by the symptoms of major depression. Therefore, both primary care physicians and psychiatrists should be aware that one disorder may resemble the other, and because the treatment regimens may be very different, accurate diagnosis is important for optimal clinical outcomes (Sherrell and Buckwalter 1997).

Medical Illness

There are several implications of medical illness that clinicians should consider in the psychiatric treatment of older men. First, clinicians should be aware of a patient's medical history, current conditions, current prescriptions, and lifestyle behaviors, such as smoking, exercise, and diet. All of these factors may influence the likelihood of a patient experiencing a psychiatric disorder, will shape the most medically appropriate treatment plan, and may affect overall prognosis. Older men who have not received routine medical care recently and who are seen by mental health clinicians should be referred for such care to rule out underlying or undiagnosed physical problems. Second, clinicians should be aware that although some psychiatric symptoms may result from physical illness, patients may still benefit from treatment within a psychiatric setting. Appropriate medical treatment of a physical disorder may not only reduce psychiatric symptoms but also reveal underlying psychiatric problems that are better handled by a mental health professional. Third, mental health professionals, when possible, should integrate physical health concerns into the psychiatric treatment of older men. As discussed later, men in general have poorer health habits than women, whether seeking help, adhering to treatment regimens, or maintaining healthy behaviors. Mental health professionals have the opportunity to improve both the physical and mental health of older male patients by assisting in and reinforcing better health habits. In addition, with the higher illness burden in older men compared with women, mental health professionals may be useful in helping patients to adjust to the chronic illnesses and increasing restrictions related to normal aging.

PREVALENCE ESTIMATES OF PSYCHIATRIC DISORDERS

With medical comorbidity as a complicating factor, assessing the true prevalence of psychiatric disorders among older men is difficult. Large epidemiological studies of psychiatric disorders in the community such as the National Comorbidity Survey have excluded potential respondents older than age 55. The Epidemiologic Catchment Area study, conducted in the early 1980s, found that lifetime rates of any psychiatric disorder among men older than 65 were 21% for white men, 39% for black men (which was significantly higher than for black women), and 30% for Hispanic men (Robins et al. 1991). For men and women, the rate of active psychiatric disorder (including cognitive impairment) was 13% among respondents older than age 65 and about 7% not including cognitive impairment (Weissman et al. 1985). The most common disorders were depression, anxiety, and cognitive impairment or dementia.

Other surveys have assessed psychiatric symptoms and found that 15% of older adults reported severe depressive symptoms; rates were lower among men (10%–12%) except in the oldest group, where 17%–23% of men older than age 80 reported severe depressive symptoms (Federal Interagency Forum on Aging-Related Statistics 2000). Although prevalent, psychiatric symptoms were often not recognized or treated appropriately in the elderly (Mulsant and Ganguli 1999), and this feature has important implications for training primary care physicians in the accurate diagnosis and treatment of psychiatric symptoms in medical settings (Pincus et al. 2001; Von Korff et al. 2001).

CHANGES IN SOCIAL ROLES

Numerous changes in social roles occur with normal aging. However, two seminal events may particularly impact older men: retirement and bereavement.

Retirement

In the current generation of elders, because of the nature of the workforce until the 1960s, men are more likely than women to experience retirement as a significant life event. Gender differences in labor force participation have changed dramatically since the 1960s: labor force participation among men age 65 and older has declined, whereas participation among women age 65 and older has steadily increased. In 1999, 30% of men ages 65–69 and 15% of men age 70 and older were still working, whereas the corresponding rates among women were 20% and 7%, respectively (Federal Interagency Forum on Aging-Related Statistics 2000). These data indicate that a substantial proportion of men retire from the workforce by the age 65.

The mental health effects of retirement vary substantially from person to person. In general, little evidence indicates that men respond more negatively to retirement than women (Quick and Moen 1998). However, data suggest that preretirement variables such as age at retirement (e.g., younger than age 65 vs. age 65 or later), reasons for retirement (e.g., forced vs. voluntary), and spouse retirement status all have an effect on adjustment to retirement (Bosse et al. 1990; Mutran and Reitzes 1981; Szinovacz and Davey 2004). Transitions out of the workforce can result in a reduction in social ties, changes in feelings of self-worth (particularly if self-identity concepts are particularly tied to employment), and depression (Bosse et al. 1990). However, data also indicate that some factors may buffer the potential negative effects of retirement; these factors include strong family ties, maintaining active lifestyles through community participation, and maintaining the size of social networks, either through contact with former coworkers or by expanding networks into new social circles (Siebert et al. 1999).

Although little evidence indicates that retirement is a universal risk to mental health, for some individuals, retirement represents a traumatic transition (Szinovacz and Davey 2004). Retirement may be a precipitating event that drives older men to seek mental health care; for example, some men who have used work as a defense against chronic depression or anxiety may find that such feelings become overwhelming and debilitating (Sternbach 2001; Szinovacz and Davey 2004). Men also have differing reactions to the transition to retirement; for example, men who worked in higher-status jobs may have more difficulty dealing with the loss of job-related power and control, whereas retired blue-collar workers may welcome not working but be anxious about meager postretirement income (Quick and Moen 1998). Finally, the role of the spouse or partner, if one exists, may change after retirement. Wives or partners who continue to work after their husbands retire become family breadwinners, thus potentially changing the household dynamic. Couples in which wives do not work or are also retired often need to adjust to spending more time together. After their husbands' retirement, wives may become more aware of, or more vocal about, the husband's problems related to drinking, aggression, depression, or emotional withdrawal (Mutran and Reitzes 1981; Sternbach 2001; Szinovacz and Davey 2004). Mental health professionals seeing older men should inquire about labor force participation, work history, and time and conditions of retirement and should be aware of the potential negative impact of retirement on mental health.

Bereavement

Although older women experience bereavement more often than men, evidence suggests that the effects of bereavement may be more debilitating in older men than in older women. In contrast to retirement, bereavement is more frequently a direct threat to mental health—particularly for men. Men report higher rates of depression after bereavement than do women (Byrne and Raphael 1999; Fry 2001; van Grootheest et al. 1999), and men grieve for longer periods of time following their spouse's death. Bereavement also appears to increase the frequency and quantity of alcohol use more in men and may be associated with alcohol abuse and dependence (Byrne et al. 1999; van Grootheest et al. 1999). The mental health effects of bereavement in men may be either direct or mediated through other variables. For example, symptoms of depression may be a direct result of the loss and may persist longer than usual in men who have a past history of depression, undiagnosed persistent dysthymia, or alcohol abuse or dependence. Alternatively, psychiatric symptoms may result indirectly from bereavement as a result of loss of social ties and support, loneliness, or failing physical health. For example, older bereaved men report fewer depressive symptoms if they continue to be employed, which provides them with a social network and consistent activity (Fitzpatrick and Bosse 2000).

Psychiatric symptoms immediately after the loss are considered natural, and under normal circumstances these symptoms would resolve within a relatively short time period. Despite the relative normalcy of such a reaction, however, there are still distinct dangers of suicide (Erlangsen et al. 2004) and alcohol abuse (Byrne et al. 1999) that should be monitored by both primary care and mental health professionals. For patients who present beyond about 6 months postloss, clinicians should consider the presence of persistent depression or anxiety, which in older men may manifest as unexplained somatic symptoms.

HEALTH BEHAVIORS

Patterns of engagement in multiple health-promoting or health-risking behaviors differ in older men and older women. These behaviors include rates of smoking, alcohol use, obesity, sedentary lifestyles, vaccinations, dental care, vegetable and fruit consumption, and regular medical care. Older men are more likely than older women to smoke, use more than moderate amounts of alcohol, be overweight, consume less than adequate amounts of fruits and vegetables, and not have a regular source of medical care (Janes et al. 1999; Kamimoto et al. 1999). However, they are less likely than women to report a sedentary lifestyle and are more likely to be appropriately vaccinated (Federal Interagency Forum on Aging-Related Statistics 2000; Janes et al. 1999).

Healthy behaviors such as physical activity, a proper diet, and regular preventive medical care can influence mental health either 1) directly by reducing symptoms or preventing the onset of psychiatric disorders (Huijbregts et al. 1998) or 2) indirectly through the impact of these healthy behaviors on physical health (Milani and Lavie 1998; Warr et al. 2004). More importantly, older men receiving mental health care should be encouraged to increase such healthy behaviors and may find the assistance of a mental health professional helpful in making positive health changes.

HEALTHY AGING

Although factors linked to healthy aging have been mentioned (e.g., better mental health in old age), it is worth emphasizing that these areas represent potential targets amenable to intervention by a mental health professional. Factors of healthy aging include maintaining an appropriate level of physical activity given one's physical health, maintaining or strengthening social networks, and remaining an active member of the community.

Physical activity has been repeatedly shown to be beneficial to both physical and mental health even among the oldest old and with the most seriously ill (van Gelder et al. 2004; Visser et al. 2002). Physical activity reduces symptoms of depression, increases circulation (which may affect cognitive function and the speed of cognitive decline), increases feelings of well-being, and increases the stamina needed to maintain other activities and remain independent (van Gelder et al. 2004; Visser et al. 2002; Warr et al. 2004). Likewise, strong social networks have been shown to buffer difficult transitions such as retirement and bereavement and to improve recovery from both acute and chronic physical illnesses (Berkman et al. 2003; Paterniti et al. 2002). Related to social networks but still a distinct concept, participation in community activities (e.g., volunteering, religious participation) has been associated with higher morale, less depression, stronger feelings of self-worth, and longer amounts of time remaining independent (Greenfield and Marks 2004; Morrow-Howell et al. 2003; Shmotkin et al. 2003). Although mental health professionals may encourage such activities with patients of all ages, benefits of participating in these activities appear particularly salient to older patients.

GETTING OLDER MEN INTO MENTAL HEALTH TREATMENT

The majority of psychiatric symptoms seen among older men will first be noticed in a primary care setting (Charney et al. 2003). This situation represents a serious problem because many psychiatric symptoms will go unnoticed until they become severe. Even when symptoms are noticed in a general medical setting, primary care physicians are often resistant to implementing evidence-based treatment protocols for psychiatric symptoms such as depression (Bartels et al. 2002; Charney et al. 2003; Pincus et al. 2001). Older men are less likely than older women to have a regular source of care and are more likely to delay receiving care. All these findings imply that there is likely a substantial undiagnosed burden of psychiatric problems in older men (Janes et al. 1999).

Models of treatment seeking have often emphasized several classes of factors that influence the likelihood that an individual will receive psychiatric treatment. These factors include measures of need for care, individual help-seeking styles, accessibility of care, and palatability of care. Older men face challenges in each of these areas. Even when an individual perceives the need for help and is willing to seek care for mental health problems, he may be faced with limited or unpalatable health care options and stigma associated with mental illness, older age, or physical illness.

Despite recent policy efforts, a disparity persists in health insurance coverage for physical versus mental health problems. Under Medicare, a 20% copayment is required for outpatient physical health care and a 50% copayment for outpatient mental health care (Coviello and Glaun 2003), and this option is offered only through Medicare Part B, which many people cannot afford to purchase. Medicare also frequently does not cover community mental health services such as substance abuse treatment centers or psychiatric rehabilitation programs and has a 190-day lifetime cap on inpatient psychiatric care, with substantial deductibles (Coviello and Glaun 2003). Seniors living on restricted incomes may thus find mental health care either unpalatable due to cost or unaffordable and thus inaccessible.

Limited research exists regarding the best ways to get seniors into mental health care, assuming an appropriate level of insurance coverage. Available data indicate that seniors prefer integrated treatment strategies in which mental health professionals work as a team with primary care and other physicians (Bartels et al. 2004). Such settings increase ease of access by locating services in closer proximity and thus reducing the burden of traveling for appointments. These settings also provide a more integrated treatment approach in which both physical and psychiatric issues are treated simultaneously (Bartels et al. 2004). Integrating services may also reduce the stigma associated with mental health problems.

Elders with psychiatric problems experience stigma on several fronts, including those associated with mental health, older age, and physical illness (Graham et al. 2003). Stigma seriously affects multiple stakeholders. Stigma reduces self-esteem and treatment seeking among people with a need for care, as well as their families. Stigma also influences relationships between clinicians and patients and the availability of appropriate mental health services in the community for elders (De Mendonca Lima 2004; Von Korff et al. 2001). The discussion of stigma is covered in more detail in Chapter 17 ("Overcoming Stigma and Barriers to Mental Health Treatment"); for older men the stigma of mental illness appears particularly salient. Negative attitudes about mental illness seem more pronounced in older men (Sternbach 2001), and the stigma associated with physical illness may compound the problem due to the higher illness burden in this group.

UNIQUE PSYCHIATRIC TREATMENT ISSUES

Several books review psychotherapy and counseling for older men (Collison 1987; Sternbach 2001). Some issues important for older men compared with younger men and for men compared with women are reviewed here briefly, including the therapist's understanding of the male patient's culture and context, exposure to combat, view of the "traditional male" role, and attitudes about alcohol.

Older patients have a longer life history. Thus they may have been affected by major world events that a younger therapist may not have experienced and thus may not realize the implications of (Sternbach 2001). These events include 1) the worldwide flu epidemic of 1918, which killed more people, including the young and otherwise healthy, than did World War I and may have killed parents or siblings; 2) the Great Depression of the 1930s, in which many families experienced severe and prolonged poverty; and 3) forced migrations from all over the world, in which families or individuals entered this country as (not always welcome) refugees. These events in an older man's life may have profoundly impacted his relationships with family, particularly his father, and may have been the source of significant trauma (Aarts and Op den Velde 1998). Sternbach (2001) has suggested that older patients deeply appreciate a younger therapist who realizes the potential impact of such events and takes the time to explore them.

In addition to the events just mentioned, the major military conflicts of the past century have had a substantial effect on older Americans, particularly men. In 2000, 65% of men over age 65 had a history of military service and almost 25% of men over age 55 were combat veterans (U.S. Census Bureau 2000). The three major conflicts relevant to older men (World War II and the Korean and Vietnam Wars) transpired in very different social and cultural circumstances. World War II veterans were warmly welcomed home, but the traumatic effects of combat were not well understood or tolerated, resulting in many veterans becoming emotionally withdrawn and experiencing decades of undiagnosed posttraumatic stress disorder (Spiro et al. 1994). The veterans of the Korean War, often called the "forgotten war," experienced trauma related both to combat and to operating in conditions of extreme cold and faced similar cultural attitudes about the appropriateness of talking about war experiences (Sternbach 2001). By contrast, veterans of the Vietnam War returned to a largely hostile society and may have faced profound conflict related to their war experiences and their attitude toward the war. Even men who were not drafted or who resisted the draft may have been emotionally impacted by a conflict that created large rifts in families and institutions (Kulka et al. 1990). Because military service represents a pervasive experience for this generation of elders, mental health professionals should assess the nature of the experience and determine the extent to which potential traumatic effects persist into older age (Spiro et al. 1994). On the other hand, prior military experience may also represent a source of pride or positive self-esteem for older men, thus warranting physician acknowledgment or recognition in health care interactions.

Along with the major world events of the past century, there have also been large cultural changes in American society that could affect mental health and the context that older men bring to a therapeutic relationship. Many older men came of age in a culture that was racist, anti-Semitic, antigay, and sexist. The civil rights and women's movements each challenged traditional men's roles, attitudes, and sense of self in profound ways (Brooks 1998). The traditional man, who was the powerful head of a household and primary breadwinner, was expected to keep emotions under control and be tough enough not to need much emotional or physical care. Although it is now recognized that such roles and attitudes have negative physical and psychological effects (Harrison 1978), many older men find it difficult to adapt to changing societal expectations and continue to struggle to make sense of these changes (Brooks 1998). Mental health professionals should be aware of the cultural context that affected their patients most as well as the patients' potential negative and positive influences. For example, negative factors might include greater societal prejudice in prior decades, and positive factors might relate to self-esteem derived from societal, occupational, and familial roles. Mental health practitioners may also consider group therapy modalities that are age and gender specific to make older men feel more comfortable.

One aspect of the traditional male role involves attitudes toward alcohol. Many older men came of age at a time when heavy drinking among men was both sanctioned and expected (Byrne et al. 1999). Older men may not recognize the lifelong negative effects of heavy alcohol use or abuse or the links between alcohol consumption and symptoms of depression, anxiety, or cognitive decline (Kamimoto et al. 1999). Similarly, media attention to recent evidence that indicates that moderate alcohol consumption may protect against some chronic conditions may indirectly condone continued or excessive alcohol use in older men (Whelan 1995). Alcohol-related treatment programs, particularly cognitive-behavioral approaches, have been found to be effective for many older men (Whelan 1995). However, as mentioned earlier, entry into treatment may be hampered by cost, availability, or the stigma attached to such treatment. For those unwilling to quit drinking, harm-reduction approaches may prove helpful.

CONCLUSION

The burden of psychiatric illness in the elderly is substantial, although often undiagnosed, and influences both their quality of life and physical health. Mental health clinicians who treat older men should be aware of these patients' 1) physical health status, including medication use; 2) health-risk and health-promotion behaviors such as smoking, alcohol use, and physical activity; 3) marital status, social support, employment status, and level of community involvement; 4) veteran status and combat experience; and 5) other major life experiences and the influence of large cultural changes since the 1950s. Placing these factors into context will assist the clinician in prescribing the best medication regimen for the patient, if appropriate; developing a therapeutic relationship; and working with male patients to improve their mental health and quality of life in their later years.

KEY POINTS

- Older men, compared with older women, are more likely to have poor health habits, a greater burden of medical illness, and a greater burden of undiagnosed psychiatric illness.

- There are substantial barriers to older men receiving mental health care, including financial concerns, stigma associated with mental illness, and resistance to treatment for psychiatric problems.

- Once in mental health treatment, older men have unique life experiences that may affect their ability to benefit from such treatment, including comorbid medical conditions, medication regimens, negative and ingrained attitudes about mental illness and the "appropriate" roles for men in society, and life experiences such as exposure to combat.

PRACTICE GUIDELINES

1. It is crucial that medical and psychiatric symptoms be differentiated from each other and treated accordingly, but with proper attention paid to comorbidity. This approach may require integration of medical and mental health care through, at minimum, close communication between providers.

2. Both primary care and mental health professionals should be aware of major life events in an older man's life (e.g., retirement, bereavement, major medical illness or disability) as potential threats to mental health and should monitor, refer, and treat potential psychiatric symptoms accordingly.

3. Mental health professionals should be sensitive to and appreciative of the wealth of life experiences offered by their older patients but should also be aware that some of these experiences may have profoundly affected mental health in ways that may not be immediately obvious, particularly to a younger therapist.

REFERENCES

Aarts P, Op den Velde W: Prior traumatization and the process of aging: theory and clinical implications, in Traumatic Stress: The Effects of Overwhelming Experience on Mind, Body, and Society. Edited by van der Kolk BA, McFarlane AC, Weisaeth L. New York, Guilford, 1998, pp 359–377

American Cancer Society: Cancer Facts and Figures 2003. Washington, DC, American Cancer Society, 2003

Ansong KS, Lewis C, Jenkins P, et al: Epidemiology of erectile dysfunction: a community-based study in rural New York State. Ann Epidemiol 10:293–296, 2000

Asthana S, Bhasin S, Butler RN, et al: Masculine vitality: pros and cons of testosterone in treating the andropause. J Gerontol A Biol Sci Med Sci 59:461–465, 2004

Bartels SJ, Dums AR, Oxman TE, et al: Evidence-based practices in geriatric mental health care. Psychiatr Serv 53:1419–1431, 2002

Bartels SJ, Coakley EH, Zubritsky C, et al: Improving access to geriatric mental health services: a randomized trial comparing treatment engagement with integrated versus enhanced referral care for depression, anxiety, and at-risk alcohol use. Am J Psychiatry 161:1455–1462, 2004

Berkman LF, Blumenthal J, Burg M, et al: Effects of treating depression and low perceived social support on clinical events after myocardial infarction: the Enhancing Recovery in Coronary Heart Disease Patients (ENRICHD) Randomized Trial. JAMA 289:3106–3116, 2003

Blanker MH, Bosch JL, Groeneveld FP, et al: Erectile and ejaculatory dysfunction in a community-based sample of men 50 to 78 years old: prevalence, concern, and relation to sexual activity. Urology 57:763–768, 2001

Borson S, Claypoole K, McDonald GJ: Depression and chronic obstructive pulmonary disease: treatment trials. Semin Clin Neuropsychiatry 3:115–130, 1998

Bosse R, Aldwin CM, Levenson MR, et al: Differences in social support among retirees and workers: findings from the Normative Aging Study. Psychol Aging 5:41–47, 1990

Brooks GR: A New Psychotherapy for Traditional Men. San Francisco, CA, Jossey-Bass, 1998

Burg MM, Abrams D: Depression in chronic medical illness: the case of coronary heart disease. J Clin Psychol 57:1323–1337, 2004

Byrne GJ, Raphael B: Depressive symptoms and depressive episodes in recently widowed older men. Int Psychogeriatr 11:67–74, 1999

Byrne GJ, Raphael B, Arnold E: Alcohol consumption and psychological distress in recently widowed older men. Aust N Z J Psychiatry 33:740–747, 1999

Charney DS, Reynolds CF 3rd, Lewis L, et al: Depression and Bipolar Support Alliance consensus statement on the unmet needs in diagnosis and treatment of mood disorders in late life. Arch Gen Psychiatry 60:664–672, 2003

Collison B: Counseling aging men, in Handbook of Counseling and Psychotherapy With Men. Edited by Scher M, Stevens M, Good G, et al. Newbury Park, CA, Sage, 1987, pp 165–177

Coviello A, Glaun K: Medicare mental health coverage. Issue Brief Cent Medicare Educ 4:1–6, 2003

De Mendonca Lima CA: The reduction of stigma and discrimination against older people with mental disorders: a challenge for the future. Arch Gerontol Geriatr Suppl (9):109–120, 2004

Desai AK: Use of psychopharmacologic agents in the elderly. Clin Geriatr Med 19:697–719, 2003

Desai MM, Zhang P, Hennessy CH: Surveillance for morbidity and mortality among older adults—United States, 1995–1996. MMWR CDC Surveill Summ 48:7–25, 1999

Erlangsen A, Jeune B, Bille-Brahe U, et al: Loss of partner and suicide risks among oldest old: a population-based register study. Age Ageing 33:378–383, 2004

Farre JM, Fora F, Lasheras MG: Specific aspects of erectile dysfunction in psychiatry. Int J Impot Res 16(suppl):S46–S49, 2004

Federal Interagency Forum on Aging-Related Statistics: Older Americans 2000: Key Indicators of Well-Being. Washington, DC, Federal Interagency Forum on Aging-Related Statistics, 2000

Fitzpatrick TR, Bosse R: Employment and health among older bereaved men in the Normative Aging Study: one year and three years following a bereavement event. Soc Work Health Care 32:41–60, 2000

Frasure-Smith N, Lesperance F, Talajic M: Depression and 18-month prognosis after myocardial infarction. Circulation 91:999–1005, 1995

Fry PS: Predictors of health-related quality of life perspectives, self-esteem, and life satisfactions of older adults following spousal loss: an 18-month follow-up study of widows and widowers. Gerontologist 41:787–798, 2001

Graham N, Lindesay J, Katona C, et al: Reducing stigma and discrimination against older people with mental disorders: a technical consensus statement. Int J Geriatr Psychiatry 18:670–678, 2003

Greenfield EA, Marks NF: Formal volunteering as a protective factor for older adults' psychological well-being. J Gerontol B Psychol Sci Soc Sci 59:S258–S264, 2004

Hafez B, Hafez ES: Andropause: endocrinology, erectile dysfunction, and prostate pathophysiology. Arch Androl 50:45–68, 2004

Harrison J: Warning, the male sex role may be dangerous to your health. J Soc Issues 34:65–86, 1978

Hedon F: Anxiety and erectile dysfunction: a global approach to ED enhances results and quality of life. Int J Impot Res 15(suppl):S16–S19, 2003

Herrmann N, Black SE, Lawrence J, et al: The Sunnybrook Stroke Study: a prospective study of depressive symptoms and functional outcome. Stroke 29:618–624, 1998

Hershey SC, Hales RE: Psychopharmacologic approach to the medically ill patient. Psychiatr Clin North Am 7:803–816, 1984

Hijazi RA, Cunningham GR: Andropause: is androgen replacement therapy indicated for the aging male? Annu Rev Med 56:117–137, 2005

Huijbregts PP, Feskens EJ, Rasanen L, et al: Dietary patterns and cognitive function in elderly men in Finland, Italy and the Netherlands. Eur J Clin Nutr 52:826–831, 1998

Jakobsson L, Loven L, Hallberg IR: Micturition problems in relation to quality of life in men with prostate cancer or benign prostatic hyperplasia: comparison with men from the general population. Cancer Nurs 27:218–229, 2004

Janes GR, Blackman DK, Bolen JC, et al: Surveillance for use of preventive health-care services by older adults, 1995–1997. MMWR CDC Surveill Summ 48:51–88, 1999

Kamimoto LA, Easton AN, Maurice E, et al: Surveillance for five health risks among older adults—United States, 1993–1997. MMWR CDC Surveill Summ 48:89–130, 1999

Kulka RA, Schlenger WE, Fairbank JA, et al: Trauma and the Vietnam War Generation. New York, Brunner/Mazel, 1990

Lesperance F, Frasure-Smith N: Depression in patients with cardiac disease: a practical review. J Psychosom Res 48:379–391, 2000

Milani RV, Lavie CJ: Prevalence and effects of cardiac rehabilitation on depression in the elderly with coronary heart disease. Am J Cardiol 81:1233–1236, 1998

Monga M, Rajasekaran M: Erectile dysfunction: current concepts and future directions. Arch Androl 49:7–17, 2003

Morley JE: Testosterone and behavior. Clin Geriatr Med 19:605–616, 2003

Morley JE, Perry HM 3rd: Andropause: an old concept in new clothing. Clin Geriatr Med 19:507–528, 2003

Morrow-Howell N, Hinterlong J, Rozario PA, et al: Effects of volunteering on the well-being of older adults. J Gerontol B Psychol Sci Soc Sci 58:S137–S145, 2003

Mulhall JP: Current concepts in erectile dysfunction. Am J Manag Care 6:S625–S631, 2000

Mulsant BH, Ganguli M: Epidemiology and diagnosis of depression in late life. J Clin Psychiatry 60(suppl):9–15, 1999

Mutran E, Reitzes DC: Retirement, identity and well-being: realignment of role relationships. J Gerontol 36:733–740, 1981

Nys GM, van Zandvoort MJ, van der Worp HB, et al: Early depressive symptoms after stroke: neuropsychological correlates and lesion characteristics. J Neurol Sci 228:27–33, 2005

Olsen RB, Gydesen SU, Kristensen M, et al: Psychotropic medication in the elderly: a survey of prescribing and clinical outcome. Dan Med Bull 37:455–459, 1990

Paterniti S, Verdier-Taillefer MH, Dufouil C, et al: Depressive symptoms and cognitive decline in elderly people: longitudinal study. Br J Psychiatry 181:406–410, 2002

Pincus HA, Pechura CM, Elinson L, et al: Depression in primary care: linking clinical and systems strategies. Gen Hosp Psychiatry 23:311–318, 2001

Quick HE, Moen P: Gender, employment, and retirement quality: a life course approach to the differential experiences of men and women. J Occup Health Psychol 3:44–64, 1998

Robins LN, Locke BZ, Regier DA: An overview of psychiatric disorders in America, in Psychiatric Disorders in America: The Epidemiologic Catchment Area Study. Edited by Robins LN, Regier DA. New York, Free Press, 1991, pp 328–366

Shabbir M, Mikhailidis DM, Morgan RJ: Erectile dysfunction: an underdiagnosed condition associated with multiple risk factors. Curr Med Res Opin 20:603–606, 2004

Sherrell K, Buckwalter KC: Geropsychiatry: barriers to follow-up studies with the chronically mentally ill elderly in long-term care settings. J Gerontol Nurs 23:37–40, 1997

Shmotkin D, Blumstein T, Modan B: Beyond keeping active: concomitants of being a volunteer in old-old age. Psychol Aging 18:602–607, 2003

Siebert DC, Mutran EJ, Reitzes DC: Friendship and social support: the importance of role identity to aging adults. Soc Work 44:522–533, 1999

Spiro A, Schnurr PP, Aldwin CM: Combat-related posttraumatic stress disorder symptoms in older men. Psychol Aging 9:17–26, 1994

Sternbach J: Psychotherapy with the young older man, in The New Handbook of Psychotherapy and Counseling With Men. Edited by Brooks GR, Good GE. San Francisco, CA, Jossey-Bass, 2001, pp 464–480

Strik JJ, Honig A, Maes M: Depression and myocardial infarction: relationship between heart and mind. Prog Neuropsychopharmacol Biol Psychiatry 25:879–892, 2001

Szinovacz ME, Davey A: Honeymoons and joint lunches: effects of retirement and spouse's employment on depressive symptoms. J Gerontol B Psychol Sci Soc Sci 59:P233–P245, 2004

U.S. Census Bureau: Data tables, 2000 census. Washington, DC, U.S. Census Bureau. Available at: http://www.va.gov/vetdata/Census2000/CenData/agesexdata.pdf. Accessed May 11, 2006.

van Gelder BM, Tijhuis MA, Kalmijn S, et al: Physical activity in relation to cognitive decline in elderly men: the Fine study. Neurology 63:2316–2321, 2004

van Grootheest DS, Beekman AT, Broese van Groenou MI, et al: Sex differences in depression after widowhood: do men suffer more? Soc Psychiatry Psychiatr Epidemiol 34:391–398, 1999

Visser M, Pluijm SM, Stel VS, et al: Physical activity as a determinant of change in mobility performance: the Longitudinal Aging Study Amsterdam. J Am Geriatr Soc 50:1774–1781, 2002

Von Korff M, Katon W, Unutzer J, et al: Improving depression care: barriers, solutions, and research needs. J Fam Pract 50:E1, 2001

Warr P, Butcher V, Robertson I: Activity and psychological well-being in older people. Aging Ment Health 8:172–183, 2004

Weissman MM, Myers JK, Tischler GL, et al: Psychiatric disorders (DSM-III) and cognitive impairment among the elderly in a U.S. urban community. Acta Psychiatr Scand 71:366–379, 1985

Whelan G: Alcohol-related health problems in the elderly. Med J Aust 162:325–327, 1995

Yoshimura K, Terada N, Matsui Y, et al: Prevalence of and risk factors for nocturia: analysis of a health screening program. Int J Urol 11:282–287, 2004

Zlotta AR, Schulman CC: BPH and sexuality. Eur Urol 36(suppl):107–112, 1999

PART II

PSYCHIATRIC DISORDERS IN MEN

Assessment and Treatment

4

ANXIETY DISORDERS

CARLOS BLANCO, M.D., PH.D.
ORIANA VESGA LÓPEZ, M.D.

Case Vignette 1

Whenever Ben leaves his house, and before he goes to bed at night, he is plagued with doubts about whether he has switched off the oven or other electrical appliances and locked the doors and windows. Ben is horrified that if the oven is left on accidentally, it might start a fire or some other terrible thing might happen. He does not want to be responsible for harm befalling his family and thus checks the switches frequently to be certain that the appliances are turned off. He stares at each knob on the stove to be sure it is aligned in the "off" position and says to himself "it's off" over and over again.

Case Vignette 2

Two months ago, Connor received a promotion at his company and was anxious about the extra demands being placed on him. As a manager, he was now required to make presentations to other divisions in the company and to prospective new clients. He was starting to use alcohol regularly to relieve the pressure and to try to relax at the end of the day. Connor had always been concerned that he was not performing his duties at the level people expected of him. Now he was feeling even more self-conscious, particularly in situations in which he had to be the center of attention. Although he had previously found meetings quite stressful, now he was very uncomfortable in anticipation of meetings and avoided attending them on multiple occasions. He did not understand what was happening to him and was considering requesting an extended leave from his employer or requesting a return to his previous position.

PREVALENCE

Anxiety disorders are among the most common psychiatric disorders in the United States (Kessler et al. 2005a, 2005b). Large-scale epidemiological studies indicate that anxiety disorders affect 15.7 million people in the United States each year and more than 30 million people at some point during their lifetimes (Kessler et al. 1994). Four epidemiological studies have described lifetime prevalence data for anxiety disorders in the United States: the Epidemiologic Catchment Area (ECA) study, the National Comorbidity Survey (NCS), the National Comorbidity Survey Replication (NCS-R), and the National Epidemiologic Survey on Alcohol and Related Conditions (NESARC). The ECA study estimated the lifetime prevalence rate for anxiety disorders in the U.S. population at 15%. Phobic disorders, obsessive-compulsive disorder (OCD), and panic disorder were among the seven most frequently diagnosed psychiatric disorders in the United States (Regier et al. 1990). The NCS estimated past-year prevalence rates of anxiety disorders at 17%, consistent with the results of the ECA study (Kessler et al. 1994). More recently, the NCS-R confirmed that anxiety disorders are very common in the United States. The lifetime prevalence estimate for anxiety disorders was 28.8%, compared with 20.8% for mood disorders, 24.8% for impulse control disorders, and 14.6% for substance use disorders (Kessler et al. 2005a). The 12-month prevalence estimate for anxiety disorders was 18.1%, also higher than those for mood, impulse control, and substance use disorders (Kessler et al. 2005b). Median age at onset was found to be earlier for anxiety disorders (11 years) than for other DSM-IV-TR disorders (American Psychiatric Association 2000; Kessler et al. 2005a).

EPIDEMIOLOGY AND COMORBIDITY

Epidemiological studies consistently indicate that men are half as likely as women to experience an anxiety disorder during their lives (Kessler et al. 1994, 2005a; Regier et al. 1990). Approximately 6% of men, compared with 13% of women, met 6-month criteria for a DSM-III (American Psychiatric Association 1980) anxiety disorder in the ECA study

(Regier et al. 1990). Similarly, the NCS data also found women to be at increased risk for anxiety disorders compared with men. The NCS estimates provided strong evidence that anxiety disorders are much less prevalent in men than in women: panic disorder (2.0% vs. 5.0%), post-traumatic stress disorder (PTSD; 6.0% vs. 11.3%), specific phobia (6.7% vs. 15.7%), generalized anxiety disorder (GAD; 3.6% vs. 6.6%), and agoraphobia (3.5% vs. 7.0%). The smallest difference was found in social phobia (11.1% vs. 15.5%) (Kessler et al. 1994).

Although gender-specific data are not available from epidemiological studies, data from clinical populations indicate that men with anxiety disorders appear to be more likely than women to have a comorbid substance use disorder (Yonkers et al. 1996). Anxiety disorders in both men and women are associated with an increased risk for subsequent major depressive disorder.

FACTORS IN GENDER-RELATED DIFFERENCES IN ANXIETY DISORDERS

Several genetic, developmental, and environmental factors have been implicated in the lower prevalence of anxiety disorders in men. Sex-role socialization and hormonal influences are likely to contribute. However, little is presently known regarding the specific sex-related mechanisms associated with differential risks for experiencing anxiety disorders observed in men and women.

Genetics

Familial aggregation resulting from genetic risk factors has been documented for all of the major anxiety disorders (Hettema et al. 2001, 2005; Kendler et al. 1995). Twin studies have been used to extensively investigate the potential role of genetic factors in the development of certain anxiety disorders in women and men. These studies suggest that vulnerability to anxiety disorders may be more heavily influenced by genetic factors in women than in men (Kendler et al. 1995). A twin study (Hettema et al. 2005) of the structure of genetic risk factors for anxiety disorders found that genes predispose to two broad groups of disorders: 1) panic disorder, GAD, and agoraphobia; and 2) specific phobias. Common genetic factors accounted for less than 5% of the variance of GAD, panic disorder, and agoraphobia. The total proportion of variance explained by genetic factors was estimated to be approximately 25%–35% for all the disorders except social phobia, in which genetic factors accounted for 10% of the total variance. The remaining associations between the disorders were largely explained by unique environmental factors shared across the disorders and, to a lesser extent, common shared environmental factors, which accounted for approximately 10% or less of the variance for any of the disorders. No difference in the underlying structure of the genetic risk factors for the anxiety disorders has been found between men and women (Hettema et al. 2001, 2005).

Development

Gender differences in the prevalence of anxiety disorders may derive, in part, from sex differences in socialization. Socially conferred gender labels pervade multiple levels of social experience (Feingold 1994). These social processes may explain gender-specific personality traits and assumptions about social relations and thus influence the processing of cognitive-emotional stimuli that may impact response to stress. Ultimately, the differential socialization of males and females may result in behavioral gender differences that alter thresholds for vulnerability to psychopathology, possibly by increasing the potential for specific psychiatric symptoms viewed by society as compatible with the individual's gender role (Seeman 1997). The gender-based social factors linked to the increased vulnerability of women to depression, such as discrimination in the workplace (Lennon 1995), power imbalances in relationships, childhood adversity (Gold et al. 1998), and response to violence and trauma, might contribute to the higher prevalence of anxiety disorders in females as compared with males.

Environment

Studies concerning the relationship between triggering events and prevalence of anxiety disorders have found that the presence of stressful events like perinatal trauma, early separation, and mourning are significantly more frequent in males than in females with OCD (Bogetto et al. 1999). Childhood trauma, including childhood physical or sexual abuse, has been implicated in an increased risk of developing anxiety disorders during adulthood in both genders. Childhood abuse has been strongly related to the presence of panic disorder, social phobia, GAD, and PTSD (Safren et al. 2002). Some data suggest that men, compared with women, are less vulnerable to psychopathology after childhood abuse (Breslau et al. 1991; Thompson et al. 2004). For example, a history of childhood trauma appears to predict more reliably PTSD in women than in men (Breslau et al. 1991). Furthermore, gender has been proposed to have a substantial impact on the specific anxiety disorder that may develop following chronic environmental stress.

TREATMENT SEEKING AND TREATMENT RESPONSE

Research has consistently shown that, despite the availability of effective treatments, a high proportion of people with anxiety disorders in the United States are untreated, resulting in substantial distress and impairment (Lepine 2002; Wang et al. 2005a, 2005b). Recent data from the NCS-R suggest that the vast majority of people with anxiety disorders will eventually make treatment contact. Men had significantly lower odds of treatment contact than did women, particularly men with social phobia. Furthermore, when men with anxiety disorders seek treatment, they tend to do so later than women (Wang et al. 2005a), consistent with general gender-related treatment-seeking patterns (see Chapter 17, "Overcoming Stigma and Barriers to Mental Health Treatment"). However, men who seek treatment are more likely than treatment-seeking women to use mental health services, resulting in men having a considerably higher probability of receiving adequate treatment than women (Wang et al. 2005a, 2005b).

Although the prevalence and role of etiological factors in anxiety disorders are different in men and women (Kessler et al. 2005a, 2005b; Regier et al. 1990), very few studies have examined the impact of gender on treatment response in patients with anxiety disorders. Pharmacotherapy studies have not identified significant gender differences in response to selective serotonin reuptake inhibitors (SSRIs; Denys et al. 2003; Marshall et al. 2001; Van Ameringen et al. 2004; Van der Kolk et al. 2001), anticonvulsants (Pande et al. 1998), or reversible monoamine oxidase A inhibitors (Connor et al. 2001). Treatment response for each anxiety disorder is discussed in greater detail in the following sections; however, for a discussion of PTSD, please see Chapter 10, "Posttraumatic Stress Disorder."

GENERALIZED ANXIETY DISORDER

The DSM-IV-TR criteria for GAD include both somatic and cognitive manifestations. Cognitive features include impaired concentration, worry, and apprehension. Physical manifestations include restlessness, fatigue, irritability, sleep disturbances, and muscle tension. Recent population surveys estimate that the lifetime prevalence rate for GAD is between 5% and 6% (Kessler et al. 2005a), with a 12-month prevalence rate of 3.1% (Kessler et al. 2005b). GAD is associated with significant disability and dysfunction in both community and primary care samples (Gater et al. 1998).

Prevalence and Comorbidity

Men have approximately one-half to one-third the risk for developing GAD compared with women. Population surveys report 12-month GAD prevalence rates of 2.4% for men and 5% for women (Wittchen et al. 1994). Men also have significantly later age of onset (Steiner et al. 2005), a slightly less chronic course, and milder symptom severity (Bruce et al. 2005; Wittchen et al. 1994; Yonkers et al. 1996). In clinical samples, men are less likely to have a lifetime history of a comorbid anxiety disorder (80% vs. 95%). In particular, men appear less likely to experience panic disorder with agoraphobia (Bruce et al. 2005; Yonkers et al. 1998, 2003). Comorbidity rates of major depressive disorder, however, have been found to be equivalent for men and women (Brawman-Mintzer et al. 1993). In clinical samples, men with GAD report less functional impairment and are at lower risk of suicide than women with GAD (Yonkers et al. 1996), a finding that might be explained in part by the lower rates of other comorbid anxiety disorders. This lower rate of comorbidity and less severe symptom presentation may explain why men with GAD are less likely to seek treatment with a health care professional (Brawman-Mintzer et al. 1993).

Etiological Factors

In a large population-based sample of male and female twins, Hettema et al. (2001) found evidence for a modest genetic contribution to GAD. The genetic contributions to GAD were similarly robust in men and women, in the range of 15%–20%, with data suggesting that largely identical genetic factors contribute to the risk for GAD in men and women. Gender differences have not been identified in neurobiological or neuroimaging investigations conducted in patients with GAD, perhaps because existing studies have not focused on the potential impact of gender.

Clinical Course

Although complete remission of GAD symptoms is rare, the majority of patients report a stable but symptomatic presentation. In addition, approximately one-half of individuals with GAD continue to experience symptoms associated with a comorbid anxiety disorder (Bruce et al. 2005; Yonkers et al. 1996, 2003). Analysis of data from a 12-year follow-up from the Harvard-Brown Anxiety Research Program (HARP) revealed that the probability of remission for GAD was 0.15 after 1 year and 0.25 after 2 years. The probability of becoming completely asymptomatic was only 0.08 (Bruce et al. 2005). However, unlike other anxiety disorders, the clinical course of GAD appears similar for men and women, with the risks for remission and relapse being approximately equivalent (Bruce et al. 2005).

Treatment Response

Despite the findings of gender differences in prevalence, comorbidity, and treatment seeking, there is limited information on the impact of gender on treatment response in GAD. Pollack et al. (2003) analyzed pooled data from 1,839 patients in five individual placebo-controlled studies of extended-release venlafaxine for GAD. These investigators found that men receiving venlafaxine were significantly less likely than women receiving venlafaxine to achieve remission after 24 weeks of treatment (odds ratio [OR] = 0.79). After 8 weeks in the study, men in the placebo group were relatively more likely to remit than were women (OR = 1.57). In contrast, Steiner et al. (2005) recently found no gender differences in efficacy of or tolerability to sertraline treatment in a sample of 167 men and 203 women. The patients were randomized to 12 weeks of double-blind treatment with sertraline (n = 182) or placebo (n = 188). Although no interaction between gender and treatment with sertraline was observed, the response rates to sertraline as compared with placebo were significantly different (men, 64% vs. 40%; women, 62% vs. 34%). To date, no study has examined gender difference in response to cognitive-behavioral therapy, and further examination of gender differences in response to specific pharmacological and behavioral interventions for GAD is warranted.

PANIC DISORDER AND AGORAPHOBIA

DSM-IV-TR defines panic disorder as the presence of panic attacks that are persistent, unexpected, and followed by 1 month or more of constant concern about having additional attacks, substantial behavioral changes related to the attacks, and worry about the implications and consequences of the attacks. Panic attacks are sudden paroxysms that include four or more of a list of physical and cognitive symptoms. The somatic features include tingling sensations, dizziness, abdominal discomfort, chest pain, shortness of breath, palpitations, sweating, and trembling and flushing, whereas the cognitive manifestations are often related to an irrepressible fear of losing control or dying and feelings of unreality or depersonalization. DSM-IV-TR criteria for panic disorder with agoraphobia include anxiety about being in places or situations from which escape might be difficult or not available in the face of developing paniclike symptoms. Patients most commonly present with panic disorder in medical rather than mental health settings, often with prominent cardiovascular, respiratory, or gastrointestinal complaints, although presentation in mental health clinics is not unusual either.

Both the ECA study and the NCS identified panic disorder as a common psychiatric condition with a lifetime prevalence rate estimated between 2.2% and 3.5% (Kessler et al. 1994; Regier et al. 1990). Slightly higher lifetime (4.7%) and 12-month (2.7%) prevalence estimates were reported by the NCS-R (Kessler et al. 2005a, 2005b). Data from clinical samples suggest that agoraphobia in the absence of panic disorder is rare. Lifetime prevalence of agoraphobia without panic attacks was estimated at 1.4%, in contrast with the 4.7% lifetime prevalence for panic disorder reported by the NCS-R (Kessler et al. 2005a).

Epidemiology

The ECA study found that men are almost four times less likely than women to meet criteria for panic disorder (0.9% vs. 3.4%; Regier et al. 1990). ECA data estimate the rate for panic disorder with agoraphobia in men is approximately half that in women (3.7% vs. 7.9%) (Regier et al. 1990).

Biological Factors

Gender differences in vulnerability to panic disorder and in clinical presentations of the disorder may be explained in part by the influences of estrogen on norepinephrine at the α_2-adrenergic receptor (Stahl 1997). Estrogen decreases responsiveness of the α_2-adrenergic receptor, thereby enhancing norepinephrine release in the synaptic terminal and neurotransmission (Stahl 1997). Studies examining β-adrenergic receptor sensitivity indicate that women with panic disorder have significantly lower sensitivity to stimulation of the β-adrenergic receptor than do healthy female volunteers. Interestingly, male subjects with panic disorder do not show differences in sensitivity to stimulation of the β-adrenergic receptor compared with healthy male volunteers (Kim et al. 2004). These results suggest a mechanism for gender differences in the pathophysiology of panic disorder. The interaction between biological factors and social roles and traumatic experiences as contributing to gender differences in the development of panic disorder has yet to be systematically investigated.

Symptomatology

Clinical studies have identified gender differences in the symptomatology of panic disorder with agoraphobia, particularly in three main dimensions: agoraphobic avoidance, cognitions, and body sensations (Starcevic et al. 1998; Turgeon et al. 1998). Turgeon et al. (1998) compared 96 women and 58 men with panic disorder with agoraphobia and assessed various clinical features associated with the disorder. The investigators found that men reported less severe agoraphobic avoidance when facing situations or places alone, related fewer catastrophic thoughts, and judged their body sensations to be significantly less frightening. These findings are consistent with studies in which men were found to avoid fewer public situations and less frequently become completely homebound and dependent. Men are less likely to seek help and request to be accompanied in agoraphobic situations by the spouse or the children (Starcevic et al. 1998).

Trembling and shaking during panic attacks are reported less frequently and with less intensity in men as compared with women (Starcevic et al. 1998). Compared with women with the disorder, men with panic disorder with agoraphobia are more afraid of having a heart attack or a physical illness, leaving home alone, or being in crowded places (Starcevic et al. 1998; Turgeon et al. 1998).

Comorbidity

Evidence suggests that men with panic disorder are less likely to have a second anxiety disorder (55% vs. 66%; Turgeon et al. 1998). Results from clinical samples indicate that the most frequent comorbid anxiety disorders are GAD (38% of men vs. 44% of women), specific phobia (21% vs. 25%), PTSD (9% vs. 23%), and social phobia (7% vs. 17%) (Turgeon et al. 1998). Comorbid alcohol abuse and dependence, mitral valve prolapse, and hyperthyroidism are each associated more frequently with panic disorder in men than in women. No significant gender differences have been reported regarding the co-occurrence of lifetime major depressive disorder with panic disorder (Starcevic et al. 1998).

Clinical Course

Data suggest that the clinical course and outcome of panic disorder with agoraphobia differ by gender. In a prospective study, the probability of remission of panic disorder with or without agoraphobia was 0.41 for men compared with 0.38 in women (Yonkers et al. 1998). However, the cumulative probability of recurrence for panic disorder with agoraphobia was 0.39 in men versus 0.65 in women. In terms of the symptoms that were more likely to recur, panic attacks, not agoraphobic fear, were almost invariably the trigger for clinical worsening in both groups (Yonkers et al. 1998).

Treatment Seeking and Treatment Response

Data from the HARP study found no gender differences in the prescription of psychoactive medications (Blanco et al. 2004; Yonkers et al. 2003). Both genders have been found to have virtually identical rates of treatment with benzodiazepines, tricyclic antidepressants, monoamine oxidase inhibitors, and serotonin reuptake inhibitors. No gender differences were found regarding the intensity of treatment received or number of weeks of medication use (Yonkers et al. 1998).

Most patients with panic disorder respond acutely to pharmacological treatment. In clinical trials, approximately 60%–70% of patients have a positive response to treatment, although only 30%–40% experience complete remission (Roy-Byrne and Cowley 1998). Male gender is a weak predictor of poor outcome in patients with panic disorder (Yonkers et al. 1998). However, no published research has systematically examined the differential antipanic efficacy of SSRIs in patients at high risk for poor outcome. Analysis of data pooled ($N=664$) from four double-blind, placebo-controlled studies of the efficacy of sertraline for the treatment of panic disorder found no gender difference in treatment response. The study examined the predictive value of five other clinical variables (panic severity, presence of agoraphobia, comorbid depression, comorbid personality disorder, and duration of illness) in the response to sertraline (Pollack et al. 2000). Similar findings were reported by a clinical trial examining the predictors of treatment response in a primary care setting of 115 patients with DSM-IV-TR panic disorder with and without agoraphobia. Patients were randomly assigned either to pharmacotherapy with the SSRI paroxetine along with a patient-targeted multifaceted intervention or to no pharmacological intervention and standard care by a primary care physician. The study included 82 women and 33 men and found no relationship between gender and response to paroxetine over 1 year of follow-up (Roy-Byrne et al. 2003).

Cognitive-behavioral therapy is well established as an effective treatment for panic disorder. To date, few studies have examined the potential impact of gender on treatment response in panic disorder. Martinsen et al. (1998) compared the outcome of 27 men and 56 women with panic disorder who received 4-hour cognitive-behavioral therapy sessions conducted once a week for 11 weeks. The study found no gender-related differences in response over a 1-year follow-up. In conjunction with the results of pharmacotherapy studies, these findings suggest that the tendency to a poorer outcome observed in female patients with panic disorder is not explained by a gender-related difference in response to pharmacotherapy with SSRIs or to cognitive-behavioral therapy. Nonetheless, further research is needed to elucidate the potential impact of gender in response to specific pharmacotherapies and psychotherapies for panic disorder patients.

SPECIFIC PHOBIAS

Phobias represent irrational fears of specific objects, circumstances, or situations. Either the presence or the anticipation of the phobic entity elicits severe distress in an affected person and produces conscious avoidance of the feared subject. Specific phobias encompass a wide range of fears, including situation-related phobias (claustrophobia, acrophobia), animal-related phobias (fear of spiders, insects, snakes), and health care–related phobias (e.g., fear of injections, blood, dental procedures).

Data from the NCS-R suggest that specific phobia is the third most prevalent psychiatric disorder. The lifetime prevalence rate is 12.5%, and the 12-month prevalence rate is 8.7% (Kessler et al. 2005a, 2005b). Most studies suggest that specific phobia begins during adolescence, with a mean age at onset of approximately 15 years (Fredrickson et al. 1996). Situational phobias represent the most common specific phobias (13.2%), followed by animal-related phobia (8%), and then health care–related phobia (3%). Monosymptomatic phobias appear more common than multiple phobias (Fredrickson et al. 1996).

Epidemiology and Clinical Presentation

Men have less than half the lifetime risk for specific phobia than do women (12% vs. 26%; Fredrickson et al. 1996). Men also appear less likely than women to meet criteria for situational phobias (8.5% vs. 17%) and animal phobias (3% vs. 12%) and less frequently experience fears related to objects and situations. In contrast, health care–related phobias have largely similar prevalence rates in men and women (2.7% vs. 3.2%; Fredrickson et al. 1996). Gender differences in the frequency of both monosymptomatic and multiple phobias have been documented, with 11% of men having a single specific phobia and 1.5% having multiple phobias, compared with rates of 21% and 5%, respectively, for women (Fredrickson et al. 1996).

Etiological Factors

Phobias aggregate in families (Fyer et al. 1995; Stein et al. 1998). Epidemiological studies indicate gender differences in the prevalence of specific phobias, and twin studies report significant genetic influence (Fyer et al. 1995; Stein et al. 1998). An investigation involving more than 3,000 twin pairs found that situational and medical phobias had a slightly lower heritability estimate in males than females. By contrast, the model suggested equal heritability in males and females for animal phobias. No evidence was found for an impact of family environment on vulnerability to these fears or phobias (Kendler et al. 2002). These findings suggest that the overall etiological impact of genes is similar in males and females with situational and health care–related fears or phobias, with no significant etiological role for family environment (Kendler et al. 2002). Although numerous reports have found that men have lower prevalence rates of specific phobia compared with women, little additional information is available concerning gender differences in the clinical features or course of specific phobia. Similarly, despite the high prevalence of phobias among the general population, to date little is known about gender-related differences in response to pharmacotherapy or cognitive-behavioral therapy in phobic patients, suggesting an area in need of future research.

SOCIAL PHOBIA

DSM-IV-TR defines social phobia as the persistent fear of social situations in which an individual may be open to scrutiny by others. Individuals with social phobia fear being the focus of attention of a crowd or an individual or the possibility of behaving in an embarrassing or humiliating way. Exposure to the situation almost invariably provokes anxiety manifested as blushing, shaking, or gastrointestinal symptoms. As a result, a pattern of avoidance of social situations often emerges.

Data from the NCS-R indicate that social anxiety disorder is the fourth most prevalent psychiatric lifetime disorder, with a 12.1% lifetime prevalence rate and a 6.8% 12-month prevalence rate (Kessler et al. 2005a, 2005b). The NCS-R also found that social phobia shows a later mean age at onset (13 years) than do specific phobias. Data from a 12-year prospective study examining the recovery and recurrence rates of GAD, social phobia, and panic disorder indicate that patients with social phobia have the lowest probability of achieving recovery (0.37) among the examined anxiety disorders (Bruce et al. 2005). These findings suggest that overall social phobia has a more chronic course than do other anxiety disorders.

Epidemiology

Social phobia is less prevalent in men than in women. Early epidemiological studies estimated the lifetime prevalence rates were 2.0% for men and 3.1% for women (Regier et al. 1990). However, the NCS data reported higher lifetime prevalence estimates (11.1% in men and 15.5% in women; Kessler et al. 1994). These findings are reconciled by the fact that the NCS assessed a wider spectrum of social situations than did earlier studies.

Etiological Factors

Data from clinical samples examining the potential association between the onset of phobias and the occurrence of adverse experiences during childhood indicate that the onset of social phobia is often associated with the occurrence of two adverse experiences during childhood: sexual assault and chronic exposure to verbal outbursts between parents (Safren et al. 2002). In examining gender differences in the etiology of social phobia, it seems important to look beyond differences in overall severity of fear. A study of gender differences in social anxiety disorder using a clinical sample found that men report less distress displaying negative feelings and less anxiety about public oration, speaking in front of small groups of familiar people, talking to strangers, and meeting new people. However, men report more reluctance to display behavior related to expression of and dealing with personal limitations (Turk et al. 1998). Taken together, these findings suggest that gender differences in social behavior in specific situations might explain in part gender differences in the situational and performance fears associated with social phobia.

Symptomatology

A study of a clinical sample with social phobia found that men tend to have less severe symptoms than do women (Turk et al. 1998). Significant differences in phenomenology were also reported. As compared with women, men were more likely to report anxiety related to urinating in public bathrooms and returning goods to a store and less likely to acknowledge anxiety related to talking to authority figures; acting, performing, speaking, or working in front of others or while being observed; being the center of attention; expressing disagreement or disapproval to unfamiliar people; and hosting parties (Turk et al. 1998).

Comorbidity

Turk et al. (1998) found that men and women with social phobia were equally likely to receive a comorbid diagnosis of a mood disorder (21.9% in men vs. 27.3% in women), an additional anxiety disorder (38.4% vs. 48.5%), or any mood or anxiety disorder (47.9% vs. 56.1%). These findings contrast with data from the HARP study, in which men were found to have significantly lower rates of comorbid panic disorder with agoraphobia (28% in men vs. 50% in women) and specific phobia (9% vs. 24%) (Bruce et al. 2005; Yonkers et al. 2001). Data from the same report indicate that men were more likely to have a diagnosis of current or past alcohol or drug abuse or dependence.

Clinical Course

Few studies have investigated potential gender differences in the clinical course of social phobia. Available data indicate that the chronicity of social phobia is strikingly high for both men and women (Bruce et al. 2005; Yonkers et al. 2003). No significant differences have been found for relapse or remission rates between genders. Using data from the HARP study, Yonkers et al. (2003) compared the clinical course of subjects with social phobia after 8 years of follow-up. Only 32% of the men and 38% of the women experienced full remission. No gender differences in full or partial remission rates were detected.

Altogether, study findings suggest that men are less likely than women to meet lifetime criteria for social phobia. Men with social phobia have fewer social anxiety–related fears and less overall symptom severity. However, they are more likely to seek treatment, possibly due to higher interference of the symptoms in their lives (Weinstock 1999).

Treatment Response

Data support the efficacy of multiple treatments for social phobia, including cognitive-behavioral therapy, social skills training (Heimberg et al. 1998), monoamine oxidase inhibitors, reversible inhibitors of monoamine oxidase A, benzodiazepines, anticonvulsants, and SSRIs (Van Ameringen et al. 2001). SSRIs are considered the first-line treatments for social phobia (Van Ameringen et al. 2001). However, little is known about gender differences in treatment response in social phobia.

A recent clinical trial examined the influence of age at onset on the response to treatment in 204 subjects with social phobia. Subjects were randomly assigned to sertraline or placebo for a 20-week treatment period. Men composed 56% of the sample. Men and women showed equivalent improvement in response to 20 weeks of sertraline treatment. Women assigned to placebo showed a superior improvement slope compared with men receiving placebo (Van Ameringen et al. 2004). Smaller clinical samples have shown a similar pattern of response. A trial involving 69 patients and evaluating the efficacy and safety of gabapentin found that placebo-treated men showed lower response rates than did placebo-treated women. However, male and female patients did not differ in their rates of response to 14 weeks of treatment with gabapentin (Pande et al. 1998). These findings might reflect the slightly higher remission rates observed in clinical studies in women with social anxiety disorder. However, further research is warranted to elucidate the clinical impact of these findings.

OBSESSIVE-COMPULSIVE DISORDER

Obsessions and compulsions are the core features of OCD. According to DSM-IV-TR, an *obsession* is defined as a recurrent intrusive and excessive thought, impulse, or image that causes marked distress. *Compulsions* are repetitive behaviors or mental acts that the person feels driven to perform in response to an obsession and that are aimed at preventing or reducing distress. However, compulsions are not fully connected with what they are designed to neutralize or prevent. Regardless of how vivid and persuasive the obsessive idea or impulse is, the person usually recognizes its irrationality and thus constantly attempts to ignore or suppress such objects. The patient with OCD can present with a wide range of symptoms, but the most common obsessive symptoms relate to aggression, contamination, symmetry, saving or collecting, sexual impulses, or religious matters, and the most common compulsive rituals include checking, cleaning, counting, ordering, and hoarding rituals.

The recently published NCS-R estimated the 12-month prevalence of OCD to be 1%, with a lifetime prevalence of 1.6% (Kessler et al. 2005a, 2005b). Onset of OCD is early, usually during adolescence or young adulthood. Mean age at onset appears to range from ages 18 to 29 years, closely followed by ages 30–44 years (Bogetto et al. 1999; Kessler et al. 2005a). Most patients with OCD experience a chronic clinical course characterized by waxing and waning of symptoms without complete remissions and with constant functional impairment between exacerbations (Bogetto et al. 1999; Lenzi et al. 1996).

Epidemiology

Data estimate that the lifetime prevalence of OCD is 0.5%–2.5% in men and 0.9%–3.4% in women (Bogetto et al. 1999; Lenzi et al. 1996). Men tend to have an earlier, more insidious onset and more chronic course (Bogetto et al. 1999). Onset of OCD before age 10 is associated with male gender, tic disorder, and a positive family history. Male OCD patients appear more likely to remain single. However, these findings may be confounded by the age of the patients at index evaluation as well as age at onset of the disorder (Lenzi et al. 1996). Analyses from epidemiological samples are needed to confirm these findings.

Etiological Factors

Despite recent advances, there are gaps in the understanding of the etiology of OCD. Concerning the relationship between triggering events and the onset of the disorder, Lenzi et al. (1996) found stressful life events in association with the onset of OCD in 64.2% of the patients in their sample and noted that the more common antecedent events before onset of the disorder were undesirable events such as losing a loved one, severe medical illness, or major financial difficulties. Negative events, such as separation and mourning, before the onset of the disorder were more frequent in males than females. Men had higher percentages of at least one negative life event before the onset of the disorder. Data from the same report indicate that men who have early-onset OCD have a significantly greater history of perinatal trauma (e.g., application of forceps, breech presentation, or prolonged hypoxia). These results are in contrast with findings by Bogetto et al. (1999), who found that females more frequently report stressful life events in the year preceding OCD onset. However, males with at least one severe event before OCD onset had a lower mean age at onset. These discrepancies may in part reflect the different criteria to classify stressful events in the studies.

Symptomatology

Gender differences have been observed in OCD symptoms. Men generally less frequently acknowledge aggressive and contamination obsessions and cleaning rituals and more frequently report obsessions involving slowness, sex, exactness, symmetry, and odd rituals (Bogetto et al. 1999; Lenzi et al. 1996).

Comorbidity

Among clinical samples, more than 50% of OCD patients receive concurrent psychiatric diagnoses (Bogetto et al. 1999; Lenzi et al. 1996). Higher lifetime prevalences of social phobia, hypomanic episodes, and depersonalization disorder have been reported in male compared with female patients in clinical samples (Lenzi et al. 1996). A higher proportion of males also report that social phobia and specific phobia precede the onset of OCD. Rates of major depressive disorder, GAD, and panic disorder appear not to differ between men and women with OCD (Bogetto et al. 1999; Lenzi et al. 1996).

Clinical Course

A study of 160 patients with OCD found that men as compared with women had a more insidious onset and chronic course, with greater fluctuations in symptoms and persistence of social and occupational impairment between exacerbations (Bogetto et al. 1999). In contrast, Lenzi et al. (1996) did not observe gender differences in the percentage of subjects with chronic or episodic courses of OCD.

Treatment Response

Studies of gender differences in treatment response have yielded mixed results. One study of 50 subjects with OCD (24 men) who were randomly assigned to 10 weeks of either clomipramine or fluvoxamine after failing to respond to single-blind intravenous clomipramine found that men had a poorer response to serotonergic agents (Mundo et al. 1999). Similarly, a study of 159 OCD subjects (88 men) undergoing a 12-week standardized treatment with fluvoxamine, clomipramine, citalopram, or paroxetine found that female gender was a positive predictive variable of response only for those subjects treated with clomipramine (Erzegovesi et al. 2001).

Other authors have not identified gender differences in treatment response. Denys et al. (2003) studied the treatment response of 150 OCD subjects (57 men) who were randomly assigned to receive either paroxetine or extended-release venlafaxine for 12 weeks in a double-blind, parallel-group study. The study failed to detect an association between gender and treatment response.

Gender-related differences in response to psychotherapy have not been reported to date. However, clinical trials have examined the predictors of treatment response to cognitive-behavioral therapy in patients with OCD. One clinical trial evaluated 49 inpatients with OCD treated over 3 years. Treatment consisted of inpatient exposure, occasionally combined with other interventions individually tailored to the patient's specific difficulties. The study reported an approximately 40% reduction in rituals in 31 (63.3%) of these chronic patients. These gains were maintained at an average 19-month follow-up. Checking rituals were more likely to be associated with good outcome. Women had a later onset of the disorder and a slight tendency to better prognosis. No other predictors of outcome were found (Ackerman et al. 1998).

CONCLUSION

A substantial body of literature consistently indicates that anxiety disorders are less prevalent in men. Although the etiological factors implicated in the genesis of anxiety disorders are not entirely understood, it appears that men are less vulnerable to the impact of traumatic exposure on the development of an anxiety disorder, despite the higher prevalence of traumatic events in this population.

Gender differences in the clinical presentation of DSM-IV-TR anxiety disorders have been extensively documented, but the impact of these differences on the performance of the social roles historically conferred to male gender, quality of life, and treatment seeking remains to be elucidated. Little is known about gender differences in treatment response. The available evidence suggests that in most cases gender is generally not a predictor of response to pharmacological treatments for anxiety disorders. Further research is needed to confirm this finding and to examine the extent to which it extends to psychotherapy treatments.

REFERENCES

Ackerman DL, Greenland S, Bystritsky A: Clinical characteristics of response to fluoxetine treatment of obsessive-compulsive disorder. J Clin Psychopharmacol 18:459–465, 1998

American Psychiatric Association: Diagnostic and Statistical Manual of Mental Disorders, 3rd Edition. Washington, DC, American Psychiatric Association, 1980

American Psychiatric Association: Diagnostic and Statistical Manual of Mental Disorders, 4th Edition, Text Revision. Washington, DC, American Psychiatric Association, 2000

KEY POINTS

- Men have a substantially lower risk of developing lifetime anxiety disorders compared with women. In addition, researchers have generally observed a decreased symptom severity, less chronic course, and lower functional impairment in men with anxiety disorders compared with women.

- Men with anxiety disorders have a lower lifetime risk compared with women for developing comorbid psychiatric disorders in general and certain comorbid disorders in particular. The smaller prevalence of comorbid disorders in men with panic disorder may result in a less chronic and severe course of the illness than in women.

- To date, evidence of gender differences in treatment response to different anxiety disorders is scarce and remains mostly inconclusive.

PRACTICE GUIDELINES

1. Attempt early recognition of initial indicators of a primary or comorbid anxiety disorder, keeping in mind that on average the clinical presentation tends to be less severe.

2. Assess the impact of the symptoms on the social roles conferred traditionally to male gender.

3. Estimate appropriateness for pharmacological versus behavioral interventions.

Blanco C, Goodwin R, Liebowitz M, et al: Use of psychotropic medications for patients with office visits who receive a diagnosis of panic disorder. Med Care 42:1242–1253, 2004

Bogetto F, Venturello S, Albert U, et al: Gender-related clinical differences in obsessive-compulsive disorder. Eur Psychiatry 14:434–441, 1999

Brawman-Mintzer O, Lydiard R, Emmanuel N: Psychiatric comorbidity in patients with generalized anxiety disorder. Am J Psychiatry 150:1216–1218, 1993

Breslau N, Davis GC, Andreski P, et al: Traumatic events and posttraumatic stress disorder in an urban population of young adults. Arch Gen Psychiatry 48:216–222, 1991

Bruce S, Yonkers K, Otto M, et al: Influence of psychiatric comorbidity on recovery and recurrence in generalized anxiety disorder, social phobia, and panic disorder: a 12-year prospective study. Am J Psychiatry 162:1179–1187, 2005

Connor K, Hidalgo R, Crockett B, et al: Predictors of treatment response in patients with posttraumatic stress disorder. Prog Neuropsychopharmacol Biol Psychiatry 25:337–345, 2001

Denys D, Burger H, Megen H, et al: A score for predicting response to pharmacotherapy in obsessive-compulsive disorder. Int Clin Psychopharmacol 18:315–322, 2003

Erzegovesi E, Cavallini MC, Cavedini P, et al: Clinical predictors of drug response in obsessive compulsive disorder. J Clin Psychopharmacol 21:488–492, 2001

Feingold A: Gender differences in personality: a meta-analysis. Psychol Bull 116:429–456, 1994

Fredrickson M, Annas P, Hakan F, et al: Gender differences in the prevalence of specific fears and phobias. Behav Res Ther 34:33–39, 1996

Fyer A, Manuzza S, Chapman TF, et al: Specificity in familial aggregation in phobic disorders. Arch Gen Psychiatry 52:554–573, 1995

Gater R, Tansella M, Korten A, et al: Sex differences in the prevalence and detection of depressive and anxiety disorders in general health care settings: report from the World Health Organization Collaborative Study on Psychological Problems in General Health Care. Arch Gen Psychiatry 55:405–413, 1998

Gold SN, Lucenko B, Elhai JD, et al: A comparison of psychological/psychiatric symptomatology of women and men sexually abused as children. Child Abuse Negl 23:683–692, 1998

Heimberg RG, Liebowitz MR, Hope DA: Cognitive behavioral group therapy vs phenelzine therapy for social phobia: 12-week outcome. Arch Gen Psychiatry 55:1133–1141, 1998

Hettema J, Prescott C, Kendler K: A population-based twin study of generalized anxiety disorder in men and women. J Nerv Ment Dis 189:413–420, 2001

Hettema J, Prescott C, Myers J, et al: The structure of genetic and environmental risk factors for anxiety disorders in men and women. Arch Gen Psychiatry 62:182–189, 2005

Kendler KS, Walters EE, Neale MC: The structure of the genetic and environmental risk factors for six major psychiatric disorders in women: phobia, generalized anxiety disorder, panic disorder, bulimia, major depression, and alcoholism. Arch Gen Psychiatry 52:374–383, 1995

Kendler KS, Jacobson KC, Myers J, et al: Sex differences in genetic and environmental risk factors for irrational fears and phobias. Psychol Med 32:209–217, 2002

Kessler R, McGonagle K, Zhao S: Lifetime and 12-month prevalence of DSM-III-R psychiatric disorders in the United States: results from the National Comorbidity Survey. Arch Gen Psychiatry 51:8–19, 1994

Kessler R, Berglund P, Demler O, et al: Lifetime prevalence and age-of-onset distributions of DSM-IV disorders in the National Comorbidity Survey Replication. Arch Gen Psychiatry 62:593–602, 2005a

Kessler R, Chiu W, Demler O, et al: Prevalence, severity, and comorbidity of 12-month DSM-IV disorders in the National Comorbidity Survey Replication. Arch Gen Psychiatry 62:617–627, 2005b

Kim Y, Kil Min S, Yu B: Differences in beta-adrenergic receptor sensitivity between women and men with panic disorder. Eur Neuropsychopharmacol 14:515–520, 2004

Lennon MC: Work conditions as explanations for the relation between socioeconomic status, gender and psychological disorders. Epidemiol Rev 17:120–127, 1995

Lenzi P, Cassano G, Correddu G, et al: Obsessive-compulsive disorder: family developmental history, symptomatology, comorbidity and course with special reference to gender-related differences. Br J Psychiatry 169:101–107, 1996

Lepine J: The epidemiology of anxiety disorders: prevalence and societal costs. J Clin Psychiatry 63 (suppl 14):4–8, 2002

Marshall R, Beebe K, Oldham M, et al: Efficacy and safety of paroxetine treatment for chronic PTSD: a fixed-dose, placebo-controlled study. Am J Psychiatry 158:1982–1988, 2001

Martinsen E, Olsen T, Tonset E, et al: Cognitive-behavioral group therapy for panic disorder in the general clinical setting: a naturalistic study with 1-year follow-up. J Clin Psychiatry 59:437–442, 1998

Mundo E, Bareggi S, Pirola R, et al: Effect of acute intravenous clomipramine and antiobsessional response to proserotonergic drugs: is gender a predictive variable? Biol Psychiatry 45:290–294, 1999

Pande A, Davidson J, Jefferson J, et al: Treatment of social phobia with gabapentin: a placebo-controlled study. J Clin Psychopharmacol 19:341–348, 1998

Pollack MH, Rapaport MH, Clary CM, et al: Sertraline treatment of panic disorder: response in patients at risk for poor outcome. J Clin Psychiatry 61:922–927, 2000

Pollack MH, Meoni P, Otto M, et al: Predictors of outcome following venlafaxine extended-release treatment of DSM-IV generalized anxiety disorder: a pooled analysis of short-term and long-term studies. J Clin Psychopharmacol 23:250–259, 2003

Regier D, Narrow W, Rae D: The epidemiology of anxiety disorders: the Epidemiologic Catchment Area (ECA) experience. J Psychiatr Res 24 (suppl 2):3–14, 1990

Roy-Byrne P, Cowley DS: Clinical approach to treatment-resistant panic disorder, in Panic Disorder and Its Treatment. Edited by Rosenbaum JF, Pollack MH. New York, Marcel Dekker, 1998, pp 205–227

Roy-Byrne P, Russo J, Cowley D, et al: Unemployment and emergency room visits predict poor treatment outcome in primary care panic disorder. J Clin Psychiatry 64:383–389, 2003

Safren S, Gershuny B, Marzol P, et al: History of childhood abuse in panic disorder, social phobia, and generalized anxiety disorder. J Nerv Ment Dis 190:453–456, 2002

Seeman MV: Psychopathology in women and men: focus on female hormones. Am J Psychiatry 154:1641–1647, 1997

Stahl S: Reproductive hormones as adjuncts to psychotropic medication in women. Essent Psychopharmacol 2:147–164, 1997

Starcevic V, Djordjevic A, Latas M, et al: Characteristics of agoraphobia in women and men with panic disorder with agoraphobia. Depress Anxiety 8:8–13, 1998

Stein MB, Chartier MJ, Hazen AL, et al: A direct interview family study of generalized social phobia. Am J Psychiatry 155:90–97, 1998

Steiner M, Allgulander C, Ravindran A, et al: Gender differences in clinical presentation and response to sertraline treatment of generalized anxiety disorder. Hum Psychopharmacol 20:3–13, 2005

Thompson MP, Kingree JB, Desai S: Gender differences in long-term health consequences of physical abuse of children: data from a nationally representative survey. Am J Public Health 94:599–604, 2004

Turgeon L, Marchand A, Dupuis G: Clinical features in panic disorder with agoraphobia: a comparison of men and women. J Anxiety Disord 12:539–553, 1998

Turk C, Heimberg R, Orsillo S, et al: An investigation of gender differences in social phobia. J Anxiety Disord 12:209–223, 1998

Van Ameringen MA, Lane RM, Walker JR, et al: Sertraline treatment of generalized social phobia: a 20-week, double blind, placebo controlled study. Am J Psychiatry 158:275–281, 2001

Van Ameringen MA, Michael M, Oakman J, et al: Predictors of response in generalized social phobia: effect of age of onset. J Clin Psychopharmacol 24:42–48, 2004

Van der Kolk B, Dreyfuss D, Michaels M, et al: Fluoxetine in posttraumatic stress disorder. J Clin Psychiatry 55:517–522, 2001

Wang P, Berglund P, Olfson M, et al: Failure and delay in initial treatment contact after first onset of mental disorders in the National Comorbidity Survey Replication. Arch Gen Psychiatry 62:603–613, 2005a

Wang P, Lane M, Olfson M, et al: Twelve-month use of mental health services in the United States. Arch Gen Psychiatry 62:629–640, 2005b

Weinstock L: Gender differences in the presentation and management of social anxiety disorder. J Clin Psychiatry 60(suppl):9–13, 1999

Wittchen H, Zhao S, Kessler R, et al: DSM-III-R generalized anxiety disorder in the National Comorbidity Survey. Arch Gen Psychiatry 51:355–364, 1994

Yonkers K, Warshaw M, Massion A, et al: Phenomenology and course of generalised anxiety disorder. Br J Psychiatry 168:308–313, 1996

Yonkers K, Zlotnick C, Allsworth J, et al: Is the course of panic disorder the same in women and men? Am J Psychiatry 155:596–602, 1998

Yonkers K, Dyck I, Keller M: An eight-year longitudinal comparison of clinical course and characteristics of social phobia among men and women. Psychiatr Serv 52:637–643, 2001

Yonkers K, Bruce S, Dyck I, et al: Chronicity, relapse and illness course of panic disorder, social phobia and generalized anxiety disorder: findings in men and women from 8 years of follow-up. Depress Anxiety 17:173–179, 2003

5

DEPRESSION

YAEL LEVIN, B.A.
GERARD SANACORA, M.D., PH.D.

Case Vignette

Albert, a 45-year-old divorced white male, presented with a chief complaint of fatigue. On questioning, he also reported disturbed sleep, recent weight loss, difficulty functioning at work, and recent problems with erectile dysfunction. Although Albert appeared reserved and showed some signs of psychomotor retardation, he denied any significant problems with mood, anxiety, or social functioning outside work.

He reported a history of alcohol abuse and occasional excessive drinking at present. He was a high school graduate and described being very quiet and withdrawn throughout school. Albert married at age 21, and he had been divorced several months before seeking treatment. He had been at the same job for years but described a significant decrease in his work performance and an increase in work-related stressors over the past year. His family history was notable for a father who had mood difficulties throughout his life and who passed away when Albert was a teenager.

The authors would like to acknowledge Carolyn Mazure, Ph.D., for her generous assistance with this chapter.

Albert's physical examination revealed no gross abnormalities. Laboratory tests showed that thyroid function, electrolytes, complete blood count, and testosterone were within normal limits. Liver function tests revealed a slight elevation of γ-glutamyltransferase, aspartate aminotransferase, and alanine aminotransferase. No abnormalities were noted on an electrocardiogram, and Albert denied any cardiac symptoms.

Albert was treated with cognitive-behavioral therapy, in which both his depressive symptoms and excessive alcohol consumption were targeted. He responded well and, after 12 weeks of therapy, showed significant improvements in his fatigue, sleep, weight, and sexual symptoms.

Major depression is among the most commonly occurring and widely debilitating mental disorders worldwide (World Health Organization 2001). Although women are diagnosed with depression nearly twice as often as men (Kuehner 2003; Weissman and Klerman 1977; Weissman et al. 1991), the psychological, biological, and social ramifications of this disorder are no less striking in men who have it. In addition, depressed men exhibit higher rates of comorbid alcohol abuse and dependence than women (Kessler et al. 1997), face an elevated risk of heart disease (Angst et al. 2002a; Ferketich et al. 2000; Hippisley-Cox et al. 1998; Roose 2003), and present alarmingly high rates of completed suicides, taking their own lives approximately four times more often than women (Möller-Leimkühler 2003; Murphy 2000).

Yet depression may be less adequately identified and treated in males. Men with depression frequently endorse fewer diagnostic symptoms than women (Angst et al. 2002a; Kessler et al. 1993), and men may be more hesitant to seek treatment (Angst et al. 2002a). Even among those seeking treatment, men may less frequently be diagnosed with depression than women with similar symptoms, especially in primary care settings. In one study of men and women presenting to a primary care clinic with similarly severe ratings on the Beck Depression Inventory (Beck et al. 1961), 33% of women were diagnosed with depression as compared with only 13.9% of men ($P=0.0295$; Bertakis et al. 2001). Although gender has not always been found to affect the likelihood of being diagnosed with depression (Gater et al. 1998; Olfson et al. 2001), several studies have found that women do appear more likely to be prescribed antidepressant medications than men (Angst et al. 2002a; Hohmann 1989), even when diagnosis and health status are controlled for. This finding may not reflect adequate dosing or even the most appropriate clinical choices in all cases, but it does highlight the disparate treatment given to men and women with similar symptoms of depression.

Despite such potential differences between men and women in the presentation and diagnosis of depression, however, only limited data are available directly examining these gender differences. To date, most studies of depression report relatively little information on gender, and most of the reports that do were not specifically designed to examine these differences. Because women are more commonly diagnosed with depression than men, they are more robustly represented in research studies and have thus accounted for much of the current knowledge about this disorder. However, depression remains a serious and debilitating disorder among men as well. On average, men with depression endorse fewer of its diagnostic symptoms than depressed women, making identification of men with depression more difficult. Men with depression may also exhibit distinct features and seem to respond preferentially to particular antidepressant and hormonal treatments, perhaps due to different underlying precipitants of their depression. Current knowledge of gender differences in depression remains incomplete and further research is essential; however, current findings underscore the importance of accurately identifying and diagnosing depression in men to best treat this disorder. Toward this end, the National Institute of Mental Health has launched an outreach campaign to educate men and mental health clinicians about the signs, symptoms, and treatment of male depression (http://menanddepression.nimh.nih.gov).

DEPRESSION AS EXPRESSED IN MEN

Some estimates suggest that as many as 21.4% of American men in a primary care sample have had a depressive episode in their lifetime (Maier et al. 1999). Larger community samples have been more conservative. The Epidemiologic Catchment Area study reported the lifetime prevalence of major depression among all men to be 2.6%, with the lifetime risk of any depressive episode estimated at 3.6% (Weissman et al. 1991). The subsequent National Comorbidity Survey (NCS) made an effort to elicit more complete information regarding past episodes of depression and as a result estimated this rate to be 12.7% (Kessler et al. 1994b). The NCS also determined that 7.7% of men had had a major depressive episode in the preceding 12 months, with the highest prevalence of 9.5% among men ages 15–24 years (Kessler et al. 1993). Although reported rates of depression vary substantially across cultures and between samples, epidemiological findings in community, primary care, and psychiatric populations consistently indicate that beginning at puberty (Angold et al. 1998; Kessler et al. 1993), men meet the diagnostic criteria for both current and lifetime episodes of depression only half as often as women (Angst et al. 2002a; Gater et al. 1998; Kessler et al. 1993; Kuehner 2003; Maier et al.

1999; Nolen-Hoeksema 1987; Weissman and Klerman 1977; Weissman et al. 1991, 1993). However, there are indications that the diagnosis of depression among men is increasing. An analysis of the Epidemiologic Catchment Area data suggests that prevalence rates for those born after World War II have been rising consistently in men but have become relatively stable in women (Wolk and Weissman 1995), and a similar trend has been reported worldwide (Weissman et al. 1993). Although the NCS did not find such a change in the gender ratio of depression over time, investigators did find that the lifetime rates of depression were increasing in both men and women in more recent birth cohorts (Kessler et al. 1994a), highlighting this disorder as an increasingly prominent health concern for men.

Efforts have been made to understand whether the manifestation of depression in men is distinctly different from that of women, composed of a unique symptom profile and lifetime presentation. Such differences in course and diagnostic tendencies would aid tremendously in the identification and treatment of depression in men. However, major depression remains a heterogeneous disorder, encompassing a wide and disparate range of symptoms (American Psychiatric Association 2000). Although certain diagnostic and descriptive trends have emerged in the study of male depression, no consistent grouping of characteristically male depressive symptoms has yet been identified.

Symptoms of Male Depression

Several groups of symptoms have been suggested to describe the manifestation of depression in men. Although these symptoms remain contentious, the most consistent findings seem to indicate that depressed men endorse fewer of the current diagnostic symptoms of depression than depressed women, particularly in community-based samples (Hildebrandt et al. 2003b). Because current diagnostic criteria define increasing severity in part by a greater number of symptoms (American Psychiatric Association 2000), it could be thought that, on average, men simply have a less severe form of depression than many women. However, this finding may also suggest that the current diagnostic criteria do not adequately embody the symptoms that men present or, alternatively, that men presenting with this more limited range of depressive symptoms do not have the same disorder as women, who more frequently meet the full criteria. Men and women often endorse similar rates of sadness or depressed mood, yet men less frequently experience or report the other diagnostic symptoms of depression (Bogner and Gallo 2004; Hildebrandt et al. 2003b; Kessler et al. 1993). Among individuals presenting with only three or four depressive symptoms, as opposed to the five symptoms currently required for a full diagnosis of major depression (American Psychiatric Association 2000), Chen et al. (2000) found the female-to-male ratio to be 1.18:1 and not statistically significant. In those individuals presenting with five or six symptoms, the gender ratio increased to 2.28:1 ($P=0.01$), and when seven or more symptoms were considered, women were an astoundingly 9.34 times more likely to fulfill this criteria than men ($P=0.001$). The NCS (Kessler et al. 1993) similarly reported the gender ratio to be 1.26:1 when considering only symptoms of depressed mood or loss of interest, whereas the addition of each symptom required in excess of this core increased the gender ratio. This ratio reached 1.68:1 when four additional symptoms were required, as in the current diagnostic criteria; 1.95:1 when five additional symptoms were necessary; and a peak of 2.5:1 when all nine diagnostic symptoms were used. Similar trends have commonly been reported (Angst et al. 2002a; Ernst and Angst 1992; Maier et al. 1999; Young et al. 1990a), and although not universal (Kockler and Heun 2002), particularly in clinical samples (Hildebrandt et al. 2003a), it does appear that depressed men are often less likely to endorse as many depressive symptoms as depressed women. Because the current diagnostic criteria for major depression do require the presence of five or more symptoms (American Psychiatric Association 2000), the fewer symptoms reported by men may affect the likelihood of their receiving a diagnosis of depression. Whether this finding is indicative of fewer men truly presenting with depression or whether this finding highlights the need for a different diagnostic threshold for men remains to be seen. However, this difference may contribute to gender disparity seen in current rates of diagnosed depression and therefore emphasizes the need to more closely examine male patients who report only a limited number of symptoms.

Particular groups of symptoms have commonly been suggested to represent a unique form of depression in men. Pollack (1998) hypothesized a male type of major depression identified in part by a withdrawal from relationships, an avoidance of help, an overinvolvement with work, angry outbursts, an inability to cry, increased use of psychoactive substances, and changes in concentration, sleep, weight and sexual interest.

The possibility that men are more likely to endorse feelings of irritability and aggressiveness and to have low impulse control as a part of their depression resulted in the proposal of a similar male depressive syndrome by Walinder and Rutz (2001), expressed primarily through anxiety and aggression. The Gotland Male Depression Scale evolved from the identification of these symptoms and a concern with an underdiagnosis of depression in men (Rutz 1999). This scale probes for symptoms putatively associated with the expression of depression in men, such as a reduced stress threshold, increased aggression, irritability, increased substance use, and restlessness as expressed through an increase in work or exercise.

Efforts to empirically validate these proposed symptoms of depression in men have met with varying levels of success. For example, after Möller-Leimkühler et al. (2004) examined the validity of the male depressive syndrome, they found that symptoms of the syndrome were not shown to be any more prevalent in men with depression than in women with depression. Fava et al. (1995) did show that depressed men score higher on measures of trait but not state hostility, but other researchers have found depressed men less likely to express anger than depressed women (Frank et al. 1988) and men to report significantly lower levels of hostility, anxiety (Scheibe et al. 2003), anger, and somatization (Ernst and Angst 1992; Scheibe et al. 2003). These and other symptoms have commonly been found less prevalent among men. Among outpatients with chronic depression, fewer men than women experienced anxiety, somatization, sleep problems, or psychomotor retardation (Kornstein et al. 2000a). Other studies also have shown men to endorse fewer appetite, sleep, and energy abnormalities than women (Angst and Dobler-Mikola 1984; Young et al. 1990a), and although decreased levels of sexual satisfaction are often associated with male depression, Nofzinger et al. (1993) reported that actual rates of sexual activity in men may be unaffected. More limited symptom profiles in men may contribute to the challenge of identifying male depression, but some symptoms have been found to be more prevalent among men. Weight loss (Frank et al. 1988) and insomnia (Khan et al. 2002) may be more common among men, along with increased restlessness (Líndal and Stefánsson 1991) and agitation (Khan et al. 2002).

Significant differences have also been noted in the way men and women respond to their depressive feelings. Depressed men report significantly more impairment at work than depressed women (Angst et al. 2002a; Carter et al. 2000; Kornstein et al. 2000a). To a lesser extent, men also report more impairment in social activities and interpersonal behavior (Carter et al. 2000), whereas they show less impairment in their marital roles and levels of physical functioning, bodily pain, and vitality (Kornstein et al. 2000a). Earlier findings suggest that men are less likely to tell others of their depression, to express their emotions, to cry, or to refer to themselves using the word "depressed." Instead, men more often tell people that they are physically sick or that they are tired in an effort to conceal their depression (Warren 1983). Depressed men have also been found to exhibit more alexithymia, or an inability to verbalize their emotions, than depressed women (Honkalampi et al. 1999). Nolen-Hoeksema (1987) found that in response to a depressed mood, men would be more likely to avoid thinking about why they were depressed, to take drugs, or to do something physical, whereas women would try to determine why they were depressed, talk to others about how they were feeling, or cry. These responses have been confirmed more recently with findings that depressed women turn more often to friends, family, religion, laughter, or crying in response to their depression, whereas men turn more often to sports, hobbies, or alcohol (Angst et al. 2002a).

It may not be surprising, therefore, that men with major depression commonly present with past or current substance abuse or dependence (Fava et al. 1996), particularly involving alcohol. Of men with alcohol dependence, 24.3% have a lifetime history of depression (Kessler et al. 1997), and depressed men report a greater lifetime history of excessive alcohol use than depressed women (Fava et al. 1996; Gratzer et al. 2004; Reynolds et al. 1990; Simpson et al. 1997). Depressed men also report a greater need for alcohol (Angst et al. 2002a) and appear to drink more and to have more alcohol-related problems than men who have never been depressed or than depressed women (Pettinati et al. 1997). Many depressed men with alcohol-related problems report the onset of their depression only after they experience alcohol abuse or dependence (Kessler et al. 1997). Given the high comorbidity of depression and alcoholism in men, and the fact that excessive consumption of alcohol substantially increases the risk of suicide (Kung et al. 2003), it seems warranted to assess men with one of these disorders for the presence of the other.

The most alarming aspect of male depression may be the exceptionally high rate of completed suicide associated with it. Although women are twice as likely as men to be diagnosed with depression and may attempt suicide more often (Weissman et al. 1993), 7% of men with major depression will ultimately take their own lives as compared with 1% of depressed women. The suicide risk for those with major depression has been calculated to be as much as 10 times higher for men younger than 25 than for women of this age group (Blair-West et al. 1999), and men often prefer more violent means such as firearms rather than drug overdoses to achieve these ends (Cochran and Rabinowitz 2000; Isometsä et al. 1994). In addition, a large proportion of men who commit suicide seem to have received inadequate care (Isometsä et al. 1994). Therefore, some researchers argue that major depression may be underdiagnosed in men and that their elevated risk of suicide may warrant lowering the threshold for the treatment of depression in men, particularly in those exhibiting signs of substance abuse (Blair-West et al. 1999).

Depressive Subtypes and Male Depression

Although men suffer distinct risks associated with their depression, they do not manifest an entirely unique form of this disorder. Instead they appear to share common symptoms and even incidence rates with a subset of depressed women. The difference between men and women in depressive symptoms and prevalence rates may then be explained in part by a specific subtype of depression that is diagnosed much more frequently in women. Two such subtypes will be examined: depression with melancholic features and depression with atypical features.

Melancholic Features

Despite women being diagnosed with major depression twice as often as men, rates of the melancholic subtype (Carter et al. 2000; Ernst and Angst 1992; Young et al. 1990b), or endogenous depression (Reynolds et al. 1990) have generally been very similar between depressed men and women and have even been found by some researchers to be higher among males (Hildebrandt et al. 2003b). This melancholic subtype is characterized by loss of mood reactivity or pleasure along with at least three of the following symptoms: distinct quality of mood, mood worsening in the morning, early morning awakening, psychomotor changes, decreased appetite or weight, or excessive guilt (American Psychiatric Association 2000).

Atypical Features

Unlike the similar gender rate for melancholic depression, the rate for depression with atypical features is lower in men than in women. The prevalence of this subtype, defined by mood reactivity, reversed neurovegetative symptoms, rejection sensitivity, and leaden paralysis (American Psychiatric Association 2000), much more consistently parallels and often exceeds the 2:1 gender ratio commonly reported for the rates of depression overall. Atypical depression has been reported to be from 1.7 (Benazzi 2000) to 4 (Angst et al. 2002b) and 5 times more common in women than in men (Carter et al. 2000). Depressed women are also more likely than men to report increased appetite and weight gain associated with their depression (Ernst and Angst 1992; Frank et al. 1988), as well as an increase in carbohydrate cravings, actual food consumption, and interpersonal sensitivity, all associated with the atypical subtype (Scheibe et al. 2003).

Comparison of Subtypes and Symptoms

The majority of depressed individuals may not meet the full diagnostic criteria for either the melancholic or atypical subtype, and the rates of atypical depression may not be sufficient to account for the full gender disparity in the overall prevalence of depression. However, these trends do suggest that depression with melancholic features may represent a more gender-neutral disorder, whereas depression with atypical features could be a more commonly female illness.

Findings by Silverstein (1999, 2002) divide depressed individuals into different groupings that show a very similar trend and may help to explain the differences observed in the number of depressive symptoms presented by men and women. One group, dubbed *somatic depression*, is defined by a diagnosis of major depression along with somatic complaints of fatigue, either insomnia or hypersomnia, and either increased or decreased appetite. The second group, designated *pure depression*, is made up of individuals who did not endorse these somatic complaints. In a reanalysis of data from the NCS using this categorization (Silverstein 1999), no substantial gender differences were found in either 6-month or lifetime prevalences of pure depression, whereas somatic depression proved more than twice as common in women as in men. Similar results were found when examining data from the Epidemiologic Catchment Area study (Silverstein 2002). Although further validation of these findings is necessary, other investigators have similarly reported that men less commonly present with symptoms of fatigue (Líndal and Stefánsson 1991; Young et al. 1990a), and sleep (Kornstein et al. 2000a; Young et al. 1990a) and appetite disturbances (Young et al. 1990a), as is consistent with men's endorsement of fewer symptoms overall.

Onset, Course, and Severity

Although the general incidence of depression is lower in men than in women, for those men who do develop depression the course of the illness appears quite similar to the course of depression in women. Men and women share the same likelihood of developing depression when no stressful life events occur in the month before onset (Maciejewski et al. 2001), but when stressful life events do precede a depressive episode, men seeking treatment are significantly more likely to attribute their depression to problems at work (Angst et al. 2002a; Kendler et al. 2001) than to an illness or a death in the family (Angst et al. 2002a; Maciejewski et al. 2001), and men's depression is more likely to be accompanied by divorce or separation (Kendler et al. 2001). Genetic factors may also contribute differentially to the development of depression in men and women. Depressed men are less likely to report a family history of affective disorders than depressed women (Kornstein et al. 2000a; Rapaport et al. 1995), and some investigators have found depression to be less heritable in men than in women (Bierut et al. 1999), although a meta-analysis did not support these findings (Sullivan et al. 2000).

A later onset of depression in men than in women has commonly been reported (Fava et al. 1996; Kornstein et al. 2000a; Reynolds et al. 1990), but this finding has not been confirmed in the NCS (Kessler et al. 1993), in a cross-national survey (Weissman et al. 1993), or by others (Benazzi 2000; Carter et al. 2000; Frank et al. 1988; Maier et al. 1999; Rapaport et al. 1995; Scheibe et al. 2003; Thase et al. 1994). Kornstein et al. (2000a) suggested that this discrepancy may be due to the common exclusion of men with excessive alcohol use from clinical studies, because Klein et al. (1988) reported a younger age at depressive onset for depressed patients with comorbid substance abuse, particularly in depressed patients with a history of dysthymia. This supposition of later onset of depression in men also may be an artifact of the greater rates of atypical depression among women, because atypical depression appears to manifest at an earlier age than nonatypical depression (Angst et al. 2002b), whereas the melancholic subtype of depression commonly manifests later than nonmelancholic depression (Parker et al. 2001). Although estimates vary substantially, the NCS reported the average age at onset for a first depressive episode to be 24.04 for men and 23.53 for women (Kessler et al. 1993). However, NCS data also suggest that 69.3% of depressed men report the onset of their depression only after another psychiatric disorder, as compared with 57.5% of women, and that only 18.6% of men with a lifetime history of depression carry no other psychiatric diagnosis (Kessler et al. 1996).

A number of studies have reported that men may have a less recurrent form of depression than women (Ernst and Angst 1992; Lewinson et al. 1989; Merikangas et al. 1994). Yet several other studies have reported no gender differences in the likelihood of relapse (Coryell et al. 1991; Simpson et al. 1997), in rates of recurrent or chronic episodes of depression (Carter et al. 2000; McCullough et al. 2003), or in the overall number of depressive episodes (Kornstein et al. 2000a; Rapaport et al. 1995; Scheibe et al. 2003; Thase et al. 1994). In the NCS sample, Kessler et al. (1993) reported equal ratios of 12-month to lifetime prevalence of depression among men and women, suggesting similar rates of recurrence, and a trend was actually observed for more chronic depressive episodes in males. Other findings support that men who have experienced one episode of depression are as likely as women to experience more (Wainwright and Surtees 2002), with no significant differences in the length of each depressive episode (Ernst and Angst 1992; Kornstein et al. 2000a).

The fewer depressive symptoms often reported in men have been used to suggest that men have less severe depressive episodes than women (Chen et al. 2000), but reports of gender differences in the severity of depressive episodes have been inconsistent. Although self-report measures of depression severity such as the Beck Depression Inventory often elicit higher scores in depressed women than in depressed men (Frank et al. 1988; Kornstein et al. 2000a), in several samples no significant gender differences were seen in clinician-rated reports such as the Montgomery-Åsberg Depression Rating Scale or the Hamilton Rating Scale for Depression (Ham-D) (Benazzi 2000; Carter et al. 2000; Frank et al. 1988; M. Hamilton 1967; Kornstein et al. 2000a; Martényi et al. 2001; Montgomery and Åsberg 1979; Simpson et al. 1997). Interestingly, one study (Frank et al. 1988) reported no significant gender differences in Ham-D scores but did observe the emergence of a higher mean score among women when the scale was revised to include reversed neurovegetative symptoms such as increased appetite, weight gain, and hypersomnia, among others consistent with the atypical subtype.

TREATMENT OF MALE DEPRESSION

The differences in prevalence rates and symptom profiles between men and women may suggest that treatment response should vary between the genders, and this variation has in fact been the case in some treatment modalities. Although no differences have been reported in placebo response between men and women (Casper et al. 2001; Quitkin et al. 2002), patterns have emerged suggesting that some men and women may indeed respond differently to particular interventions.

Psychotherapy

Relatively few studies have addressed gender differences in response to psychotherapy, but most of those that have report that men and women respond equally well to empirically validated psychotherapies such as cognitive-behavioral therapy (CBT), with no significant gender differences in the rates of remission or treatment failure (Bruder et al. 1997; Jarrett et al. 1991; Sotsky et al. 1991; Thase et al. 1991a). A compilation of several studies by Thase et al. (1994) found that 55% of men treated with CBT met remission criteria as compared with 48% of women. Although these findings suggest that CBT may be somewhat less effective in more severely depressed individuals, the investigators found that among these more severely depressed patients, men tended to respond more positively to CBT than did severely depressed women ($P=0.03$), even though men attended fewer therapy sessions on average. Some evidence indicates that group sessions of CBT may be as effective for men as for women (Peterson and Halstead 1998). Mahalik (1999) highlighted certain cognitive distortions that may be particularly common among men, such as "I must be successful to be happy and fulfilled"; "For things to go right, I have to be in charge"; and "If I can't do it myself, people will think I'm inept."

Other forms of psychotherapy also appear to be effective in the treatment of depression in men. No gender differences were found in the response of depressed individuals to interpersonal psychotherapy, with 46% of men and 49% of women achieving remission after an average of 12.6 weekly sessions (Thase et al. 1997). Sotsky et al. (1991) also did not find gender to be a significant predictor of response to interpersonal psychotherapy. In addition, several psychodynamic strategies have been developed to particularly address depression in men. Pollack (1998) suggested a treatment of male depression focusing on an empathetic resolution to the sense of loss he views as prominent in men as they develop, which may contribute to depression later in life. Krugman (1998) developed a similar therapy based on resolving underlying feelings of shame. However, the efficacy of such therapies has not been empirically validated and therefore remains unclear.

Pharmacotherapy

Although recent attention has been given to gender differences in response to pharmacological antidepressant treatment, findings have been complicated by the interaction of age, depressive subtype, and gender that has arisen in the literature. The most commonly reported findings suggest a superior response to tricyclic antidepressants (TCAs) among men. Raskin (1974) first reported that imipramine was more effective than placebo for men, whereas the monoamine oxidase inhibitor (MAOI) phenelzine was less effective, particularly in men under age 40. Although perhaps influenced by a relatively low phenelzine dosage of 45 mg/day (Thase et al. 2000), these findings proved similar in women over age 40 but were reversed in younger females, who responded well to phenelzine but no better to imipramine than to placebo (Raskin 1974).

A meta-analysis of gender differences in response to imipramine between 1957 and 1991 (J.A. Hamilton et al. 1996) found statistically significant gender differences, with 62% of men responding to imipramine as compared with 51% of women ($P=0.001$). However, men's superior response to TCAs has not been consistently replicated. Although controversial, Quitkin et al. (2002) reanalyzed the data examined by J.A. Hamilton et al. (1996) and suggested that the studies used may have been small in size and underpowered, resulting in a smaller advantage of imipramine in men than that reported (Quitkin et al. 2002). A prospective study by Parker et al. (2003) concluded that men fared no better with TCAs than with selective serotonin reuptake inhibitors (SSRIs) in either clinical improvement or self-report measures, and in a review of 30 studies using TCAs in nearly 4,000 subjects, Wohlfarth et al. (2004) found no consistent difference in TCA response between males and females. Upon examination of outpatient data collected over 20 years, Quitkin et al. (2002) noted no significant gender differences in response to TCAs or to fluoxetine but did suggest that men respond somewhat less robustly than women to MAOIs ($P=0.009$).

The inconsistency regarding men's superior response to TCAs may be due in part to the confounding effects of both age and depressive subtype on antidepressant response.

In a comparison of patients with chronic depression taking either the TCA imipramine or the SSRI sertraline, a small but significant interaction of gender and treatment was found, with men across all age groups showing a more favorable response to imipramine than to sertraline ($P=0.04$) and male responders to imipramine also responding more quickly than women. Women, conversely, responded more often to sertraline than to imipramine ($P=0.02$), but this result was due to a superior response to sertraline only in premenopausal subjects ($P=0.01$) or those younger than 40 that was absent in postmenopausal subjects ($P=0.88$) and those older than 40 (Kornstein et al. 2000b). This difference in response between younger and older women may bias findings of antidepressant efficacy in studies that have compared men with women of all ages.

Depressive subtypes similarly complicate current understanding of antidepressant response. Hildebrandt et al. (2003c) reported a superior response for both men and women to the TCA clomipramine as compared with the SSRIs citalopram and paroxetine and with the MAOI moclobemide, with no gender-specific differences in response or remission. However, this sample was primarily composed of melancholic inpatients, suggesting that perhaps this melancholic subtype predicts response to treatment with clomipramine in both males and females. A retrospective examination by Parker et al. (2003) supports this finding, because although it failed to show any overall gender differences in response rates to either SSRIs or TCAs, the results did vary by subtype. In melancholic patients, TCAs were again somewhat more effective than SSRIs in both males and females. However, in nonmelancholic patients, women of all ages were more likely to report effectiveness from a TCA than were men, but no gender differences were noted in response to an SSRI. Baca et al. (2004) found no significant differences in the response or dropout rates of nonmelancholic men between sertraline and imipramine, suggesting that perhaps the benefit of TCAs in men may be greatest in men with melancholic features. Fava et al. (1997) reported that melancholic depression may respond less robustly to SSRIs, albeit only in 17-item Ham-D measures and not in other ratings attained in the study. Preliminary findings in patients with atypical features, more commonly represented by women, suggest that patients with this subtype respond better to fluoxetine than to imipramine, whereas patients without symptoms of atypical depression show a trend toward a better response to imipramine (Reimherr et al. 1984). Patients with atypical depression also appear to fare no better with TCAs than placebo (Sotsky and Simmens 1999; Stewart et al. 1998) but are likely to respond to MAOIs (Quitkin et al. 1988; Thase et al. 1991b). The greater number of women with atypical depression than men may in part confound findings of gender differences in antidepressant response when these subtypes are not taken into account.

Specific effects of other antidepressants on men have been studied to a lesser extent. In a meta-analysis, venlafaxine was found to be more effective than SSRIs in the treatment of depressed men (Entsuah et al. 2001), whereas no difference has been observed between response to fluoxetine and the tetracyclic norepinephrine reuptake inhibitor maprotiline in men (Martényi et al. 2001). Bruder et al. (2004) found that a reduced right-hemisphere advantage on a dichotic tone task may predict response to fluoxetine specifically in men, consistent with previous findings of brain laterality in depression and perhaps indicative of a type of depression in men that is characterized by decreased right-hemisphere processing and superior response to SSRIs.

Androgen Replacement Therapy

The role of testosterone in male depression has yet to be fully elucidated, but some studies have shown significant antidepressant effects with androgen replacement in depressed men. Low testosterone levels have been manifested in several somatic and psychological symptoms, such as dysphoria, fatigue, irritability, anorexia, and decreased libido, similar to those commonly seen in major depression (Seidman and Walsh 1999), and hypogonadal men treated with testosterone have shown an improvement in these symptoms (Wang et al. 1996). A meta-analysis determined the mean testosterone level among all adult males to be 479 ng/dL (Gray et al. 1991), with hypogonadism commonly defined as levels below 200 or 300 ng/dL (Seidman and Walsh 1999). These levels naturally decline with age, and this decline has been more evident in depressed men than in nondepressed men in some (Rubin et al. 1989; Seidman and Walsh 1999) but not all (Kaneda and Fujii 2002; Schweiger et al. 1999) samples.

Some studies suggest that depressed men may have lower levels of testosterone (Booth et al. 1999; Schweiger et al. 1999), but the majority of depressed men seem to exhibit testosterone levels that are indistinguishable from those of healthy control subjects (Kaneda and Fujii 2002; Levitt and Joffe 1988; Rubin et al. 1989; Seidman et al. 2002; Undén et al. 1988). Booth et al. (1999) suggested that men with below-average testosterone levels and men with above-average testosterone levels may be more likely to be diagnosed with depression. The direct relationship between testosterone and depression disappears in men with above-average testosterone levels after controlling for the absence of marriage and employment and the presence of high rates of antisocial and risky behavior. This finding may account for some of the inconclusive data regarding testosterone levels and depression. Several examinations have found no correlations between testosterone levels and depression severity ratings (Kaneda and Fujii 2002; Levitt and Joffe 1988; Rubin et al. 1989), although such correlations have been found in some men with melancholic depression (Davies et al. 1992). Although it does not appear that low levels of testosterone alone can account for depression in most men, hypogonadal men do have an increased risk for developing the disorder. Over a 2-year period, 21.7% of hypogonadal men over age 45 (total testosterone levels ≤ 200 ng/dL) were diagnosed with major depression, as compared with only 7.1% of eugonadal men. In this sample, all testosterone levels below 280 ng/dL increased the likelihood of developing a major depressive episode (Shores et al. 2004).

Androgen replacement therapy may be an effective treatment for depression in some men. Vogel et al. (1985) reported the synthetic androgen mesterolone to be as effective as the TCA amitriptyline in the treatment of depressed men, with mesterolone producing significantly fewer side effects. These investigators also found that 11 of the 13 chronically depressed eugonadal men responded to an open trial of mesterolone (Vogel et al. 1978). In another study, Seidman and Rabkin (1998) found that 5 subjects with SSRI-refractory depression exhibiting plasma testosterone levels in the low normal range (200–350 ng/dL) all showed significant improvement ($P=0.01$) when intramuscular testosterone enanthate injections were added to their current SSRI treatment for 8 weeks. When the testosterone treatments of 4 of the 5 men were discontinued in a single-blind manner, 3 of the 4 men relapsed, suggesting that androgen replacement may potentially enhance the efficacy of SSRI medications in some hypogonadal depressed men. Among men still meeting criteria for depression after at least 4 weeks of antidepressant treatment, 43% were found to have low or borderline morning serum testosterone levels between 100 and 350 ng/dL, and these men responded significantly better to a 1% testosterone gel than to a placebo, at least as measured by overall Ham-D scores ($P=0.0004$), but not by the Beck Depression Inventory ($P=0.15$; Pope et al. 2003).

Other investigations have not been as conclusive. In a 6-week randomized trial, Itil et al. (1984) found no difference in response rates between placebo and treatment with 450 mg/day of mesterolone in hypogonadal depressed men. Rabkin et al. (2004) also found no significant difference among placebo, testosterone, and fluoxetine in improving mood in human immunodeficiency virus (HIV)–positive depressed men, although testosterone did improve fatigue symptoms significantly more than the other treatments. Seidman et al. (2001) found no significant differences among mildly hypogonadal depressed men (testosterone level ≤350 ng/dL) in response either to 200-mg weekly injections of testosterone enanthate or to placebo, with both showing a response rate of approximately 40%. However, several nonresponders subsequently treated with a higher weekly dose of 400 mg of testosterone enanthate did show a significantly better response.

Although some initial findings using testosterone in depressed men appear promising, particularly in men with some level of hypogonadism, sample sizes in these studies have generally been small, and further evidence is needed to elucidate the antidepressant efficacy of testosterone. There are also risks associated with androgen administration, including erythropoiesis and stimulation of prostate adenocarcinoma, that should be taken into account before testosterone use is considered (Seidman and Walsh 1999).

CONCLUSION

Men meet the current diagnostic criteria for depression only half as often as women, yet depression remains a very serious threat to men's health. Approximately 1 in 10 men will have a major depressive episode in their lifetime, and these episodes are likely to be as severe and as recurrent as those of women. In men, depression is also associated with greater risks of heart disease, alcoholism, and completed suicide than in women. Accurately diagnosing this disorder in men is essential for treatment. However, depressed men commonly present with fewer symptoms than women and may be more hesitant to verbalize or share their emotions, making depression more difficult to identify in men.

The causes for the gender disparity in depression are not entirely understood, and further research in the field is essential. To date, very little of our knowledge about gender differences in depression has emerged from studies directly designed to investigate them, and the need for more targeted research is clear. Yet current findings have highlighted salient manifestations of depression that may be more common in men, such as fewer symptoms, a greater tendency for melancholic than atypical features, and increased risk of excessive alcohol use. Men with depression may also benefit more from particular pharmacological interventions than do women, as well as from androgen replacement therapy. A growing knowledge of the complicated interactions between hormonal, genetic, and psychosocial factors in depression may in time shed light on these gender differences and greatly improve our ability to diagnose and treat depression in men as well as women. However, until these factors are better understood, treating this disorder in men and preventing its devastating consequences will continue to require vigilance in assessing and correctly identifying the manifestation of depressive symptoms.

KEY POINTS

- Although men are diagnosed with major depression only half as often as women, this disorder is no less burdensome and disabling in men who have it.

- Men and women with depression show a similar course and severity of the illness, but depressed men have higher rates of comorbid alcohol abuse, heart disease, and completed suicide.

- Men often report fewer symptoms of depression than women and may therefore be more difficult to identify and diagnose.

PRACTICE GUIDELINES

1. Because men with depression may endorse fewer symptoms than women, it is important to carefully assess men for major depression even if they do not report the full range of symptoms traditionally described by diagnostic criteria.

2. Men being assessed for depression should be thoroughly evaluated for suicidal ideation, access to weapons, alcohol and substance abuse, and cardiac risk factors.

3. In treating depression, psychotherapy is as effective in men as it is in women.

4. Men, particularly those with the melancholic subtype of depression, may respond more robustly to TCAs than to MAOIs.

5. Some men, especially those with low baseline testosterone levels, may benefit from testosterone therapy as well.

REFERENCES

American Psychiatric Association: Diagnostic and Statistical Manual of Mental Disorders, 4th Edition, Text Revision. Washington, DC, American Psychiatric Association, 2000

Angold A, Costello EJ, Worthman CM: Puberty and depression: the roles of age, pubertal status and pubertal timing. Psychol Med 28:51–61, 1998

Angst J, Dobler-Mikola A: Do the diagnostic criteria determine the sex ratio in depression? J Affect Disord 7:189–198, 1984

Angst J, Gamma A, Gastpar M, et al: Gender differences in depression: epidemiological findings from the European DEPRES I and II studies. Eur Arch Psychiatry Clin Neurosci 252:201–209, 2002a

Angst J, Gamma A, Sellaro R, et al: Toward validation of atypical depression in the community: results of the Zurich cohort study. J Affect Disord 72:125–138, 2002b

Baca E, Garcia-Garcia M, Porras-Chavarino A: Gender differences in treatment response to sertraline versus imipramine in patients with nonmelancholic depressive disorders. Prog Neuropsychopharmacol Biol Psychiatry 28:57–65, 2004

Beck AT, Ward CH, Mendelson M, et al: An inventory for measuring depression. Arch Gen Psychiatry 4:561–571, 1961

Benazzi F: Female vs. male outpatient depression: a 448-case study in private practice. Prog Neuropsychopharmacol Biol Psychiatry 24:475–481, 2000

Bertakis KD, Helms LJ, Callahan EJ, et al: Patient gender differences in the diagnosis of depression in primary care. J Womens Health Gend Based Med 10:689–698, 2001

Bierut LJ, Heath AC, Bucholz KK: Major depressive disorder in a community-based twin sample: are there different genetic and environmental contributions for men and women? Arch Gen Psychiatry 56:357–563, 1999

Blair-West GW, Cantor CH, Mellsop GW, et al: Lifetime suicide risk in major depression: sex and age determinants. J Affect Disord 55:171–178, 1999

Bogner HR, Gallo JJ: Are higher rates of depression in women accounted for by differential symptom reporting? Soc Psychiatry Psychiatr Epidemiol 39:126–132, 2004

Booth A, Johnson DR, Granger DA: Testosterone and men's depression: the role of social behavior. J Health Soc Behav 40:130–140, 1999

Bruder GE, Stewart JW, Mercier MA, et al: Outcome of cognitive-behavioral therapy for depression: relation to hemispheric dominance for verbal processing. J Abnorm Psychol 106:138–144, 1997

Bruder GE, Stewart JW, McGrath PJ, et al: Dichotic listening tests of functional brain asymmetry predict response to fluoxetine in depressed women and men. Neuropsychopharmacology 29:1752–1761, 2004

Carter JD, Joyce PR, Mulder RT, et al: Gender differences in the presentation of depressed outpatients: a comparison of clinical variables. J Affect Disord 61:59–67, 2000

Casper RC, Tollefson GD, Nilsson ME: No gender differences in placebo responses of patients with major depressive disorder. Biol Psychiatry 49:158–160, 2001

Chen L, Eaton WW, Gallo JJ, et al: Understanding the heterogeneity of depression through the triad of symptoms, course and risk factors: a longitudinal, population-based study. J Affect Disord 59:1–11, 2000

Cochran SV, Rabinowitz FE: The murder of the self: men and suicide, in Men and Depression: Clinical and Empirical Perspectives. Edited by Cochran SV, Rabinowitz FE. San Diego, CA, Academic Press, 2000, pp 135–164

Coryell W, Endicott J, Keller MB: Predictors of relapse into major depressive disorder in a nonclinical population. Am J Psychiatry 148:1342–1358, 1991

Davies RH, Harris B, Thomas DR, et al: Salivary testosterone levels and major depressive illness in men. Br J Psychiatry 161:629–632, 1992

Entsuah AR, Huang H, Thase ME: Response and remission rates in different subpopulations with major depressive disorder administered venlafaxine, selective serotonin reuptake inhibitors, or placebo. J Clin Psychiatry 62:869–877, 2001

Ernst C, Angst J: The Zurich study: sex differences in depression. Evidence from longitudinal epidemiological data. Eur Arch Psychiatry Clin Neurosci 241:222–230, 1992

Fava M, Nolan S, Kradin R, et al: Gender differences in hostility among depressed and medical outpatients. J Nerv Ment Dis 183:10–14, 1995

Fava M, Abraham M, Alpert J, et al: Gender differences in Axis I comorbidity among depressed outpatients. J Affect Disord 38:129–133, 1996

Fava M, Uebelacker LA, Alpert JE, et al: Major depressive subtypes and treatment response. Biol Psychiatry 42:568–576, 1997

Ferketich AK, Schwartzbaum JA, Frid DJ, et al: Depression as an antecedent to heart disease among women and men in the NHANES I study. Arch Intern Med 160:1261–1268, 2000

Frank E, Carpenter LL, Kupfer DJ: Sex differences in recurrent depression: are there any that are significant? Am J Psychiatry 145:41–45, 1988

Gater R, Tansella M, Korten A, et al: Sex differences in the prevalence and detection of depressive and anxiety disorders in general health care settings. Arch Gen Psychiatry 55:405–413, 1998

Gratzer D, Levitan RD, Sheldon T, et al: Lifetime rates of alcoholism in adults with anxiety, depression, or co-morbid depression/anxiety: a community survey of Ontario. J Affect Disord 79:209–215, 2004

Gray A, Berlin JA, McKinlay JB, et al: An examination of research design effects on the association of testosterone and male aging: results of a meta-analysis. J Clin Epidemiol 44:671–684, 1991

Hamilton JA, Grant M, Jensvold MF: Sex and treatment of depressions: when does it matter? in Psychopharmacology and Women: Sex, Gender, and Hormones. Edited by Jensvold MF, Halbreich U, Hamilton JA. Washington, DC, American Psychiatric Press, 1996, pp 241–260

Hamilton M: Development of a rating scale for primary depressive illness. Br J Soc Clin Psychol 6:278–296, 1967

Hildebrandt MG, Stage KB, Kragh-Soerensen P: Gender and depression: a study of severity and symptomatology of depressive disorders (ICD-10) in general practice. Acta Psychiatr Scand 107:197–202, 2003a

Hildebrandt MG, Stage KB, Kragh-Soerensen P: Gender differences in severity, symptomatology and distribution of melancholia in major depression. Psychopathology 36:204–221, 2003b

Hildebrandt MG, Steyerberg EW, Stage KB, et al: Are gender differences important for the clinical effects of antidepressants? Am J Psychiatry 160:1643–1650, 2003c

Hippisley-Cox J, Fielding K, Pringle M: Depression as a risk factor for ischaemic heart disease in men: population based case-control study. BMJ 316:1714–1719, 1998

Hohmann AA: Gender bias in psychotropic drug prescribing in primary care. Med Care 27:478–490, 1989

Honkalampi K, Saarinen P, Hintikka J, et al: Factors associated with alexithymia in patients suffering from depression. Psychother Psychosom 68:270–275, 1999

Isometsä ET, Henriksson MM, Aro HM, et al: Suicide in major depression. Am J Psychiatry 151:530–536, 1994

Itil TM, Michael ST, Shapiro DM, et al: The effects of mesterolone, a male sex hormone, in depressed patients (a double-blind controlled study). Methods Find Exp Clin Pharmacol 6:331–337, 1984

Jarrett RB, Eaves GG, Grannemann BD, et al: Clinical, cognitive, and demographic predictors of response to cognitive therapy for depression: a preliminary report. Psychiatry Res 37:245–260, 1991

Kaneda Y, Fujii A: No relationship between testosterone levels and depressive symptoms in aging men. Eur Psychiatry 17:411–413, 2002

Kendler KS, Thornton LM, Prescott CA: Gender differences in the rates of exposure to stressful life events and sensitivity to their depressogenic effects. Am J Psychiatry 158:587–593, 2001

Kessler RC, McGonagle KA, Swartz M, et al: Sex and depression in the National Comorbidity Survey, I: lifetime prevalence, chronicity, and recurrence. J Affect Disord 29:85–96, 1993

Kessler RC, McGonagle KA, Nelson CB, et al: Sex and depression in the National Comorbidity Survey, II: cohort effects. J Affect Disord 30:15–26, 1994a

Kessler RC, McGonagle KA, Zhao S, et al: Lifetime and 12-month prevalence of DSM-III-R psychiatric disorders in the United States. Arch Gen Psychiatry 51:8–19, 1994b

Kessler RC, Nelson CB, McGonagle KA, et al: Comorbidity of DSM-III-R major depressive disorder in the general population: results from the U.S. National Comorbidity Survey. Br J Psychiatry 168:17–30, 1996

Kessler RC, Crum RM, Warner LA, et al: Lifetime co-occurrence of DSM-III-R alcohol abuse and dependence with other psychiatric disorders in the National Comorbidity Survey. Arch Gen Psychiatry 54:313–321, 1997

Khan AA, Gardner CO, Prescott CA, et al: Gender differences in the symptoms of major depression in opposite-sex dizygotic twin pairs. Am J Psychiatry 159:1427–1429, 2002

Klein DN, Taylor EB, Dickstein S, et al: Primary early-onset dysthymia: comparison with primary nonbipolar nonchronic major depression on demographic, clinical, familial, personality, and socioenvironmental characteristics and short-term outcome. J Abnorm Psychol 97:387–398, 1988

Kockler M, Heun R: Gender differences of depressive symptoms in depressed and nondepressed older persons. Int J Geriatr Psychiatry 17:65–72, 2002

Kornstein SG, Schatzberg AF, Thase ME, et al: Gender differences in chronic major and double depression. J Affect Disord 60:1–11, 2000a

Kornstein SG, Schatzberg AF, Thase ME, et al: Gender differences in treatment response to sertraline versus imipramine in chronic depression. Am J Psychiatry 157:1445–1452, 2000b

Krugman S: Men's shame and trauma in therapy, in New Psychotherapy for Men. Edited by Pollack WS, Levant RF. New York, Wiley, 1998, pp 167–190

Kuehner C: Gender differences in unipolar depression: an update of epidemiological findings and possible explanations. Acta Psychiatr Scand 108:163–174, 2003

Kung H, Pearson JL, Liu X: Risk factors for male and female suicide decedents ages 15–64 in the United States: results from the 1993 National Mortality Followback Survey. Soc Psychiatry Psychiatr Epidemiol 38:419–426, 2003

Levitt AJ, Joffe RT: Total and free testosterone in depressed men. Acta Psychiatr Scand 77:346–348, 1988

Lewinson PM, Zeiss AM, Duncan EM: Probability of relapse after recovery from an episode of depression. J Abnorm Psychol 98:107–116, 1989

Líndal E, Stefánsson JG: The frequency of depressive symptoms in a general population with reference to DSM-III. Int J Soc Psychiatry 37:233–241, 1991

Maciejewski PK, Prigerson HG, Mazure CM: Sex differences in event-related risk for major depression. Psychol Med 31:593–604, 2001

Mahalik JR: Incorporating a gender role strain perspective in assessing and treating men's cognitive distortions. Prof Psychol Res Pr 30:333–340, 1999

Maier W, Gänsicke M, Gater R, et al: Gender differences in the prevalence of depression: a survey in primary care. J Affect Disord 53:241–252, 1999

Martényi F, Dossenbach M, Mraz K, et al: Gender differences in the efficacy of fluoxetine and maprotiline in depressed patients: a double-blind trial of antidepressants with serotonergic or norepinephrinergic reuptake inhibition profile. Eur Neuropsychopharmacol 11:227–232, 2001

McCullough JP, Klein DN, Borian FE, et al: Group comparisons of DSM-IV subtypes of chronic depression: validity of the distinctions, part 2. J Abnorm Psychol 112:614–622, 2003

Merikangas KR, Wicki W, Angst J: Heterogeneity of depression: classification of depressive subtypes by longitudinal course. Br J Psychiatry 164:342–348, 1994

Möller-Leimkühler AM: The gender gap in suicide and premature death or: why are men so vulnerable? Eur Arch Psychiatry Clin Neurosci 253:1–8, 2003

Möller-Leimkühler AM, Bottlender R, Straub A, et al: Is there evidence for a male depressive syndrome in inpatients with major depression? J Affect Disord 80:87–93, 2004

Montgomery SA, Åsberg M: A new depression scale designed to be sensitive to change. Br J Psychiatry 134:382–389, 1979

Murphy SL: Deaths: final data for 1998. Natl Vital Stat Rep 48:1–105, 2000

Nofzinger EA, Thase ME, Reynolds CF 3rd, et al: Sexual function in depressed men: assessment by self-report, behavioral, and nocturnal penile tumescence measures before and after treatment with cognitive behavior therapy. Arch Gen Psychiatry 50:24–30, 1993

Nolen-Hoeksema S: Sex differences in unipolar depression: evidence and theory. Psychol Bull 101:259–282, 1987

Olfson M, Zarin DA, Mittman BS, et al: Is gender a factor in psychiatrists' evaluation and treatment of patients with major depression? J Affect Disord 63:149–157, 2001

Parker G, Roy K, Hadzi-Pavlovic D, et al: The differential impact of age on the phenomenology of melancholia. Psychol Med 31:1231–1236, 2001

Parker G, Parker K, Austin MP, et al: Gender differences in response to differing antidepressant drug classes: two negative studies. Psychol Med 33:1473–1477, 2003

Peterson AL, Halstead TS: Group cognitive behavior therapy for depression in a community setting: a clinical replication series. Behav Ther 29:3–18, 1998

Pettinati HM, Pierce JD Jr, Wolf AL, et al: Gender differences in comorbidly depressed alcohol-dependent outpatients. Alcohol Clin Exp Res 21:1742–1746, 1997

Pollack WS: Mourning, melancholia and masculinity: recognizing and treating depression in men, in New Psychotherapy for Men. Edited by Pollack WS, Levant RF. New York, Wiley, 1998, pp 147–166

Pope HG, Cohane GH, Kanayama G, et al: Testosterone gel supplementation for men with refractory depression: a randomized, placebo-controlled trial. Am J Psychiatry 160:105–111, 2003

Quitkin FM, Stewart JW, McGrath PJ, et al: Phenelzine versus imipramine in the treatment of probably atypical depression: defining syndrome boundaries of selective MAOI responders. Am J Psychiatry 145:306–311, 1988

Quitkin FM, Stewart JW, McGrath PJ, et al: Are there differences between women's and men's antidepressant responses? Am J Psychiatry 159:1848–1854, 2002

Rabkin JG, Wagner GJ, McElhiney MC, et al: Testosterone versus fluoxetine for depression and fatigue in HIV/AIDS: a placebo-controlled trial. J Clin Psychopharmacol 24:379–385, 2004

Rapaport MH, Thompson PM, Kelsoe JR, et al: Gender differences in outpatient research subjects with affective disorders: a comparison of descriptive variables. J Clin Psychiatry 56:67–72, 1995

Raskin A: Age-sex differences in response to antidepressant drugs. J Nerv Ment Dis 159:120–130, 1974

Reimherr FW, Wood DR, Byerley B, et al: Characteristics of responders to fluoxetine. Psychopharmacol Bull 20:70–72, 1984

Reynolds CF III, Kupfer DJ, Thase ME, et al: Sleep, gender, and depression: an analysis of gender effects on the electroencephalographic sleep of 302 depressed outpatients. Biol Psychiatry 28:673–684, 1990

Roose SP: Depression: links with ischemic heart disease and erectile dysfunction. J Clin Psychiatry 64:26–30, 2003

Rubin RT, Poland RE, Lesser IM: Neuroendocrine aspects of primary endogenous depression VIII: pituitary-gonadal axis activity in male patients and matched control subjects. Psychoneuroendocrinology 14:217–229, 1989

Rutz W: Improvement of care for people suffering from depression: the need for comprehensive education. Int Clin Psychopharmacol 14:S27–S33, 1999

Scheibe S, Preuschhof C, Cristi C, et al: Are there gender differences in major depression and its response to antidepressants? J Affect Disord 75:223–235, 2003

Schweiger U, Deuschle M, Weber B, et al: Testosterone, gonadotropin, and cortisol secretion in male patients with depression. Psychosom Med 61:292–296, 1999

Seidman SN, Rabkin JG: Testosterone replacement therapy for hypogonadal men with SSRI-refractory depression. J Affect Disord 48:157–161, 1998

Seidman SN, Walsh BT: Testosterone and depression in aging men. Am J Geriatr Psychiatry 7:18–33, 1999

Seidman SN, Spatz E, Rizzo C, et al: Testosterone replacement therapy for hypogonadal men with major depressive disorder: a randomized, placebo-controlled clinical trial. J Clin Psychiatry 62:406–412, 2001

Seidman SN, Araujo AB, Roose SP, et al: Low testosterone levels in elderly men with dysthymic disorder. Am J Psychiatry 159:456–459, 2002

Shores MM, Sloan KL, Matsumoto AM, et al: Increased incidence of diagnosed depressive illness in hypogonadal older men. Arch Gen Psychiatry 61:162–167, 2004

Silverstein B: Gender differences in the prevalence of clinical depression: the role played by depression associated with somatic symptoms. Am J Psychiatry 156:480–482, 1999

Silverstein B: Gender differences in the prevalence of somatic versus pure depression: a replication. Am J Psychiatry 159:1051–1052, 2002

Simpson HB, Nee JC, Endicott J: First-episode major depression: few sex differences in course. Arch Gen Psychiatry 54:633–639, 1997

Sotsky SM, Simmens SJ: Pharmacotherapy response and diagnostic validity in atypical depression. J Affect Disord 54:237–247, 1999

Sotsky SM, Glass DR, Shea MT, et al: Patient predictors of response to psychotherapy and pharmacotherapy: findings in the NIMH Treatment of Depression Collaborative Research Program. Am J Psychiatry 148:997–1008, 1991

Stewart JW, Garfinkel R, Nunes EV, et al: Atypical features and treatment response in the National Institute of Mental Health Treatment of Depression Collaborative Research Program. J Clin Psychopharmacol 18:429–434, 1998

Sullivan PF, Neale MC, Kendler KS: Genetic epidemiology of major depression: review and meta-analysis. Am J Psychiatry 157:1552–1562, 2000

Thase ME, Bowler K, Harden T: Cognitive behavior therapy of endogenous depression, part 2: preliminary findings in 16 unmedicated inpatients. Behav Ther 22:469–477, 1991a

Thase ME, Carpenter L, Kupfer DJ, et al: Clinical significance of reversed vegetative subtypes of recurrent major depression. Psychopharmacol Bull 27:17–22, 1991b

Thase ME, Reynolds CF III, Frank E, et al: Do depressed men and women respond similarly to cognitive behavioral therapy? Am J Psychiatry 151:500–505, 1994

Thase ME, Buysse DJ, Frank E, et al: Which depressed patients will respond to interpersonal psychotherapy? the role of abnormal EEG sleep profiles. Am J Psychiatry 154:502–509, 1997

Thase ME, Frank E, Kornstein SG, et al: Gender differences in response to treatments of depression, in Gender and Its Effects on Psychopathology. Edited by Frank E. Washington, DC, American Psychiatric Press, 2000, pp 103–129

Undén F, Ljunggren JG, Beck-Friis J, et al: Hypothalamic-pituitary-gonadal axis in major depressive disorders. Acta Psychiatr Scand 78:138–146, 1988

Vogel W, Klaiber EL, Broverman DM: Roles of the gonadal steroid hormones in psychiatric depression in men and women. Prog Neuropsychopharmacol Biol Psychiatry 2:487–503, 1978

Vogel W, Klaiber EL, Broverman DM: A comparison of the antidepressant effects of a synthetic androgen (mesterolone) and amitriptyline in depressed men. J Clin Psychiatry 46:6–8, 1985

Wainwright NWJ, Surtees PG: Childhood adversity, gender and depression over the life-course. J Affect Disord 72:33–44, 2002

Walinder J, Rutz W: Male depression and suicide. Int Clin Psychopharmacol 16:S21–S24, 2001

Wang C, Alexander G, Berman N, et al: Testosterone replacement therapy improves mood in hypogonadal men: a clinical research center study. J Clin Endocrinol Metab 81:3578–3583, 1996

Warren LW: Male intolerance of depression: a review with implications for psychotherapy. Clin Psychol Rev 3:147–156, 1983

Weissman MM, Klerman GL: Sex differences and the epidemiology of depression. Arch Gen Psychiatry 34:98–111, 1977

Weissman MM, Bruce ML, Leaf PJ, et al: Affective disorders, in Psychiatric Disorders in America: The Epidemiologic Catchment Area Study. Edited by Robins LN, Regier DA. New York, Free Press, 1991, pp 53–80

Weissman MM, Bland RC, Joyce PR, et al: Sex differences in the rates of depression: cross-national perspectives. J Affect Disord 29:77–84, 1993

Wohlfarth T, Storosum JG, van Zwieten BJ, et al: Response to tricyclic antidepressants: independent of gender? Am J Psychiatry 161:370–372, 2004

Wolk SI, Weissman MM: Women and depression: an update, in Review of Psychiatry, Vol 14. Edited by Oldham JM, Riba MB. Washington, DC, American Psychiatric Press, 1995, pp 227–259

World Health Organization: Burden of mental and behavioural disorders: impact of disorders, in The World Health Report 2001—Mental Health: New Understanding, New Hope. Geneva, Switzerland, World Health Organization, 2001. Available at: http://www.who.int/whr/2001/chapter2/en/index3.html. Accessed December 2, 2004.

Young MA, Fogg LF, Scheftner WA, et al: Sex differences in the lifetime prevalence of depression: does varying the diagnostic criteria reduce the female/male ratio? J Affect Disord 18:187–192, 1990a

Young MA, Scheftner WA, Fawcett J, et al: Gender differences in the clinical features of unipolar major depressive disorder. J Nerv Ment Dis 178:200–203, 1990b

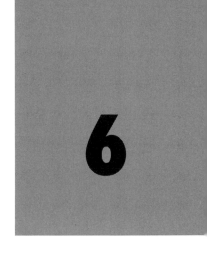

SUBSTANCE USE DISORDERS

N. WILL SHEAD, M.SC.
DAVID C. HODGINS, PH.D.

Case Vignette

Mike, age 24 years, worked intermittently as an electrician. His father, a police officer, organized an assessment for Mike through his Employee Assistance Program (EAP). Mike recently was charged with impaired and dangerous driving while using a company truck and lost his job. He could not afford his apartment and returned to live with his father and stepmother on the condition that he get treatment for alcohol, cocaine, and cannabis problems.

Mike started smoking cannabis in high school at age 16. He and his friends soon became daily users, often smoking at lunchtime. He had always struggled with the academic requirements of school despite average intellectual abilities, finding it difficult to maintain his interest and focus. He often forgot about or did not complete homework assignments and frequently skipped classes. Mike was more successful with sports, especially hockey, and played on numerous sports teams. During the last 2 years of high school, he and his friends typically got drunk on Friday and Saturday nights. His drinking led to considerable conflict with his parents, who were concerned about both him and his influence on his younger brothers.

Mike completed high school and, with the support of his father, began an apprenticeship as an electrician. His coworkers were frequent and heavy drinkers who introduced him to cocaine. Concurrently, his involvement with sports declined because he was no longer in school. No longer living at home, he began smoking cannabis before and during work and drinking and using cocaine after work. He often arrived at work hung over and tired but felt he could "push through" and work effectively. Mike had access to a company truck to travel to work sites outside the city. He regularly used the truck to go to the bar with his coworkers. On the night he was charged with impaired driving, he and his coworkers got into a fight with the members of a hockey team who were celebrating winning a game. Later, at about 1 A.M., Mike crashed the truck into a telephone pole and was arrested for driving while impaired.

Mike initially did not consider himself as having a substance abuse problem. His father hired a lawyer for the driving charges who recommended a residential treatment program, which Mike reluctantly agreed to when he saw the EAP counselor. Although Mike completed this program, it was years before Mike successfully embraced abstinence from alcohol and other drugs. During these years, he attended Alcoholics Anonymous (AA) intermittently, saw multiple outpatient counselors, and received another impaired driving charge. He enthusiastically quit drinking and using cocaine for brief periods but often relapsed when he returned to work and met a new group of coworkers. His prolonged abstinence coincided with his becoming seriously involved with the woman he eventually married. Mike then considered himself an "alcoholic" and the time periods between relapses increased. He attended AA regularly until his first child was born, when he was 29 years old.

Examinations of gender differences in substance abuse have generally focused on implications for women, with the supposition that substance abuse in men is more fully understood than is substance abuse in women. However, the important area of substance abuse in men has arguably received less attention. Epidemiological studies show that men have higher rates of substance abuse and dependence than do women (Brienza and Stein 2002), which makes new directions in theory, prevention, and treatment in substance use disorders very relevant to men. This chapter examines current findings in three areas of substance abuse in men: phenomenology, etiology, and treatment. Gender differences are discussed in each of these areas, with a focus on the implications for understanding and treating men with substance use disorders.

PHENOMENOLOGY

Prevalence of Substance Use Disorders in Men Versus Women

Men are more likely to use, abuse, and be dependent on substances than are women (Office of Applied Studies 2004). Comparisons across genders reveal that males are more likely than females to be dependent on or abuse a substance in all age groups except for the 12- to 17-year age group. Gender differences exist in susceptibility to problems following drug exposure. Kandel (2000) examined how the prevalence of dependence on four substances (nicotine, alcohol, marijuana, and cocaine) varied by gender after correcting for substance exposure (i.e., social use). Cocaine has a low experimentation rate, resulting in a lower rate of cocaine dependence within the total population compared with other drugs. Males who used substances in the past year were more likely than female past-year users to be dependent on alcohol (6.7% vs. 3.6%) and marijuana (9.3% vs. 6.4%) and less likely to be dependent on nicotine (26.5% vs. 29.5%). Among males, past-year substance users were four times more likely to be dependent on nicotine than alcohol, whereas among females, past-year users were eight times more likely to be dependent on nicotine than alcohol. Thus males appear to be at a lower risk than females for developing a dependence on nicotine but at a higher risk than females for becoming dependent on alcohol and marijuana. Among adolescent substance users, more than three times as many females as males were dependent on cocaine. Among adult substance users, men had higher rates of dependence than women for alcohol and marijuana. Men were almost twice as likely as women to meet criteria for past-year dependence on marijuana. In sum, males and females are differentially susceptible to different drugs, and these patterns vary with age.

Susceptibility to dependence is not necessarily equivalent to sensitivity to the effects of a substance. Women have a greater sensitivity to alcohol and increased mortality at lower levels of consumption compared with men (Brienza and Stein 2002). However, men experience higher rates of alcohol abuse and dependence than do women. A "telescoping" effect has been described wherein women tend to exhibit acceleration in the progression from alcohol use to alcohol abuse and dependence compared with men. Although differences in the physiological sensitivity to the effects of alcohol may contribute to the telescoping phenomenon, similar foreshortened patterns have been observed for a variety of addictive drugs (e.g., cocaine) and behaviors (e.g., gambling) (Lynch et al. 2002; Potenza et al. 2001; Tavares et al. 2001).

Expression of Substance Abuse in Men

Men have distinctive life experiences related to substance abuse disorders (Table 6–1), and these experiences provide helpful information for understanding men's unique challenges in substance abuse treatment. Compared with women in alcohol use treatment, men in treatment report

TABLE 6–1. Expression of substance abuse in men versus women

Earlier drinking-related accidents and arrests
More alcohol-related problems at school and work
Fewer alcohol withdrawal symptoms early in drinking career
Less professional treatment–seeking behavior
Fewer physical health problems
Fewer psychosocial stressors in their lives
Fewer self-reported family problems
Poorer coping skills
More negative social influences
More likely to drink for sensation seeking

fewer alcohol withdrawal symptoms earlier in their drinking careers, less psychological impairment, less professional treatment–seeking behavior, more alcohol-related school or work problems, and earlier drinking-related accidents and arrests due to drinking that are unrelated to driving while intoxicated (Karoll and Memmott 2001). Compared with women, on entering substance abuse treatment men acknowledge more alcohol use, less cocaine use, fewer past and current physical and mental problems, and fewer concerns with how their substance use is affecting their children (Wechsberg et al. 1998). Similarly, men with a lifetime alcohol use disorder are less likely than women to have histories of severe psychosocial stress, severe dependence on other substances, and antecedent mental health problems (Sannibale and Hall 2001). As such, men who enter substance abuse treatment may experience fewer stressors than women who enter substance abuse treatment and therefore may be better prepared to complete treatment successfully and avoid relapses. Alternatively, men may be less able or willing to identify stressors in their lives, and this situation could represent a barrier to effective treatment outcome (see Chapter 17, "Overcoming Stigma and Barriers to Mental Health Treatment").

Although men entering substance abuse treatment acknowledge fewer psychosocial stressors, they have poorer coping skills. Men recruited from substance abuse treatment programs reported poorer coping skills, more negative social influences, and more exposure to substances than did women (Walton et al. 2001). Thus men may lack both intrapsychic and extrapsychic facilities that might help them cope with psychosocial stressors.

Cohort effects can influence the expression of substance use disorders in men. People born after 1951 have high rates of alcohol dependence (Holdcraft and Iacono 2002). Among individuals with alcohol dependence, those born after 1951 have an earlier onset and longer duration of alcohol-related problems. This cohort effect is stronger for women than for men and may indicate that alcohol dependence is rising in younger generations, although less so for men than for women. Thus men over age 50 years may have a unique presentation compared with men younger than 50 years.

The motivations underlying substance use are complex. Some people appear motivated by sensation seeking and others by anxiety (Cook et al. 1994). Scourfield et al. (1996) compared sensation-seeking profiles of substance abusers with and without comorbid anxiety disorders. Male as compared with female substance abusers were more likely to drink for sensation seeking.

Regardless of comorbid psychological difficulties, men with substance abuse problems may share a common characteristic involving risk taking. This notion is consistent with efforts to subtype substance abusers according to personality and other individual characteristics (Babor et al. 1992; Ball et al. 1998; Cloninger 1987). One of the two types identified, characterized by earlier onset, family history of substance abuse, and greater likelihood and severity of polysubstance abuse, shows greater impulsivity (Ball et al. 1998) and is predominantly male (Babor et al. 1992). These individuals tend to have poorer long-term treatment outcomes (Ball et al. 1995). (The other subtype, characterized by later onset and without a family history of substance abuse, is comprised of a relatively smaller proportion of men.)

Substance use is often associated with aggressive and socially inappropriate behaviors, particularly in men. Laboratory studies have shown that men display greater levels of alcohol-induced aggression than do women (e.g., Giancola and Zeichner 1995; Hoaken and Pihl 2000). Males in treatment have higher rates of being under legal supervision and engage in more property crime compared with females in treatment (Grella 2003). These inappropriate behaviors are often attributed to alcohol's impairing influence on inhibitory behavioral responses. Under the influence of alcohol, men show greater impairment in inhibiting behavioral responses compared with women (Fillmore and Weafer 2004). Men report increased stimulation after alcohol intake, whereas women report increased sedation (Fillmore and Weafer 2004). Thus men typically exhibit more aggressive and socially inappropriate behaviors under the influence of alcohol, and this impairment of response inhibition appears related to higher alcohol-induced arousal. Consequently, men are at increased risk of performing seemingly impulsive or antisocial behaviors (e.g., committing a crime, injury) when intoxicated or high on drugs.

Men differ from women in the biological correlates of substance use. In a study of cocaine craving, cocaine-dependent men displayed relatively greater activation of amygdala, insula, orbitofrontal cortex, and ventral anterior cingulate and less activation of frontal cortex as compared with cocaine-dependent women (Kilts et al. 2004). The more robust limbic activation in men suggests sex differences in the affective processing of craving. Studies of self-reported measures of cocaine craving in men and women have generated conflicting results, with reports of increased (Evans et al. 1999) and decreased (Elman et al. 2001; Robbins et al. 1999) craving in men. Some apparent discrepancies might be accounted for by sex hormones, because progesterone, estrogen, and testosterone have been implicated in the pathophysiologies of substance use disorders (Lynch et al. 2002). For example, in women, progesterone appears to attenuate subjective responses to cocaine (Sofuoglu et al. 2002), and tobacco use or craving has been shown to vary with menstrual phase (Allen at al. 2000; Pomerleau et al. 1992). Of particular relevance to men, high levels of testosterone have been found in men with type II (i.e., genetic, male-limited) alcoholism (Stalenheim et al. 1998) and in alcoholic men who were sober (King et al. 1995), with impulsivity or sensation seeking representing possible mediating factors (Daitzman et al. 1978).

Co-occurring Symptoms

Men with substance use disorders present with additional problems when they have comorbid psychiatric diagnoses (Pettinati et al. 2000). In a study of substance abuse and schizophrenia, men had less social contact, fewer problems with victimization and medical illness, and more legal problems compared with women (Brunette and Drake 1997). Nonetheless, men and women had similar courses and severities of substance abuse.

It is often helpful clinically to determine which disorder is primary in individuals with co-occurring disorders. For example, recognizing that a major depressive episode ensued after several years of a substance use disorder may assist the clinician in case formulation and treatment plan development. In outpatient treatment-seeking individuals with co-occurring alcohol dependence and posttraumatic stress disorder (PTSD), the onset of PTSD in men more frequently followed the onset of a substance use disorder (Back et al. 2001). Although men as compared with women reported a lower frequency and intensity of PTSD avoidance symptoms, lower rates of sexual trauma, and less social impairment due to PTSD, they reported heavier alcohol use and greater social and legal impairment related to their substance use. These results suggest that substance use disorders in men may lead to traumatic experiences that evolve into co-occurring psychiatric diagnoses and that negatively influence the course of the substance use disorder.

Men with bipolar disorder appear more likely than women with the disorder to meet criteria for a lifetime alcohol use disorder (49% vs. 29%; Frye et al. 2003). However, because the base rate of alcohol use disorders in the general population is higher among men, the risk of having alcoholism is almost five times greater for women with bipolar disorder than for men with bipolar disorder. Almost half of all men with bipolar disorder will experience some substance use problems; familial factors, whether hereditary or environmental, contribute to these problems.

Substance use disorders often begin during adolescence, when individuals may experiment with substances. A confounding factor is the possibility that an adolescent has a co-occurring childhood psychiatric disorder. Latimer et al. (2002) found that attention-deficit/hyperactivity disorder and conduct disorder were more common among drug-abusing male adolescents compared with drug-abusing female adolescents. However, males exhibited lower rates of major depression compared with females. Drug-abusing males and females had equivalent rates of dysthymia, double depression (concurrent diagnoses of dysthymia and major depressive disorder), and bipolar disorder. These findings suggest that adolescent males with attentional and behavioral problems are particularly vulnerable to developing substance abuse problems. Future research is needed to examine the relationships between these disorders to determine the most common temporal sequencing. Such an understanding may assist in the development of more effective substance abuse prevention strategies for both sexes.

Personality disorders are common among individuals with substance use disorders (Koenigsberg et al. 1985). Given that the prevalence rates of specific personality disorders differ by gender (e.g., more men than women are diagnosed with antisocial personality disorder), it is important to consider how certain personality disorders may influence the course of substance use disorders. Men with substance dependence as compared with women with substance dependence appear more likely to have dependent personality disorder (Grant et al. 2004). Although not all studies find gender differences in the association between antisocial personality and substance use disorders (Grant et al. 2004), Landheim et al. (2003) found that men treated for substance use problems more frequently presented with antisocial personality disorder than did women in substance abuse treatment. These men were also less likely to present with major depression, PTSD, and eating disorders, which is consistent with other findings (e.g., Cornelius et al. 1995; Ross et al. 1988). Alcoholic males presented more often with Cluster A personality disorders (particularly schizoid personality disorder) than did all other substance abusers (Landheim et al. 2003). Men were also more likely to present in a treatment setting with substance abuse as the primary and often sole mental health concern.

In summary, the problems faced by men with substance use disorders are compounded when they experience comorbid disorders. They are more likely to have legal and social problems. Men with substance use disorders are at increased risk of exhibiting specific co-occurring conditions, including Cluster A personality disorders, attention problems, and bipolar disorder. However, substance use disorders appear most frequently to be the primary issue for men that precedes the development of other psychiatric disorders.

ETIOLOGY

The etiology and course of substance use disorders differ between men and women (Blume 1992). Factors contributing to the development of substance use disorders are clinically informative in generating a case formulation and treatment plan. For instance, recognizing that an individual's drinking problem developed as a result of coping with childhood abuse and low self-esteem allows the clinician to construct a treatment plan that addresses dealing with past trauma and building a positive self-image.

Adolescent Studies

Family processes contribute to the development of substance use problems in adolescent males. Galaif et al. (2001) reported significant associations among family processes, childhood maltreatment, and problem alcohol use for men and women in a longitudinal community sample. Men reported more problem alcohol use in adolescence and adulthood, whereas women reported more early sexual abuse.

Male adolescents entering substance abuse treatment exhibit worse school and legal problems and fewer psychological difficulties, family-related problems, and sexual abuse experiences than do females entering treatment (Hsieh and Hollister 2004). Among adolescent inpatients seeking treatment for substance use disorders, males progress more slowly to regular use of drugs, are less likely to endorse dependence symptoms, and report experiencing dependence symptoms at an older age than do adolescent females (Thomas et al. 2003). Whereas girls typically began substance use with cigarettes, boys typically began substance use with alcohol. Despite no gender-related differences on prevalence of depression or previous psychiatric treatment, boys are less likely than girls to exhibit suicidality.

Family History

Family history influences differently the development of substance use disorders in men and women. In a treatment sample, Chermack et al. (2001) found gender differences in the influence of family history of alcoholism. For men, family history of alcoholism did not account for alcohol problems and violence but was associated with drug problems. The investigators suggested that men are less affected than are women by family background variables in the development of adult problems with alcohol, drugs, and violence. This conclusion was supported by another study, which found that alcoholic males were less likely to have alcoholic parents compared with alcoholic females (T.R. Kosten et al. 1991).

Genetics

Genetic contributions to substance use disorders in men are substantial, in both use of specific drugs and common vulnerability across drugs (Bierut et al. 1998; Tsuang et al. 1996, 1998). In men, some of the shared genetic risk across major depression and substance use disorders (alcohol and marijuana dependence) appears attributable to the risk for antisocial personality disorders (Fu et al. 2002). Genetic factors contribute to multiple stages of alcohol use in men—for example, age at onset of regular use, age at diagnosis, and the transition between use and diagnosis (Liu et al. 2004). Although some studies of females and mixed-gender samples suggest that genetic influences are more evident in men than in women (Anthenelli and Schuckit 1997; Cadoret et al. 1995; van den Bree et al. 1998; Zilberman and Blume 2004), similar relationships in the genetic contributions to substance use and other mental health disorders have been reported, with gender differences mainly in the level of liability necessary to manifest clinical illness (Kendler et al. 2003).

Sociocultural Factors

Despite data suggesting a relatively weaker influence in men of family factors on the development of substance use problems, societal influences appear substantial. Intoxication is generally more accepted in men and condemned in women (Ricciardelli et al. 2001). Drinking large amounts of alcohol is often viewed as a "masculine" trait because it often involves boldness, endurance, and fearlessness. This societal view may represent a significant risk factor for men and partially account for higher rates of substance use disorders in men. High-risk-drinking college men demonstrate a less complex pattern of cognitions relating to restrained drinking than do high-risk-drinking college women (Ricciardelli et al. 2001). Men's capacities to refuse drinking are not influenced as strongly by social situations, negative emotional states, or other temptation cues as are women's capacities.

A large-scale community study showed that social support was associated with alcohol consumption in similar ways for both men and women; however, demographic characteristics, psychological well-being, and physical health and functioning differed between genders (Green et al. 2001). One result unique to men was that employed men drank less than unemployed men, and physically healthier men reported drinking more. In contrast, better psychological functioning protected against increased alcohol use in women but not in men. The authors suggested that mental health professionals monitor particularly closely alcohol consumption of men with few functional limitations and good health.

Relationship Factors

Relationship factors can influence the development and maintenance of a substance use disorder differentially in men and women. Among adults from the United Kingdom, men were more likely than women to report that someone else had tried to influence their drinking habits (Plant et al. 2002). Substance use may become a coping mechanism for relationship turmoil, which may in turn lead to more relationship difficulties. This pattern could result in a vicious circle of substance use, increased relationship problems, and more substance use. Substance use problems may then develop from a lack of positive relationships or poor social support. However, Room (1996) found that men's substance abuse is not as socially embedded as is women's, in that it appeared less likely to be influenced by a substance-abusing partner. DiNitto et al. (2002) examined individuals with co-occurring severe mental illness and substance dependence. Men were less likely than women to have experienced emotional, physical, or sexual abuse and were less bothered by psychiatric symptoms and their family or social relations. However, men reported being charged with more types of crimes and feeling less happy and close in their relationships.

Gender Roles

Gender roles influence the course of substance use disorders in men. Monk and Ricciardelli (2003) investigated the relationship among substance use in young men and three aspects of the male gender role: traditional attitudes toward men, masculine gender-role conflict, and masculine gender-role stress. Young men experiencing more gender-role conflict—as expressed by a tendency to adhere rigidly to restrictive emotionality norms—reported using more alcohol and cannabis. Men with more difficulty expressing their feelings or relating to the expression of emotion in others may use substances to cope. Those men who rigidly endorsed the antifemininity male-role norm of avoiding stereotypically feminine behaviors and attitudes had more alcohol-related problems.

TREATMENT

The telescoping effect discussed earlier suggests that women progress toward alcohol and drug abuse and dependence faster than do men, albeit with fewer years of use before treatment. This raises the possibility that men on average experience fewer negative consequences at earlier stages of their problem than do women (Brienza and Stein 2002). Given that men are less likely to seek help, a barrier to treatment exists for men compared with women. A major goal of mental health professionals in the field of addictions, therefore, is to develop early prevention and treatment strategies for men that are effective at early stages and that facilitate the help-seeking process.

Treatment outcomes data comparing men with women are inconclusive. In a study of men and women in a publicly funded substance abuse treatment system, men had significantly fewer problems at assessment, a higher 30-day retention rate, and higher treatment completion rates than did women (Arfken et al. 2001). In another study, Jarvis (1992) showed that men have worse outcomes than do women in the first year after treatment; however, men showed better outcomes in longer-term follow-ups. In a sample of treatment-seeking cocaine abusers, female patients at intake had more severe drug use problems than male patients. However, females appeared to benefit more from treatment as reflected by less cocaine use 6 months after treatment (T.A. Kosten et al. 1993). Jerrell and Ridgely (1995) found that men in treatment for substance abuse and mental health disorders had lower functioning scores, fewer psychiatric symptoms, and lower reductions in the use of acute treatment services than did women receiving similar treatment. In conclusion, significant variability exists in treatment outcomes research, suggesting the need to consider multiple aspects of substance abuse treatment for men.

Treatment-Seeking Behavior

Men generally have different reasons for entering treatment than do women. Men often cite employment and legal concerns for entering substance abuse treatment (Blume 1992). King et al. (2003) found that alcoholic females reported greater depression, anxiety, and neuroticism compared with alcoholic males. Furthermore, male problem drinkers reported significantly fewer depressive symptoms and health-related stressful events compared with female problem drinkers. Male problem drinkers resembled light drinkers on the dimensions of depression, anxiety, neuroticism, and health-related stressful events. These results suggest that women seek treatment at an earlier point in their drinking careers than men, perhaps due to a more rapid experiencing of negative effects of substance abuse or due to more general gender-related differences in help-seeking behaviors. Men's "resilience" may result in delayed entrance into treatment.

Brienza and Stein (2002) reported that men were more likely to enter treatment for alcohol problems via social programs such as drunk-driving rehabilitation and EAPs or via peer-oriented settings such as AA. The investigators reported that women, meanwhile, were more likely to present initially within a health care setting. Thus men's reasons for initially seeking care may preferentially involve resolving identifiable social concerns with substance use.

Individuals entering treatment for substance use disorders may differ in terms of initiation, duration, and completion of treatment. Although one study found that these aspects did not differ between men and women (Green et al. 2002), factors predicting these outcomes differed across gender. Several findings unique to men were reported. First, men who were employed or married were more likely to initiate treatment, whereas less educated men were less likely to initiate treatment. Second, older men were more likely to complete treatment, whereas men with worse psychiatric status and those receiving Medicaid were less likely to complete treatment. Finally, men with fewer health diagnoses, higher education, a history of being a victim of domestic abuse, and prior 12-step group attendance generally spent more time in treatment.

Help-seeking behavior is crucial to successful treatment outcome because without the individual's willingness to initiate treatment, the chances of overcoming a substance use disorder are reduced. In a sample of initially untreated men and women problem drinkers, Timko et al. (2002) examined help utilization and outcomes over 8 years. Participants were categorized into one of four self-selected groups at the 8-year follow-up: no help, AA only, formal treatment only, and formal treatment plus AA. Men were less likely to participate in AA and had shorter inpatient stays compared with women. Men also had worse outcomes at 1 and 8 years when baseline drinking and functional indices were controlled. However, type of help obtained did not differentially relate to improved outcomes for men and women. In a follow-up study of the same sample (Timko et al. 2005), a particularly strong association was found between approach-coping strategies and better drinking outcomes among men. Less drinking-to-cope and decreases in avoidance coping were more strongly associated with better drinking outcomes among men than among women. The development of these strategies appears to be related to longer attendance in AA. The authors concluded that men should be targeted for formal services or self-help groups to increase their use of approach coping to help them maintain abstinence.

Kohn et al. (2002) interviewed men and women who entered a substance abuse treatment program in a private, managed care facility. Men reported using less cognitive avoidance (avoiding thinking realistically about the problem) and less resigned acceptance compared with women. However, men sought less support and guidance while in treatment than did women.

Examining the effects of treatment among adolescent boys provides additional information about symptoms present in the early drinking careers of men. Hsieh and Hollister (2004) found that adolescent boys showed worse attendance in aftercare or self-help groups after treatment and had worse treatment outcomes compared with adolescent girls.

In sum, men seek treatment later in their substance-using careers as compared with women, often after experiencing social consequences of their substance use. Several variables influence the likelihood that men with substance use problems will seek treatment. Men who are employed, married, older, in better psychological and physical condition, more educated, and were previously involved in treatment tend to seek and fare better in treatment than do men without these characteristics.

Benefits of Treatment

The effects of treatment extend beyond the simple outcome of reductions in substance abuse. Because men experience an array of negative consequences due to substance abuse, an important goal of treatment is to improve these areas. For instance, the impact a substance use disorder has had on a man's relationships may be an important consideration in developing treatment approaches. Oggins et al. (2001) examined life changes in men and women in substance use treatment. Men made greater gains in work income than did women and over time were more likely to be employed than were women. These findings suggest that men are particularly likely to realize secondary benefits from substance use treatment, which is not necessarily surprising given that these factors were more likely to have brought them to treatment.

Grella et al. (2003) found that 6 months after entering a drug treatment center in an urban area, men had higher rates of incarceration and fewer episodes of subsequent treatment. Interestingly, whether men were living with someone else with a drug or alcohol problem did not influence their own use of substances; however, this factor was related to higher rates of substance use in women. These data suggest that men are less vulnerable than women to relapse because of having a partner who has a substance use problem, consistent with the notion that men's substance use is less socially embedded.

Substance use problems influence both the partners and the children of substance abusers. In a study by Collins et al. (2003), fathers showed higher levels of alcohol- and drug-use severity than did mothers. However, men who were more involved with their children showed less severe problems than did fathers who were less involved.

In summary, existing research, although limited, indicates that men appear particularly conducive to achieving secondary benefits from treatment for substance use disorders, such as improvements in work and family relations.

Treatment Modalities

A range of treatment modalities is available for substance abusers, and different modalities are appropriate at different phases of recovery. *Detoxification* is the first phase of recovery, and medications are often important in reducing symptoms of withdrawal. Longer-acting benzodiazepines are typically used in alcohol withdrawal, either in medical settings or on a carefully monitored outpatient basis. Opioid withdrawal can be effectively managed using methadone, clonidine, naltrexone, or buprenorphine. Most recently, "ultra rapid" detoxification from opioids has been evaluated. In this modality, withdrawal is induced with an opioid antagonist while the individual is under anesthesia, with the goal of minimizing patient discomfort. This method appears equally effective to other methods of detoxification, although the use of anesthesia poses significant safety concerns (O'Connor 2005).

The second phase of recovery is *active treatment*, which is provided in settings ranging from the least intensive (e.g., weekly outpatient counseling) to moderate intensity (ambulatory day programs) to the most restrictive (residential treatment). The content of these treatments tends to be multimodal, often using a disease or 12-step orientation supplemented with cognitive and behavioral strategies. Naltrexone, nalmefene, and acamprosate (calcium acetylhomotaurine), which help control cravings, have proven effectiveness in improving outcomes for alcohol-dependent patients receiving psychosocial treatments (Anton 2001; Mason et al. 1999; Swift 2003). Ondansetron has been shown to be effective in treating early-onset (predominantly male) alcoholism, presumably via targeting serotonergic abnormalities (Johnson et al. 2000). A large multicenter trial examining the efficacy of combining naltrexone and acamprosate is currently being performed in the United States (Mattson and Litten 2005). Methadone, naltrexone, levo-alpha-acetylmethadol (LAAM), and buprenorphine are pharmacological options for maintenance treatment of opioid dependence. Various medications have been evaluated for treatment of cocaine dependence, and disulfiram and baclofen have demonstrated early promise in randomized controlled trials (Carroll et al. 2004; Lima et al. 2002; Shoptaw et al. 2003). There are limited data supporting effective medications for the treatment of dependence on anxiolytics, sedatives, cannabis, hallucinogens, and other stimulants (Brands et al. 2000).

The third phase of recovery is the *maintenance phase*. For some individuals, highly structured environments, such as halfway houses, are helpful in promoting long-term success. For others, a continuing focus on recovery is important in the maintenance phase. Attendance at 12-step programs such as AA, Narcotics Anonymous, and Cocaine Anonymous was associated with better outcomes in numerous correlational studies (e.g., Timko et al. 2002). Alternative mutual support groups with less focus on the spiritual aspect of recovery, such as Women for Sobriety, SMART Recovery, and Rational Recovery, are increasingly available across North America (McCrady et al. 2003).

Because addiction-related disorders are associated with high rates of relapse, it is particularly crucial for mental health professionals to recognize the unique characteristics of men that make them susceptible to relapse after successful treatment. In a large-scale study of alcohol-dependent clients receiving aftercare therapy following inpatient or day hospital treatment, men had fewer abstinent days and consumed more alcohol per drinking day over the follow-up period compared with women (Project MATCH Research Group 1997). Thus men appear particularly vulnerable to relapse after extensive treatment. Hodgins et al. (1995) found that men were more likely to relapse because of intrapersonal rather than interpersonal reasons. For instance, men were more likely to begin using alcohol again after experiencing a bout of depression rather than after experiencing relationship difficulties.

Although some studies indicate that treatment type does not have differential effectiveness for men and women (Stewart et al. 2003; Timko et al. 2002), other findings reveal gender differences. For example, Sokolow et al. (1980) found more positive outcomes for men when the treatment program had a high peer group orientation. Jarvis (1992) found that men generally fared better with inpatient, traditional disease models. In another study, men who participated in group therapy showed less alcohol consumption at a 6-month posttreatment follow-up (Moos et al. 1990). However, more exposure to educational lectures and films about substance abuse was associated with increased consumption in men. It thus appears that having men discuss their substance use openly in groups is more effective than exposing them to educational tools, which may in fact be damaging. In a randomized, controlled trial of a general practitioner intervention with alcoholic patients, men showed better outcomes in brief treatment conditions than did men in control, no-treatment conditions. Women on the other hand did not show differences between the two conditions (Scott and Anderson 1990).

One factor that could influence the effectiveness of a residential treatment program for men is the gender composition. Bride (2001) investigated the effect of an agency's change from a mixed-gender treatment program to a single-gender program on client retention and treatment completion. Results showed that single-gender treatment programs did not significantly increase treatment retention and completion. Bride suggested that to improve treatment outcomes in men for substance abuse, the gender-specific treatment should do more than provide traditional treatment in a single-gender environment. Hodgins et al. (1997) suggested that men may benefit more from a treatment approach that is relatively more structured. Mixed-gender groups may be associated with more variation in the interpersonal style for men, which is assumed to have a positive impact of outcome.

More research is needed to determine the most effective treatment approaches for men with substance use disorders. Presently, several methods show promise. Inpatient, traditional disease models with high peer group orientation have shown some success. Brief treatment methods for outpatients may be particularly effective for men. Process variables, such as interpersonal style in group therapy, also require examination to determine their contributions to treatment outcomes.

Cost-Effectiveness

Research on the cost-effectiveness of substance use disorder treatments suggests that treatments for men are particularly beneficial from an economic standpoint. An examination of the cost-benefit ratio of treating men and women for substance abuse demonstrated that the savings from treatment are approximately 4.3 times the cost of treatment for women but 9.3 times the cost of treatment for men (Harwood et al. 1998). Thus the development of effective approaches for treating men with substance use disorders will prove to be financially beneficial for more than just the individual receiving treatment. The benefits of successfully treating these individuals will likely extend to family, friends, coworkers, and the greater community.

CONCLUSION

Mental health professionals should consider the unique aspects of the expression and treatment of substance use disorders in men. Compared with women, men have higher prevalence rates of substance use disorders, develop and express the disorders in different ways, have different co-occurring symptoms, seek treatment differently, exhibit different outcomes for specific treatments, and derive different benefits from treatment. Although research findings have generated a better understanding of substance use disorders in men, contributing factors should be considered within an individual context. Additional research should facilitate the development of improved prevention and treatment strategies for men with substance use disorders.

Perhaps the most important discoveries will be those that explain why men experience higher rates of substance abuse and dependence than do women. An integration of the research described here highlights the importance of considering specific social factors as major influences in the development of substance use disorders in men. An explanatory model for gender differences in the development, maintenance, and remission of substance use disorders would have significant clinical applicability.

Future research should examine the longitudinal course of substance use disorders in men, particularly the progression of substance use disorders through the following stages: experimentation, experiencing of negative consequences, help seeking, treatment, and posttreatment. There is also a need to further examine how each of these stages varies across different classes of drugs. More research is needed to explore new treatments for men with substance use disorders and to compare treatment efficacies with those of current treatment approaches. In the meantime, examining the unique issues men face in the course of substance use disorders should provide clinicians with a better understanding of the male experience and lead to more effective treatment.

KEY POINTS

- Men are more likely to use, abuse, and be dependent on substances than women.

- Men with substance use disorders report fewer psychosocial stressors but may be more likely to engage in impulsive behaviors while under the influence of substances, and such behavior may negatively influence their clinical course.

- Substance use disorders are frequently the primary issue for men that precede the development of other psychiatric disorders.

PRACTICE GUIDELINES

1. Screen men for substance use disorders.

2. Consider multiple avenues of substance abuse treatment for men.

3. Brief treatment methods for outpatients may be particularly effective for men.

4. For more severe cases, inpatient, traditional disease models with high peer group orientation may be beneficial.

REFERENCES

Allen SS, Hatsukami D, Christianson D, et al: Effects of transdermal nicotine on craving, withdrawal and premenstrual symptomatology in short-term smoking abstinence during different phases of the menstrual cycle. Nicotine Tob Res 2:231–241, 2000

Anthenelli RM, Schuckit MA: Genetics, in Substance Abuse: A Comprehensive Textbook. Edited by Lowinson JH, Ruiz P, Millman RB, et al. Baltimore, MD, Williams & Wilkins, 1997, pp 41–51

Anton RF: Pharmacologic approaches to the management of alcoholism. J Clin Psychiatry 62(suppl):11–17, 2001

Arfken CL, Klein C, di Menza S, et al: Gender differences in problem severity at assessment and treatment retention. J Subst Abuse Treat 20:53–57, 2001

Babor TF, Hofmann M, DelBoca FK, et al: Types of alcoholics, I: evidence for an empirically derived typology based on indicators of vulnerability and severity. Arch Gen Psychiatry 49:599–608, 1992

Back SE, Brady KT, Sonne SC: Gender differences in individuals with comorbid alcohol dependence and posttraumatic stress disorder. Drug Alcohol Depend 63 (suppl 1):S9, 2001

Ball SA, Carroll KM, Rounsaville BJ, et al: Subtypes of cocaine abusers: support for a type A/type B distinction. J Consult Clin Psychol 63:115–124, 1995

Ball SA, Kranzler HR, Tennen H, et al: Personality disorder and dimension differences between type A and type B substance abusers. J Personal Disord 12:1–12, 1998

Bierut LJ, Dinwiddie SH, Begleiter H, et al: Familial transmission of substance dependence: alcohol, marijuana, cocaine and habitual smoking. Arch Gen Psychiatry 55:982–988, 1998

Blume S: Women, alcohol and drugs, in Substance Abuse: A Comprehensive Textbook. Edited by Lowinson JH, Ruiz P, Millman RB, et al. Baltimore, MD, Williams & Wilkins, 1992, pp 794–807

Brands B, Kahan M, Selby P, et al: Management of Alcohol, Tobacco and Other Drug Problems: A Physician's Manual. Toronto, ON, Centre for Addiction and Mental Health, 2000

Bride BE: Single-gender treatment of substance abuse: effect on treatment retention and completion. Soc Work Res 25:223–232, 2001

Brienza RS, Stein MD: Alcohol use disorders in primary care: do gender-specific differences exist? J Gen Intern Med 17:387–397, 2002

Brunette MF, Drake RE: Gender differences in patients with schizophrenia and substance abuse. Compr Psychiatry 38:109–116, 1997

Cadoret RJ, Yates WR, Troughton E, et al: Adoption study demonstrating two genetic pathways to drug abuse. Arch Gen Psychiatry 52:42–52, 1995

Carroll KM, Fenton LR, Ball SA, et al: Efficacy of disulfiram and cognitive behavior therapy in cocaine-dependent outpatients: a randomized placebo-controlled trial. Arch Gen Psychiatry 61:264–272, 2004

Chermack ST, Stoltenberg SF, Fuller BE, et al: Gender differences in the development of substance-related problems: impact of family history of alcoholism, family history of violence and childhood conduct problems. J Stud Alcohol 61:848–852, 2001

Cloninger CR: A systematic method for clinical description and classification of personality variants: a proposal. Arch Gen Psychiatry 44:573–588, 1987

Collins CC, Grella CE, Hser YI: Effects of gender and level of parental involvement among parents in drug treatment. Am J Drug Alcohol Abuse 29:237–261, 2003

Cook BL, Winokur G, Fowler RC, et al: Classification of alcoholism with reference to comorbidity. Compr Psychiatry 35:165–170, 1994

Cornelius JR, Jarrett PJ, Thase ME, et al: Gender effects on the clinical presentation of alcoholics at a psychiatric hospital. Compr Psychiatry 36:435–440, 1995

Daitzman RJ, Zuckerman M, Sammelwitz P, et al: Sensation seeking and gonadal hormones. J Biosoc Sci 10:401–408, 1978

DiNitto DM, Webb DK, Rubin A: Gender differences in dually diagnosed clients
receiving chemical dependency treatment. J Psychoactive Drugs 34:105–
117, 2002

Elman I, Karlsgodt KH, Gastfriend DR: Gender differences in cocaine craving
among non-treatment-seeking individuals with cocaine dependence. Am J
Drug Alcohol Abuse 27:193–202, 2001

Evans SM, Haney M, Fischman MW, et al: Limited sex differences in response
to "binge" smoked cocaine use in humans. Neuropsychopharmacology
21:445–454, 1999

Fillmore MT, Weafer J: Alcohol impairment of behavior in men and women. Addiction 99:1237–1246, 2004

Frye MA, Altshuler LL, McElroy SL, et al: Gender differences in prevalence,
risk, and clinical correlates of alcoholism comorbidity in bipolar disorder.
Am J Psychiatry 160:883–889, 2003

Fu Q, Heath AC, Bucholz KK, et al: Shared genetic risk of major depression, alcohol dependence, and marijuana dependence: contribution of antisocial
personality disorder in men. Arch Gen Psychiatry 59:1125–1132, 2002

Galaif ER, Stein JA, Newcomb MD, et al: Gender differences in the prediction of
problem alcohol use in adulthood: exploring the influence of family factors
and childhood maltreatment. J Stud Alcohol 62:486–493, 2001

Giancola P, Zeichner A: An investigation of gender differences in alcohol-
related aggression. J Stud Alcohol 56:573–579, 1995

Grant BF, Stinson FS, Dawson DA, et al: Co-occurrence of 12-month alcohol and
drug use disorders and personality disorders in the United States: results
from the National Epidemiologic Survey on Alcohol and Related Conditions. Arch Gen Psychiatry 61:361–368, 2004

Green CA, Freeborn DK, Polen MR: Gender and alcohol use: the roles of social
support, chronic illness, and psychological well-being. J Behav Med 24:
383–399, 2001

Green CA, Polen MR, Dickinson DM, et al: Gender differences in predictors of
initiation, retention, and completion in an HMO-based substance abuse
treatment program. J Subst Abuse Treat 23:285–295, 2002

Grella CE: Effects of gender and diagnosis on addiction history, treatment utilization, and psychosocial functioning among a dually diagnosed sample in
drug treatment. J Psychoactive Drugs 35(suppl):169–179, 2003

Grella CE, Scott CK, Foss MA: Gender differences in drug treatment outcomes
among participants in the Chicago Target Cities Study. Eval Program Plann
26:297–310, 2003

Harwood H, Fountain D, Carothers S, et al: Gender differences in the economic
impacts of clients before, during and after substance abuse treatment.
Drugs and Society 13:251–269, 1998

Hoaken PN, Pihl RO: The effects of alcohol intoxication on aggressive responses
in men and women. Alcohol Alcohol 35:471–477, 2000

Hodgins DC, el-Guebaly N, Armstrong S: Prospective and retrospective reports of mood states before relapse to substance use. J Consult Clin Psychol 63:400–407, 1995

Hodgins DC, el-Guebaly N, Addington J: Treatment of substance abusers: single or mixed gender programs? Addiction 92:805–812, 1997

Holdcraft LC, Iacono WG: Cohort effects on gender differences in alcohol dependence. Addiction 97:1025–1036, 2002

Hsieh S, Hollister CD: Examining gender differences in adolescent substance abuse behavior: comparisons and implications for treatment. Journal of Child & Adolescent Substance Abuse 13:53–70, 2004

Jarvis TJ: Implications of gender for alcohol treatment research: a quantitative and qualitative review. Br J Addict 87:1249–1261, 1992

Jerrell J, Ridgely MS: Gender differences in the assessment of specialized treatments for substance abuse among people with severe mental illness. J Psychoactive Drugs 27:347–355, 1995

Johnson BA, Roache JD, Javors MA, et al: Ondansetron for reduction of drinking among biologically predisposed alcoholic patients. JAMA 284:963–971, 2000

Kandel DB: Gender differences in the epidemiology of substance dependence in the United States, in Gender and Its Effects on Psychopathology. Edited by Frank E. Washington, DC, American Psychiatric Press, 2000, pp 231–252

Karoll BR, Memmott J: The order of alcohol-related life experiences: gender differences. Journal of Social Work Practice in the Addictions 1:45–60, 2001

Kendler KS, Jacobson KC, Prescott CA, et al: Specificity of genetic and environmental risk factors for use and abuse/dependence of cannabis, cocaine, hallucinogens, sedatives, stimulants, and opiates in male twins. Am J Psychiatry 160:687–695, 2003

Kilts CD, Gross RE, Ely TD, et al: The neural correlates of cue-induced craving in cocaine-dependent women. Am J Psychiatry 161:233–241, 2004

King AC, Errico AL, Parsons OA: Eysenck's personality dimensions and sex steroids in male abstinent alcoholics and nonalcoholics: an exploratory study. Biol Psychol 39:103–113, 1995

King AC, Bernardy NC, Hauner K: Stressful events, personality, and mood disturbance: gender differences in alcoholics and problem drinkers. Addict Behav 28:171–187, 2003

Koenigsberg HW, Kaplan RD, Gilmore MM, et al: The relationship between syndrome and personality disorder in DSM-III: experience with 2,462 patients. Am J Psychiatry 142:207–212, 1985

Kohn CS, Mertens JR, Weisner CM: Coping among individuals seeking private chemical dependence treatment: gender differences and impact on length of stay in treatment. Alcohol Clin Exp Res 26:1228–1233, 2002

Kosten TR, Rounsaville BJ, Kosten TA, et al: Gender differences in the specificity of alcoholism transmission among the relatives of opioid addicts. J Nerv Ment Dis 179:392–400, 1991

Kosten TA, Gawin FH, Kosten TR, et al: Gender differences in cocaine use and treatment response. J Subst Abuse Treat 10:63–66, 1993

Landheim AS, Bakken K, Vaglum P: Gender differences in the prevalence of symptom disorders and personality disorders among poly-substance abusers and pure alcoholics: substance abusers treated in two counties in Norway. Eur Addict Res 9:8–17, 2003

Latimer WW, Stone AL, Voight A, et al: Gender differences in psychiatric comorbidity among adolescents with substance use disorders. Exp Clin Psychopharmacol 10:310–315, 2002

Lima MS, Soares BG, Reisser AA, et al: Pharmacological treatment of cocaine dependence: a systematic review. Addiction 97:931–949, 2002

Liu I-C, Blacker DL, Xu R, et al: Genetic and environmental contributions to the development of alcohol dependence in male twins. Arch Gen Psychiatry 61:897–903, 2004

Lynch WJ, Roth ME, Carroll ME: Biological basis of sex differences in drug abuse: preclinical and clinical studies. Psychopharmacology (Berl) 164:121–137, 2002

Mason BJ, Salvato FR, Williams LD, et al: A double-blind, placebo-controlled study of oral nalmefene for alcohol dependence. Arch Gen Psychiatry 56:719–724, 1999

Mattson ME, Litten RZ: Combining treatments for alcoholism: why and how? J Stud Alcohol Suppl 15:8–16, 2005

McCrady BS, Horvath AT, Delaney SI: Self-help groups, in Handbook of Alcoholism Treatment Approaches, 3rd Edition. Edited by Hester RK, Miller WR. Boston, MA, Allyn & Bacon, 2003, pp 165–187

Monk D, Ricciardelli LA: Three dimensions of male gender role as correlates of alcohol and cannabis involvement in young Australian men. Psychology of Men and Masculinity 4:57–69, 2003

Moos RH, Finney JW, Cronkite RC: Alcoholism Treatment: Context, Process, and Outcome. New York, Oxford University Press, 1990

O'Connor PG: Methods of detoxification and their role in treating patients with opioid dependence. JAMA 294:961–963, 2005

Office of Applied Studies: Results from the 2003 National Survey on Drug Use and Health: National Findings (DHHS Publ No SMA-04-3964, NSDUH Series H-25). Rockville, MD, Substance Abuse and Mental Health Services Administration, 2004

Oggins J, Guydish J, Delucchi K: Gender differences in income after substance abuse treatment. J Subst Abuse Treat 20:215–224, 2001

Pettinati HM, Rukstalis MR, Luck GJ, et al: Gender and psychiatric comorbidity: impact on clinical presentation of alcohol dependence. Am J Addict 9:242–252, 2000

Plant ML, Plant MA, Mason W: Drinking, smoking and illicit drug use among British adults: gender differences explored. Journal of Substance Use 7:24–33, 2002

Pomerleau CS, Garcia AW, Pomerleau OF, et al: The effects of menstrual phase and nicotine abstinence on nicotine intake and on biochemical and subjective measures in women: a preliminary report. Psychoneuroendocrinology 17:627–638, 1992

Potenza MN, Steinberg MA, McLaughlin SD, et al: Gender-related differences in the characteristics of problem gamblers using a gambling helpline. Am J Psychiatry 158:1500–1505, 2001

Project MATCH Research Group: Matching alcoholism treatments to client heterogeneity: Project MATCH posttreatment drinking outcomes. J Stud Alcohol 58:7–29, 1997

Ricciardelli LA, Connor JP, Williams RJ, et al: Gender stereotypes and drinking cognitions as indicators of moderate and high risk drinking among young women and men. Drug Alcohol Depend 61:129–136, 2001

Robbins SJ, Ehrman RN, Childress AR, et al: Comparing levels of cocaine cue reactivity in male and female outpatients. Drug Alcohol Depend 53:223–230, 1999

Room R: Gender roles and interactions in drinking and drug use. J Subst Abuse 8:227–239, 1996

Ross HE, Glaser FB, Stiasny S: Sex differences in the prevalence of psychiatric disorders in patients with alcohol and drug problems. Br J Addict 83:1179–1192, 1988

Sannibale C, Hall W: Gender-related symptoms and correlates of alcohol dependence among men and women with a lifetime diagnosis of alcohol use disorders. Drug Alcohol Rev 20:369–383, 2001

Scott E, Anderson P: Randomized controlled trial of general practitioner intervention in women with excessive alcohol consumption. Drug Alcohol Rev 10:313–321, 1990

Scourfield J, Stevens DE, Merikangas KR: Substance abuse, comorbidity, and sensation seeking: gender differences. Compr Psychiatry 37:384–392, 1996

Shoptaw S, Yang X, Rotheram-Fuller EJ, et al: Randomized placebo-controlled trial of baclofen for cocaine dependence: preliminary effects for individuals with chronic patterns of cocaine use. J Clin Psychiatry 64:1440–1448, 2003

Sofuoglu M, Babb DA, Hatsukami DK: Effects of progesterone treatment on smoked cocaine response in women. Pharmacol Biochem Behav 72:431–435, 2002

Sokolow L, Hynes G, Lyons J: Treatment-related differences between female and male alcoholics: focus on women. Journal of the Addictions and Health 1:43–56, 1980

Stalenheim EG, Eriksson E, von Knorring L, et al: Testosterone as a biological marker in psychopathy and alcoholism. Psychiatry Res 77:79–88, 1998

Stewart D, Gossop M, Marsden J, et al: Similarities in outcomes for men and women after drug misuse treatment: results from the National Treatment Outcome Research Study (NTORS). Drug Alcohol Rev 22:35–41, 2003

Swift RM: Medications, in Handbook of Alcoholism Treatment Approaches, 3rd Edition. Edited by Hester RK, Miller WR. Boston, MA, Allyn & Bacon, 2003, pp 259–281

Tavares H, Zilberman ML, Beites FJ, et al: Gender differences in gambling progression. J Gambl Stud 17:151–159, 2001

Thomas SE, Deas D, Grindlinger DR: Gender differences in dependence symptoms and psychiatric severity in adolescents with substance use disorders. Journal of Child & Adolescent Substance Abuse 12:19–34, 2003

Timko C, Moos RH, Finney JW, et al: Gender differences in help-utilization and the 8-year course of alcohol abuse. Addiction 97:877–889, 2002

Timko C, Finney JW, Moos RH: The 8-year course of alcohol abuse: gender differences in social context and coping. Alcohol Clin Exp Res 29:612–621, 2005

Tsuang MT, Lyons MJ, Eisen SA, et al: Genetic influences on abuse of illicit drugs: a study of 3,297 twin pairs. Am J Med Genet 67:473–477, 1996

Tsuang MT, Lyons MJ, Meyer JM, et al: Co-occurrence of abuse of different drugs in men: the role of drug-specific and shared vulnerabilities. Arch Gen Psychiatry 55:967–972, 1998

van den Bree MB, Svikis DS, Pickens RW: Genetic influences in anti-social personality and drug use disorders. Drug Alcohol Depend 49:177–187, 1998

Walton MA, Blow FC, Booth BM: Diversity in relapse prevention needs: gender and race comparisons among substance abuse treatment patients. Am J Drug Alcohol Abuse 27:225–240, 2001

Wechsberg WM, Craddock SG, Hubbard RL: How are women who enter substance abuse treatment different than men? a gender comparison from the Drug Abuse Treatment Outcome Study (DATOS). Drugs and Society 13:97–115, 1998

Zilberman ML, Blume SB: Drugs and women, in Substance Abuse: A Comprehensive Textbook. Edited by Lowinson JH, Ruiz P, Millman RB, et al. Philadelphia, PA, Lippincott Williams & Wilkins, 2004, pp 1064–1079

7

ANTISOCIAL PERSONALITY DISORDER, CONDUCT DISORDER, AND PSYCHOPATHY

DONALD W. BLACK, M.D.

Case Vignette

Ernie, age 18, was admitted to a psychiatric hospital in 1958 for evaluation of behavior problems. Ernie had lived a life of trouble: fights with other boys, expulsion, petty theft, and a 2-year stint in a boys' reformatory. He had entered the hospital voluntarily with the support of his adoptive parents, who had welcomed him into their home 10 years earlier. They had provided a good home in a fine neighborhood but had paid little attention to the behavior problems glossed over by officials at the adoption agency, who had blamed his troubles on an unstable living condition.

Ernie's natural father was a factory worker and alcoholic, and his mother, the man's fifth wife, was emotionally unstable. When Ernie was 6 years old, his father walked out, leaving Ernie and his two brothers with their mentally ill mother, who soon gave them up to the state. Foster care involved separation from his brothers and frequent relocations until his adoption at age 8.

Among his earliest memories were stealing from candy stores, taking cash from his father's wallet, and, after his adoption, pocketing toys from the homes of playmates. He had an IQ of 112, but low grades and misdeeds brought reprimands and punishment from teachers and his adoptive parents. As he entered his teen years, he began shoplifting clothing and records, burglarizing homes and churches, and hot-wiring

143

cars. After he was caught robbing a fellow student, he was sent by his adoptive parents to a military academy but did not last long there, and by age 16 Ernie was confined to a boys' reformatory.

Upon Ernie's admission to the psychopathic hospital, the psychiatric resident surmised that Ernie had a "sociopathic personality disturbance, antisocial type," and the attending psychiatrist described Ernie as "replete with surface phenomenon [sic] of lack of guilt and anxiety and a self-centered, uncontrolled person."

The psychiatrist found no evidence of depression, delusions, or anxiety and wrote that Ernie was "well oriented and performed well on tests of intellectual function." Ernie showed no interest in psychotherapy, insulted staff, and after 15 days announced he was leaving.

Ernie was identified 30 years later in the course of a follow-up study. He had been difficult to find because he had been using an alias, but a relative had provided his phone number. Ernie was not home for the scheduled appointment, which was later rescheduled. He acknowledged having forgotten the interview because of an alcoholic binge. Ernie was present for the next appointment and to the researcher he appeared chronically ill and much older than his 48 years. The house was dark and cold and in a decaying part of town.

Ernie related how he had spent a total of 17 years in the state penitentiary, an experience that still haunted him. He claimed to have witnessed several murders in prison and to have committed one himself. He had escaped from prison once but was later captured, although the details of the escape were not credible. He said he had been helped by his biological mother, an incident that led to a sexual relationship between the two.

Armed robbery, receiving stolen goods, using aliases, burglary, drunk driving, and attempted murder appeared on his record of more than 20 arrests. He had been in mental hospitals at least nine times, all alcohol related. In addition to his alcohol habit, he had used marijuana, amphetamines, cocaine, tranquilizers, and heroin.

He lived in a three-bedroom home with six others, including four children, his common-law wife, and a 15-year-old stepson. The wife, stepson, and oldest child earned the family's living, supplemented by illegal welfare payments and food stamps. Although he would paint cars occasionally in his garage, Ernie admitted a recent lack of work. He himself had never held a full-time job or maintained part-time work longer than 60 days, and he estimated he had held nearly 150 jobs in the previous decade. He and his common-law wife had met at a mental hospital about 5 years earlier, and Ernie noted that she took tranquilizers for an unnamed illness. The relationship was a bad one, fraught with constant fights that occasionally ended with police at the door. When drunk, Ernie sometimes beat his wife and children.

When asked about the difficulty tracking him down, Ernie smiled and noted that he liked to move and had used many different names. He had long since severed his relationship with his adoptive parents and acknowledged having no acquaintances outside of his family. He socialized only with men who patronized the local bars and the occasional Alcoholics Anonymous meetings that he attended. Ernie reported that he still lived a reckless life and "got a charge out of doing dangerous things."

Ernie's story, although sadder than the lives of many, illustrates the lifelong trajectory typical of antisocial personality disorder and its potential to severely impair function in all of life's important domains.

DEFINITION AND HISTORY OF ANTISOCIAL PERSONALITY DISORDER

Antisocial behavior has been described throughout recorded history, yet formal descriptions date only to the early nineteenth century. Philippe Pinel used the term *manie sans délire* to describe persons who were not insane but had irrational outbursts of rage and violence (Winokur and Crowe 1975). Later, German psychiatrists coined the term *psychopathy* to describe a broad range of deviant behaviors and eccentricities. The term was later used by American psychiatrist Hervey Cleckley in *Mask of Sanity*, originally published in 1941, which provided case vignettes illustrating typical symptoms and problems he associated with the disorder. He conceptualized psychopathy as a syndrome of emotional aloofness, callousness, self-serving attitudes, and impulsive antisocial behavior (Cleckley 1976).

The term *sociopathic personality disturbance* was introduced in DSM-I, published in 1952, and later was replaced by *antisocial personality disorder* in 1968 in DSM-II, a term whose use has continued to the present (American Psychiatric Association 1952, 1968). The term *antisocial* implies that the disturbance is directed against society. Diagnostic criteria were first enumerated in 1980 with DSM-III (American Psychiatric Association 1980) and were based partly on research conducted in the 1940s and 1950s by sociologist Lee Robins (1966) and her colleagues at Washington University in St. Louis, and by Sheldon and Eleanor Glueck (Glueck and Glueck 1950) at Harvard University. Both groups of researchers independently showed the continuity between childhood and adult behavior problems, both of which are required for the diagnosis. The DSM-IV-TR criteria (American Psychiatric Association 2000) are shown in Table 7–1 and describe a pattern of socially irresponsible, exploitative, and guiltless behavior beginning in childhood or early adolescence. Typical behaviors include criminality and failure to conform to the law, failure to sustain consistent employment, unprovoked aggression and violence, manipulation of others for personal gain, frequent deception of others, and a lack of empathy for others (Goodwin and Guze 1989). The definition of the disorder requires that the person be 18 years or older and have met criteria for conduct disorder before age 15 and that the disturbance not be due to schizophrenia or mania.

TABLE 7–1. DSM-IV-TR criteria for antisocial personality disorder

A. There is a pervasive pattern of disregard for and violation of the rights of others occurring since age 15 years, as indicated by three (or more) of the following:

(1) failure to conform to social norms with respect to lawful behaviors as indicated by repeatedly performing acts that are grounds for arrest

(2) deceitfulness, as indicated by repeated lying, use of aliases, or conning others for personal profit or pleasure

(3) impulsivity or failure to plan ahead

(4) irritability and aggressiveness, as indicated by repeated physical fights or assaults

(5) reckless disregard for safety of self or others

(6) consistent irresponsibility, as indicated by repeated failure to sustain consistent work behavior or honor financial obligations

(7) lack of remorse, as indicated by being indifferent to or rationalizing having hurt, mistreated, or stolen from another

B. The individual is at least age 18 years.

C. There is evidence of conduct disorder with onset before age 15 years.

D. The occurrence of antisocial behavior is not exclusively during the course of schizophrenia or a manic episode.

Source. Reprinted from American Psychiatric Association: *Diagnostic and Statistical Manual of Mental Disorders,* 4th Edition, Text Revision. Washington, DC, American Psychiatric Association, 2000. Used with permission.

Childhood antisocial acts were first acknowledged in DSM-II as *runaway reaction, unsocialized aggressive reaction,* and *group delinquent reaction.* Conduct disorder was introduced as a syndrome in 1980 with DSM-III and included four subtypes based on a 2×2 matrix on the axes of socialization and aggressivity. This scheme was derived from the work of Richard Jenkins and Herbert Quay but due to poor reliability was dropped from subsequent editions. Conduct disorder is currently classified as one of the *disruptive behavior disorders.* DSM-IV-TR specifies a childhood-onset type (before age 10 years) and an adolescent-onset type (after age 10 years) of conduct disorder and recognizes that early onset is one of the strongest predictors of poor outcome (Lahey et al. 1998). The diagnosis of conduct disorder requires that at least 3 of 15 problem behaviors be present in the past 12 months and 1 of the 3 problem behaviors be present for the past 6 months (see Table 7–2).

CLINICAL CHARACTERISTICS OF ANTISOCIAL PERSONALITY DISORDER AND CONDUCT DISORDER

The behavioral manifestations of antisocial personality disorder begin early, often during the preschool years and generally by age 8; by age 11,

---

TABLE 7–2.   DSM-IV-TR criteria for conduct disorder

A.   A repetitive and persistent pattern of behavior in which the basic rights of others or major age-appropriate societal norms or rules are violated, as manifested by the presence of three (or more) of the following criteria in the past 12 months, with at least one criterion present in the past 6 months:

Aggression to people and animals

(1)   often bullies, threatens, or intimidates others

(2)   often initiates physical fights

(3)   has used a weapon that can cause serious physical harm to others (e.g., a bat, brick, broken bottle, knife, gun)

(4)   has been physically cruel to people

(5)   has been physically cruel to animals

(6)   has stolen while confronting a victim (e.g., mugging, purse snatching, extortion, armed robbery)

(7)   has forced someone into sexual activity

Destruction of property

(8)   has deliberately engaged in fire setting with the intention of causing serious damage

(9)   has deliberately destroyed others' property (other than by fire setting)

Deceitfulness or theft

(10)   has broken into someone else's house, building, or car

(11)   often lies to obtain goods or favors or to avoid obligations (i.e., "cons" others)

(12)   has stolen items of nontrivial value without confronting a victim (e.g., shoplifting, but without breaking and entering; forgery)

Serious violations of rules

(13)   often stays out at night despite parental prohibitions, beginning before age 13 years

(14)   has run away from home overnight at least twice while living in parental or parental surrogate home (or once without returning for a lengthy period)

(15)   is often truant from school, beginning before age 13 years

B.   The disturbance in behavior causes clinically significant impairment in social, academic, or occupational functioning.

C.   If the individual is age 18 years or older, criteria are not met for antisocial personality disorder.

Code based on age at onset:

312.81   Conduct Disorder, Childhood-Onset Type: onset of at least one criterion characteristic of conduct disorder prior to age 10 years

312.82   Conduct Disorder, Adolescent-Onset Type: absence of any criteria characteristic of conduct disorder prior to age 10 years

312.89   Conduct Disorder, Unspecified Onset: age at onset is not known

TABLE 7–2.   DSM-IV-TR criteria for conduct disorder *(continued)*

Specify severity:

Mild: few if any conduct problems in excess of those required to make the diagnosis **and** conduct problems cause only minor harm to others

Moderate: number of conduct problems and effect on others intermediate between "mild" and "severe"

Severe: many conduct problems in excess of those required to make the diagnosis **or** conduct problems cause considerable harm to others

Source.   Reprinted from American Psychiatric Association: *Diagnostic and Statistical Manual of Mental Disorders,* 4th Edition, Text Revision. Washington, DC, American Psychiatric Association, 2000. Used with permission.

80% of future cases have had a first symptom (Robins and Price 1991). Childhood symptoms include fights with peers, conflicts with parents and other authority figures, stealing, vandalism, fire setting, and cruelty to animals or other children. School-related behavior problems are common, as is poor academic performance. Many antisocial children have a history of running away from home.

As the antisocial youth attains adult status, problems develop in other areas of life reflecting age-appropriate responsibilities and include uneven job performance, unreliability, frequent job changes, and losing jobs through quitting out of pique or being fired. Pathological lying and the use of aliases are common. Many antisocial persons are sexually promiscuous and become sexually active at a younger age than their peers (Robins 1966). Marriages are frequently unstable and characterized by physical or emotional abuse of the spouse, leading to high rates of separation and divorce. Clinical symptoms of conduct disorder and adult antisocial personality disorder are shown in Table 7–3.

Criminality is a frequent problem among antisocial persons, and although varied, offenses range from nonviolent disregard of property rights to acts of extreme violence, including murder (Black et al. 1995; Goodwin and Guze 1989; Robins 1966). In the military, the person with antisocial personality disorder is more likely than those without the disorder to be absent without leave, court-martialed, or dishonorably discharged (Robins 1966).

PSYCHOPATHY AND ANTISOCIAL PERSONALITY DISORDER

Psychopathy has been described as a distinct clinical construct defined by a constellation of psychological manifestations and has much in common with Cleckley's (1976) depiction in *Mask of Sanity.* Symptoms

TABLE 7–3. Problem behaviors in 206 men with antisocial personality disorder

Clinical symptoms	%
Juvenile behaviors	
Suspension/expulsion	69
Fighting	65
Truancy (more than three times per year)	63
Arrests	60
Running away	54
Stealing	43
Vandalism	42
Wanderlust	18
Adult behaviors	
Adult fighting	70
Frequent job changes	66
Being fired	63
Felony convictions	60
Traffic violations (more than three)	56
Quitting job	41
Frequent lying	36
Wanderlust	25
Adultery	25
Spouse abuse	21
Promiscuity	20
Use of alias	17
Divorces (more than two)	9
Child abuse	4
Deserting family	2

Source. Adapted from Dinwiddie and Reich 1993.

include inadequately motivated antisocial behaviors, a lack of emotional connection with others, and an incapacity for guilt or remorse (Hare 1993). In contrast, the DSM-IV-TR criteria for antisocial personality disorder are focused on observable behavioral manifestations (e.g., criminality, aggression).

Psychologist Robert Hare has been critical of the DSM approach for overemphasizing delinquent and antisocial symptoms to the exclusion of psychological traits. He created the Psychopathy Checklist, a semistructured instrument, to reliably assess the symptoms he associates with psychopathy, and although used mainly by researchers, the instrument appears to predict both criminal recidivism and parole violations (Hare 1986). Evidence suggests that the checklist also predicts violence in offenders and psychiatric patients (Hare 1999). Hare noted that most antisocial persons are not psychopaths, as defined by his instrument, although mostly all psychopaths are antisocial. Thus psychopathy may constitute a subtype of antisocial personality disorder associated with a particularly poor prognosis.

PREVALENCE AND RISK FACTORS

Antisocial personality disorder appears to be culturally universal; the disorder is found in persons around the globe and in all racial and ethnic groups. In the Epidemiologic Catchment Area (ECA) survey, conducted in five sites in the United States in the early 1980s, antisocial personality disorder was found to have an overall prevalence of 2%–4% in men and 0.5%–1% in women (Robins et al. 1984). The National Comorbidity Survey found an overall rate of 3.5% for antisocial personality disorder in the general population, based on a nationwide probability survey conducted in the United States in the early 1990s (Kessler et al. 1994). More recently, in the National Epidemiologic Survey on Alcohol and Related Conditions (NESARC), a nationally representative survey of over 40,000 respondents age 18 and older, antisocial personality disorder had a prevalence of 3.6% (Grant et al. 2004). Conduct disorder is relatively common in children and has an estimated prevalence of 2% for girls and 9% for boys (Russo and Beidel 1994).

Antisocial personality disorder has been associated with male gender, incarceration, low socioeconomic status, drug and alcohol misuse, and homelessness. Research shows that men are two to eight times more likely to have antisocial personality disorder than are women, and conduct disorder is estimated to be three to four times more likely in boys than in girls (Robins 1987). The gender difference has not been fully determined, but proposed mechanisms include both genetic (e.g., a gene predisposing to antisocial personality disorder either going unexpressed or being expressed differently in women) and cultural (e.g., women turning anger inward and men expressing it in outward actions) factors.

Studies from prison settings show that as many as 80% of incarcerated men and 65% of incarcerated women are antisocial (Guze 1976). These figures may be declining as the prison population has increased in the past decade, particularly as sentencing laws have become harsher. Likely, a smaller percentage of incarcerated persons meet antisocial personality disorder criteria now than in the past; for example, only 19% of offenders assessed with a structured instrument in a more recent prison-based study were diagnosed as antisocial (Black et al. 2004).

Antisocial personality disorder is associated with low socioeconomic status, which can be attributed in part to poor educational achievement, poor job performance, and frequent unemployment. In the NESARC, respondents with lower educational levels and lower income levels were at increased risk for antisocial personality disorder (Compton et al. 2005). According to Robins (1987), persons with antisocial personality disorder begin life at a disadvantaged level, and their adult social class continues to decline, even falling below that of their parents. Yet low social class itself is not responsible for antisocial personality disorder. In a study of black youths, Robins et al. (1971) showed that children without antisocial symptoms were not at risk for antisocial personality disorder even when they were raised in impoverished homes, but children with high rates of antisocial symptoms were at risk for antisocial personality disorder even when reared in white-collar settings.

Certain diagnostic and clinical groups are at high risk for antisocial personality disorder. The prevalence of antisocial personality disorder in alcoholic patients approaches 50% and may be even higher in heroin and other drug addicts (Hesselbrock et al. 1992). Pathological gamblers have a high prevalence of antisocial personality disorder, with rates ranging up to 40% (Argo and Black 2004). Frequency rates of antisocial personality disorder among the homeless are also high (North et al. 1993). The ECA survey showed that black respondents were more likely than whites to exhibit antisocial symptoms that could lead to arrest and incarceration (e.g., violence; Robins and Price 1991), although there was no racial difference in antisocial personality disorder prevalence. Yet in the NESARC, Native Americans were at increased risk for antisocial personality disorder, whereas Asian American and Hispanic/Latino respondents were at lower risk than whites for antisocial personality disorder (Compton et al. 2005). One explanation for these findings is that the expression of antisocial personality disorder is shaped by the person's immediate environment and peer group associations.

NATURAL HISTORY

Antisocial personality disorder is a lifelong disorder that typically begins at about age 8 with a variety of behavior problems at home and school and is fully expressed by the late 20s or early 30s (Robins and Price 1991). In younger persons, the corresponding diagnosis is conduct disorder. Although the majority of children with conduct disorder do not develop adult antisocial personality disorder, they remain at high risk, with an estimated 25% of girls with conduct disorder and 40% of boys with conduct disorder developing antisocial personality disorder (Robins 1987). The more extensive the variety and severity of childhood behavior, and the earlier the onset, the greater the likelihood is for the child to develop adult antisocial personality disorder (Robins 1966).

Once established, antisocial personality disorder is chronic, yet longitudinal studies show that persons with the disorder tend to improve as they age, and many remit. Robins (1966) conducted a follow-up study in the mid-1950s of more than 300 adults who had been treated as children at child guidance clinics in St. Louis in the 1920s. A subset of 82 subjects were retrospectively diagnosed with antisocial personality disorder, and when these subjects were reevaluated at a mean age of 45, 12% were judged to have remitted. Another 20% of subjects were improved, but the remainder (68%) were considered to be as disturbed or more so than when originally studied. In a more recent study (Black et al. 1995), 71 men diagnosed with antisocial personality disorder were followed a mean of 29 years after an index hospitalization. At a mean age of 56 years, 27% of subjects had remitted, another 31% were felt to have improved, and 42% were judged to be unimproved. Antisocial men least likely to improve were considered the most deviant at baseline, were younger at follow-up, or were still misusing substances (Black et al. 1997). The findings imply that antisocial persons tend to improve at a steady rate as they age and mature. One estimate is that antisocial personality disorder remits at the rate of about 2% per year (Perry and Vaillant 1989), which roughly approximates the rate seen in the study by Black and colleagues (1995, 1997).

The median age for improvement in the study by Robins (1966) was 35 years. She noted that there was "no age beyond which improvement seemed impossible" (p. 226). Although nearly one-third of the group with antisocial personality disorder had improved, Robins observed that symptoms remained: "Many of them report interpersonal difficulties, irritability, hostility toward wives, neighbors, and organized religion" (p. 236). When improvement or remission occurs, it often comes after years of antisocial behaviors that have limited the person's educational and work achievement, which is damage that most antisocial persons are unable to overcome (Goodwin and Guze 1989).

Another factor that may moderate outcome of childhood conduct disorder is degree of socialization. Socialized children form strong ties with a familiar group of friends, and undersocialized children do not. Henn et al. (1978) reported that socialized delinquents were less likely to have been convicted or incarcerated during a 10-year follow-up. Children who had continued to exhibit antisocial behavior did not form a group identity.

The tragic natural history of antisocial personality disorder was described as a developmental process by sociologist Clifford Shaw, who introduced Stanley, a young mugger, in his book *The Jack-Roller: A Delinquent Boy's Own Story* (Shaw 1930), and the Martin brothers in a later work, *Brothers in Crime* (Shaw 1938). Stanley was a chronic runaway by age 6, was truant by age 8, and had been in custody 38 times by age 17, including three terms at a home for incorrigible boys and 1 year each in two boys' reformatories. *Brothers in Crime* describes the life histories of the five Martin brothers, whose first official juvenile court records were established when the brothers were ages 2–8 years (Shaw 1938). The brothers' lives were traced into their early to mid-20s, and all the brothers were shown to have regularly offended throughout their lives. The book's cover illustration shows Shaw's thesis of an escalating criminal career: a staircase wherein each step represents a certain type of deviant behavior or crime and where ascending steps suggest increasingly serious criminality. The case of Stanley is particularly relevant because he was reinterviewed at age 70 years. Although no longer involved in significant criminal activity, he continued to have trouble keeping jobs, was constantly on his guard against assault by others, and took little responsibility for his own behavior (Jack-Roller et al. 1982).

Psychologist Terrie Moffitt has written extensively about antisocial behavior and distinguishes those individuals with "life-course-persistent" antisocial behavior from those with "adolescence-limited" behavior (Moffitt 1993a). The former group includes men with an early onset of antisocial behavior who had more severe and a greater variety of problems. The latter group involves those with less severe behavior that typically arises in the context of teenage peer group pressure and who have little or no history of earlier antisocial behavior and tend to spontaneously improve. Her theory posits a reasonable explanation for why most children with conduct disorder never develop antisocial personality disorder.

CO-OCCURRING DISORDERS AND BEHAVIORS

Because of their impulsivity and recklessness, antisocial persons are at high risk for traumatic injuries, accidents, and suicide attempts (Garvey and Spoden 1980; Woodruff et al. 1971). Antisocial persons often die prematurely from accidental deaths, suicides, or homicides, and at least one study has shown excessive rates of death from natural causes (Black and Braun 1998). In this study, the death rate among young antisocial men from diabetes mellitus was elevated, suggesting that some antisocial persons neglect their medical problems or fail to comply with medical treatment regimens. Risk for sexually transmitted diseases, including human immunodeficiency virus (HIV), is high, probably resulting in part from sexually promiscuous behavior (Brooner et al. 1993).

Psychiatric comorbidity is frequent among antisocial persons (Goodwin and Guze 1989). Substance use disorders have been associated with antisocial personality disorder, and in a recent study the odds ratio for a current alcohol disorder was nearly five times expectation in antisocial persons, and the risk for a current drug use disorder was nearly 12 times the expectation (Grant et al. 2004). On a lifetime basis, nearly 84% of antisocial persons surveyed in the ECA study had some form of substance abuse (Regier et al. 1990). Persons with antisocial personality disorder have high rates of other psychiatric diagnoses, including mood and anxiety disorders, sexual dysfunction, pathological gambling, and other Axis II disorders (e.g., borderline personality disorder) (Black et al. 1995; Dinwiddie and Reich 1993; Robins and Price 1991).

Conduct disorder is also associated with substantial psychiatric comorbidity, including substance use disorders, mood and anxiety disorders, and attention-deficit/hyperactivity disorder (ADHD). The latter is particularly common, and in one study of adolescent inpatients with conduct disorder, 68% met criteria for ADHD (Grilo et al. 1996). Although ADHD has been linked to later criminality, hyperactive children without conduct disorder are not at increased risk (Satterfield and Schell 1997).

ETIOLOGY AND PATHOPHYSIOLOGY

Increasing evidence suggests that antisocial personality disorder is a neuropsychiatric syndrome with multiple causes. Family, twin, and adoption studies support a genetic diathesis. A review of twin study data showed monozygotic concordance of nearly 67% compared with 31% concordance for dizygotic twins (Brennan and Mednick 1993). In an adoption study, Crowe (1974) showed that antisocial personality disorder occurred significantly more frequently among the biological relatives of antisocial probands than among the relatives of nonaffected control subjects. Cadoret et al. (1985) followed this work with a series of adoption studies. They demonstrated that the interaction of genetic and environmental variables increased the likelihood of antisocial personality disorder beyond the contribution of genetics or environmental factors alone, especially when the combination of antisocial biological relatives with dysfunctional family life in the adoptive environment was present. He and his colleagues concluded that although antisocial personality disorder may have a hereditary basis, environmental factors contribute to its expression. These findings are supported by recent molecular genetic research. Caspi et al. (2002) reported that 85% of abused children with a low-activity variant of a gene influencing levels of monoamine oxidase A (*MAOA*) developed antisocial behavior. In contrast, children who experienced similar abuse but had a high-activity variant of the gene rarely exhibited antisocial behaviors in adulthood. A study of male twins (Foley et al. 2004) showed that low activity of the *MAOA* gene increased the risk for conduct disorder in the presence of childhood adversity.

More recently, Krueger et al. (2002) explored the concept of externalizing disorders and, based on a large twin data set, linked substance use disorders, antisocial personality disorder, and "disinhibited personality," which they calculated to have a heritability of 0.81. In extending this work, Slutske et al. (2001) suggested that the spectrum of externalizing disorders might include pathological gambling. This body of work suggests that these disorders share common genetic risks and that their expressions likely involve specific nongenetic factors.

Neurobiological theories have been proposed. Hare (1986, 1993, 1999) has investigated autonomic underarousal, a condition that he proposes underlies antisocial personality disorder. It is hypothesized that antisocial persons require greater sensory input to produce normal brain functioning than do healthy subjects, possibly leading antisocial individuals to seek potentially dangerous or risky situations to raise their level of arousal to more optimal levels. Evidence supporting this theory includes the finding that antisocial adults (and youth with conduct disorder) have low resting pulse rates, low skin conductance, and increased amplitude on event-related potentials. One study of 15-year-old English schoolchildren found that those who committed crimes during the subsequent 9 years were more likely to have had at baseline a low resting pulse, reduced skin conductance, and more slow-wave electroencephalographic activity than the others (Raine et al. 1990).

Abnormal brain structure and function have been associated with antisocial behavior. One positron emission tomography study examined a group of Marine and Navy personnel who had assaulted others or made suicide attempts, and found that the most aggressive men had low glucose metabolism in the right temporal lobe (Goyer et al. 1994). Raine et al. (2000) reported that antisocial persons have reduced prefrontal gray matter. Kiehl et al. (2001) identified specific abnormalities in the processing of emotions in psychopathic criminals diagnosed with Hare's Psychopathy Checklist. On functional magnetic resonance imaging scans, the psychopathic criminals showed less affect-related activity in important limbic structures and increased activity bilaterally in the frontotemporal cortex. Because both the temporal lobes and the prefrontal cortex help to regulate mood and behavior, impulsive or poorly controlled behavior could stem from functional abnormalities in these brain regions.

The neurotransmitter serotonin may mediate some antisocial behavior. Low levels of cerebrospinal fluid 5-hydroxyindoleacetic acid, a major metabolite of serotonin, have repeatedly been associated with violent or impulsive behavior, as have other measures of central serotonin system function (Scarpa and Raine 1997). Genetic disturbances in serotonin function may predispose to impulsive and aggressive behavior (Nielson et al. 1994).

Another theory posits that antisocial personality disorder represents a neurodevelopmental disorder, as suggested by high rates of minor facial anomalies, learning disorders, persistent enuresis, and behavioral hyperactivity (Moffitt 1993b). Presence of electroencephalographic abnormalities in nearly half of antisocial persons is also consistent with a neurodevelopmental syndrome. Wakschlag et al. (1997) showed that maternal smoking during gestation predisposed offspring to antisocial behavior. These findings suggest that a subtle brain injury may have resulted from lower levels of oxygen available to the fetus or fetal exposure to chemicals generated from tobacco or their metabolites. The same research group reported that persons who were in utero during the "Dutch hunger winter" in 1944 (when the Nazis systematically starved the Dutch population) were more likely than others to exhibit antisocial behavior, possibly related to the pathological effects of malnutrition on neurodevelopment (Neugebauer et al. 1999).

FAMILY AND SOCIAL FACTORS IN ANTISOCIAL PERSONALITY DISORDER

Antisocial personality disorder runs in families, and antisocial parents are often incompetent, absent, or abusive. As such, the family environment of many individuals who later develop antisocial personality disorder is often troubled and chaotic (Robins 1987). Parents of troubled children exhibit high levels of antisocial behavior and are often alcoholic, criminal, divorced, separated, or absent (Glueck and Glueck 1950). One early theory posited that antisocial personality disorder resulted from prolonged maternal separation (Bowlby 1946). Later research showed that the absence of a significant adult relationship (not just the mother) and depriving a young child of a significant emotional bond could impair the ability to form intimate and trusting relationships later in life (Rutter 1982).

Erratic or inappropriate parental discipline and inadequate supervision have been linked with antisocial behavior in children (Loeber 1990; Reti et al. 2002). Antisocial parents are unlikely to effectively monitor their child's behavior, set rules and ensure that they are obeyed, check on the child's whereabouts, or steer the child away from troubled playmates. However, Bell and Chapman (1986) argued that the reverse may be true: the antisocial child might *induce* negative responses in parents.

Child abuse is more common in antisocial families, and persons with antisocial personality disorder are more likely than others to report histories of childhood abuse (Luntz and Widom 1994), a finding consistent with that fact that many of these persons were raised by neglectful and sometimes violent antisocial parents. Violent physical abuse can cause brain injuries (as from vigorously shaking a child), and it is possible that such abuse disrupts normal central nervous system development, increasing the potential for the child to develop antisocial behavior (Bremner et al. 1996).

Disturbed peer relationships are an important and often overlooked factor contributing to the development of antisocial behavior. Glueck and Glueck (1950) reported that 98% of the delinquent boys that were studied had delinquent friends as compared with 8% of their nondelinquent peers. This pattern typically begins during the elementary school years, wherein the "birds of a feather" phenomenon might lead "social outcasts" to associate. Unfortunately, such relationships often encourage and reward aggressive behavior and may later lead to gang membership. Gangs may be attractive to those who feel neglected by their families and peer groups.

ASSESSING FOR ANTISOCIAL PERSONALITY DISORDER

The diagnosis of antisocial personality disorder is generally based on a history of chronic and repetitive behavior problems. Patients may provide some information about their behavior, and family members and friends are often useful informants. Among children, parents and teachers are often the best sources of information about antisocial behaviors. Family history studies have shown that informants are often more accurate in describing a person's antisocial behavior than is the subject (Andreasen et al. 1986). Medical records may also provide diagnostic information—for example, a history of traumatic injuries. As in other psychiatric disorders, no specific laboratory or neuropsychological tests are confirmatory, and for that reason extensive testing is generally unnecessary. Neuropsychological and cognitive testing may be useful in assessing the patient for learning disorders. Such testing can identify specific deficits that can be targeted for intervention. The physical examination adds little to the assessment for antisocial personality disorder, although antisocial persons are more likely than others to have tattoos, often depicting violent themes (Favazza 1987).

The Minnesota Multiphasic Personality Inventory is a well-established test that yields a broad profile of personality functioning. Antisocial subjects often score highly on inventory scales 4 ("hypomania") and 9 ("psychopathic deviate"); this pattern is often referred to as the *4–9 profile* (Dahlstrom et al. 1972). Several structured interviews have been developed to identify personality disorders, including the Structured Interview for DSM-IV Personality Disorders (Pfohl et al. 1997), the Structured Clinical Interview for DSM-IV Personality Disorders (First et al. 1995), and the International Personality Diagnostic Examination (Loranger 1999), but all are used mainly in research settings.

DIFFERENTIAL DIAGNOSIS OF ANTISOCIAL PERSONALITY DISORDER AND CONDUCT DISORDER

The differential diagnosis of antisocial personality disorder includes other personality disorders (e.g., borderline personality disorder), substance use disorders, psychotic or mood disorders, intermittent explosive disorder, and medical conditions such as temporal lobe epilepsy. Chronic or intermittent alcohol or drug use can contribute to the development of antisocial behavior, either as a product of the intoxication itself or from the result of a drug habit that needs financial support. In these cases, drug-seeking behavior may develop in persons who have no history of antisocial personality disorder and have shown antisocial behavior only in the context of their drug use. Psychoses or bipolar disorder can also lead to violent or assaultive behavior and should be considered a cause of antisocial behavior. Psychotic patients occasionally offend or misbehave, but such behavior is typically the product of psychotic thought processes (e.g., "The voices told me to do it!"). Partial complex seizures can cause random outbursts of violence, and tumors, strokes, or other brain insults can lead to personality changes. With intermittent explosive disorder, the essential feature is isolated episodes of assaultive or destructive behavior, but generally neither a history of childhood conduct disorder nor other features of antisocial personality disorder, such as chronic irresponsibility, are present.

The differential diagnosis in children with conduct disorder includes oppositional defiant disorder (ODD), ADHD, pervasive developmental disorders, and psychotic and mood disorders, all of which can be associated with sporadic verbal outbursts or physical assaultiveness. Arguably the most difficult aspect of diagnosis involves distinguishing between conduct disorder and ODD. The child with ODD is difficult and uncooperative, but his or her behavior is generally not directed against others as it is with conduct disorder. With ADHD, the child may be inattentive or hyperactive but otherwise does not obviously misbehave. The two disorders can coexist, in which case both diagnoses are merited.

Both antisocial personality disorder and conduct disorder are distinguishable from normal behavior. Most children experience episodes of rambunctious behavior that could be accompanied by inappropriate language or destructive acts. Similarly, many children or adolescents engage in reckless behavior, vandalism, or even minor criminal activity such as shoplifting, with such behaviors often involving peer influences. Isolated acts of misbehavior are inconsistent with the diagnosis of either conduct disorder or antisocial personality disorder, both of which involve repetitive misbehavior over time. Adults who develop criminal or antisocial behavior but who have no evidence of childhood conduct disorder receive the DSM-IV-TR diagnosis of *adult antisocial behavior*; this is one of the V-code diagnoses that are not considered attributable to a mental illness but are a focus of clinical concern. An example of a person receiving this diagnosis is a man who becomes involved in organized crime after having a conventional childhood and adolescence.

CLINICAL MANAGEMENT OF ANTISOCIAL PERSONALITY DISORDER

Individuals with antisocial personality disorder rarely seek medical care for treatment of its symptoms (Shapiro et al. 1984). Those persons who choose to seek mental health care can generally be accommodated in outpatient settings, in which they can be offered an array of services including medication management, individual psychotherapy, and family and marital counseling. There is generally little reason to hospitalize antisocial patients, who are often disruptive to the hospital milieu (Carney 1978), unless there is co-occurring depression, suicidal behavior, violent or assaultive behavior, or substance use disorder.

There are no standard treatments for either conduct disorder or antisocial personality disorder. Clinicians should consider that many youth with conduct disorder spontaneously improve as they age and mature, as do adults with antisocial personality disorder. Therefore, any assessment of improvement must consider this developmental trajectory before the clinician can conclude that a treatment works.

Medication

No medications specifically target antisocial behavior, yet several drugs have been shown in randomized, controlled trials to reduce aggression, the chief complaint for many people with antisocial personality disorder. Lithium carbonate has been demonstrated to reduce anger and verbal and physical assaultiveness in prison settings (Sheard et al. 1976). The drug also reduces bullying, fighting, and temper outbursts in aggressive children (Campbell et al. 1995). Phenytoin, an anticonvulsant, has also been shown to reduce impulsive aggression in incarcerated men (Barrett et al. 1991), whereas divalproex reduces temper outbursts and mood lability in disruptive youth (Donovan et al. 2000).

Other medications, including carbamazepine, fluoxetine, propranolol, buspirone, and trazodone, have shown some success in treating aggression in selected populations such as individuals with brain injury or mental retardation (Corrigan et al. 1993; Davis et al. 1995), although most positive reports have involved open trials or small case series. In similar populations, antipsychotic medications have also been shown to deter aggression (Brodaty et al. 2003; Walker et al. 2003). Because first-generation antipsychotics can induce tardive dyskinesia, this potential adverse effect should be considered when prescribing them. In behaviorally disturbed children, haloperidol, in comparison with placebo, reduces aggressiveness and outbursts (Campbell et al. 1984). Although aggression and violence are among the most problematic symptoms of conduct disorder or antisocial personality disorder, they compose only one facet of the syndrome, and little evidence shows that these medications have any impact on other aspects of the disorder. Nonetheless, a medication-induced reduction in violence and assaultiveness could represent an important therapeutic outcome.

Medication may also target co-occurring psychiatric disorders and may produce the additional benefit of reducing antisocial personality disorder behavior. For example, when concurrent substance use disorder is treated, persons with antisocial personality disorder are less likely to engage in criminal conduct, have fewer family conflicts, and have fewer emotional problems (Cacciola et al. 1996). Mood and anxiety disorders may respond to treatment with antidepressant or anxiolytic medication, although avoiding the use of benzodiazepines is advisable for several reasons. First, benzodiazepines have been shown to increase acting-out behaviors (e.g., aggressive outbursts) in patients with borderline personality disorder (Cowdry and Gardner 1988) and may conceivably produce a similar response in antisocial persons. Another reason to avoid benzodiazepines is that they are potentially habit-forming medications and thus their use is unwise in a patient population prone to addiction. Co-occurring bipolar disorder can be treated with mood stabilizers such as lithium carbonate, carbamazepine, or valproate. Clinicians should be mindful that individuals with severe personality disorders, including antisocial personality disorder, are less likely to respond to conventional antidepressant treatment than those without personality disorders (Reich and Green 1991).

There is considerable overlap of antisocial personality disorder with ADHD, and stimulant medication may help improve the antisocial person's ability to focus and concentrate, although potentially addictive stimulants should be avoided. Some antisocial persons have concomitant paraphilias, and the combination of the two disorders can lead to dangerous sexual behaviors. Such individuals may benefit from selective serotonin reuptake inhibitors, although in more dangerous or aggressive persons, injections of medroxyprogesterone or the use of another testosterone-reducing agent (e.g., leuprolide) may be beneficial (Gottesman and Schubert 1993; Kafka 1994).

Psychotherapy and Counseling

Psychotherapy with the antisocial person is particularly challenging (Strasberger 1986). First, individuals with antisocial personality disorder rarely seek psychotherapy, and when seeking treatment they often do so at the behest of a spouse, a significant other, or lawyers and judges. This external impetus produces a situation wherein a person with minimal insight has little motivation to engage in treatment and may see little potential benefit. The tendency of individuals with antisocial personality disorder to blame others and to demonstrate low frustration tolerance, impulsivity, and difficulty in developing trusting relationships further erodes their ability to engage in therapy (Black 1999). Some people with antisocial personality disorder have a potential for violence that leads many mental health professionals to avoid treating them. The antisocial person's criminal or violent past can make it difficult for some therapists to act in an objective and nonjudgmental way because of negative feelings they have toward the antisocial patient. For that reason, therapists who treat antisocial persons should remain vigilant to the potential for countertransference issues to disrupt therapy.

Cognitive-behavioral therapy may be helpful to persons with mild antisocial personality disorder who possess some insight and have reason to improve—for example, those who risk losing a spouse or job if their behavior is not controlled (Davidson and Tyrer 1996). Beck and Freeman (1990) made several recommendations for applying cognitive therapy to antisocial personality disorder. These recommendations involve evaluating situations in which the patient's beliefs or behaviors interfere with functioning or success in achieving goals—for example, an explosive temper creating problems on the job or disrupting family life. A goal of therapy might be to help patients understand how they create their own problems and how their distorted perceptions prevent them from seeing themselves the way others do.

Psychotherapy with antisocial patients has been criticized by Hare (1993), who believes that the rigid personality structure of psychopathic individuals generally resists outside influence. He has observed that in therapy many often simply go through the motions and may even learn skills that help them better manipulate others. Hare is particularly skeptical of group therapy. His observations probably apply to the more severe end of the antisocial spectrum. There is no empirical evidence that therapy makes antisocial patients worse (D'Silva et al. 2004).

Apart from individual psychotherapy, family and marital therapy may be helpful for antisocial individuals with partners and families, although there are no empirical data on the success of such approaches (Black 1999). Bringing family members into the therapeutic process may help the people with antisocial personality disorder better understand how their disorder affects others. Therapists may also address trouble in maintaining enduring attachments, ineffective parenting, difficulty with honesty and responsibility, and anger and hostility that can lead to domestic violence.

With misbehaving children, one goal of treatment should be to stop the progression from conduct disorder to adult antisocial personality disorder, yet little evidence supports specific interventions. The Cambridge-Somerville study, conducted in the 1930s, involved 320 troubled boys who received intensive counseling and family therapy for up to 8 years (McCord et al. 1959). Initially, about 20% of the test subjects appeared more improved than a control group, but the benefits diminished over time. Many years later, the two groups were performing similarly. The study has been criticized because of high attrition, and the scope and quality of the study have been hard to duplicate.

Treatment programs for juvenile offenders that emphasize behavior modification or skills training may produce modest benefits and reduce recidivism (Lipsey 1992). Unsuccessful approaches have generally included traditional counseling and deterrent strategies such as "shock" incarceration. The latter gives young offenders stiff sentences that are later reduced to spur improvement. "Scared straight"–type programs, which attempt to frighten troubled youth out of crime by having them visit prisons, have also shown little success (Gibbons 1981). Recently there has been an interest in developing boot camps or wilderness programs for misbehaving children. These programs attempt to foster good behavior through encouraging cooperation and insight in isolated settings where misbehaving children are separated from their bad peers and have little or no access to drugs and alcohol. Whether these programs offer more than transitory benefit is unclear. Some evidence indicates that early adjudication is helpful and that juveniles who are apprehended, prosecuted, and punished for their first offenses are less likely to have adult convictions than those who escape penalties (Brown et al. 1987). Robins (1966) observed in her 30-year follow-up that antisocial men did better in the long run if they served brief jail sentences early in life, a finding consistent with this observation in youth.

Parental management training programs may offer the best help for dealing with misbehavior in children. In these programs, parents learn skills to help stop misbehavior before it escalates into violence, which may eventually help to reduce their child's risk for antisocial personality disorder (Kazdin 1997). These skills may include improved communication, more effective and consistent discipline, learning to better supervise the child, and learning how to steer impressionable children away from troubled peers.

CONCLUSION

Antisocial personality disorder is a common disorder that has been recognized by physicians for nearly 200 years. The disorder has an onset in childhood (or early adolescence), manifested by age-appropriate misbehavior; when childhood conduct disorder persists past age 18, the diagnosis becomes antisocial personality disorder. Although the disorder is considered chronic, some patients do improve or even remit, but for most individuals, antisocial personality disorder leads to lifelong difficulties, including criminal behavior. The cause of antisocial personality disorder is unknown, yet it appears that both genetic and nongenetic factors are responsible for its occurrence. There are no standard approaches to treatment or proven medications or therapies. A variety of psychotropic medications, including anticonvulsants, lithium, and antipsychotics, have been shown to reduce aggression, although not specifically in antisocial subjects. Treating comorbid disorders such as depression, bipolar disorder, or substance use disorders may be accompanied by a general reduction in antisocial symptoms. Cognitive-behavioral therapy has been described in antisocial subjects and may help those with milder syndromes. Prevention strategies targeting troubled children have been developed and may offer hope to parents, but these strategies' ultimate success is unknown.

KEY POINTS

- Antisocial personality disorder is widespread and has a male preponderance.
- Research suggests that both genes and environment interact to cause the disorder.
- Psychiatric comorbidity with antisocial personality disorder is the rule, not the exception.

PRACTICE GUIDELINES

1. There are no standard treatments for antisocial personality disorder.
2. Psychotropic medications may help to reduce aggression but do not target the entire syndrome.
3. Treating comorbid disorders is key and may help to reduce antisocial behavior.

REFERENCES

American Psychiatric Association: Diagnostic and Statistical Manual: Mental Disorders. Washington, DC, American Psychiatric Association, 1952

American Psychiatric Association: Diagnostic and Statistical Manual of Mental Disorders, 2nd Edition. Washington, DC, American Psychiatric Association, 1968

American Psychiatric Association: Diagnostic and Statistical Manual of Mental Disorders, 3rd Edition. Washington, DC, American Psychiatric Association, 1980

American Psychiatric Association: Diagnostic and Statistical Manual of Mental Disorders, 4th Edition, Text Revision. Washington, DC, American Psychiatric Association, 2000

Andreasen NC, Rice J, Endicott J, et al: The family history approach to diagnosis: how useful is it? Arch Gen Psychiatry 43:421–429, 1986

Argo T, Black DW: Clinical Characteristics in Pathological Gambling: A Clinical Guide to Treatment. Washington, DC, American Psychiatric Publishing, 2004, pp 39–54

Barrett ES, Kent TA, Bryant SG, et al: A controlled trial of phenytoin in impulsive aggression. J Clin Psychopharmacol 11:388–389, 1991

Beck A, Freeman A: Antisocial personality disorder, in Cognitive Therapy of Personality Disorders. New York, Guilford, 1990, pp 162–186

Bell RQ, Chapman M: Child effects in studies using experimental or brief longitudinal approaches to socialization. Dev Psychol 22:595–603, 1986

Black DW: Bad Boys, Bad Men: Confronting Antisocial Personality Disorder. New York, Oxford University Press, 1999

Black DW, Braun D: Antisocial patients: a comparison of persons with and persons without childhood conduct disorder. Ann Clin Psychiatry 10:53–57, 1998

Black DW, Baumgard CH, Bell SE: A 16- to 45-year follow-up of 71 males with antisocial personality disorder. Compr Psychiatry 36:130–140, 1995

Black DW, Monahan P, Baumgard CH, et al: Predictors of long-term outcome in 45 men with antisocial personality disorder. Ann Clin Psychiatry 9:211–217, 1997

Black DW, Arndt S, Hale N, et al: Use of the Mini International Neuropsychiatric Interview (MINI) as a screening tool in prisons: results from a preliminary study. J Am Acad Psychiatry Law 32:158–162, 2004

Bowlby J: Forty-Four Juvenile Thieves: Their Character and Home-Life. London, England, Baillere, Tindall & Cox, 1946 ·

Bremner JD, Krystal JH, Charney D, et al: Neuromechanisms in dissociative amnesia for childhood abuse: relevance to the current controversy surrounding false memory syndrome. Am J Psychiatry 153:71–82, 1996

Brennan PA, Mednick SA: Genetic perspectives on crime. Acta Psychiatr Scand Suppl 370:19–26, 1993

Brodaty H, Ames D, Snowdon J, et al: A randomized placebo-controlled trial of risperidone for the treatment of aggression, agitation, and psychosis of dementia. J Clin Psychiatry 64:134–143, 2003

Brooner RK, Greenfield L, Schmidt CW, et al: Antisocial personality disorder and HIV infection among intravenous drug abusers. Am J Psychiatry 150:53–58, 1993

Brown WK, Miller TP, Jenkins RL: The favorable effect of juvenile court adjudication of delinquent youth on the first contact with the juvenile justice system. Juv Fam Court J 38:21–26, 1987

Cacciola JS, Alterman AI, Rutherford MJ, et al: Treatment response of antisocial substance abusers. J Nerv Ment Dis 183:166–171, 1996

Cadoret RJ, O'Gorman TW, Troughton E, et al: Alcoholism and antisocial personality: interrelationships, genetic, and environmental factors. Arch Gen Psychiatry 42:161–167, 1985

Campbell M, Small AM, Green WH, et al: Behavioral efficacy of haloperidol and lithium carbonate: a comparison in hospitalized aggressive children with conduct disorder. Arch Gen Psychiatry 41:650–656, 1984

Campbell M, Adams PB, Small AM, et al: Lithium in hospitalized aggressive children with conduct disorder: double-blind and placebo controlled trial. J Am Acad Child Adolesc Psychiatry 34:445–453, 1995

Carney FL: Inpatient treatment programs, in The Psychopath: A Comprehensive Study of Antisocial Disorders and Behaviors. Edited by Reid WH. New York, Brunner/Mazel, 1978, pp 261–285

Caspi A, Moffitt TE, Mill J, et al: Role of genotype in the cycle of violence in maltreated children. Science 297:851–854, 2002

Cleckley H: Mask of Sanity: An Attempt to Clarify Some Issues About the So-called Psychopathic Personality, 5th Edition. St. Louis, MO, CV Mosby, 1976

Compton WM, Conway KP, Stinson FS, et al: Prevalence, correlates, and comorbidity of DSM-IV antisocial personality syndromes and alcohol and specific drug use disorders in the United States: results from the National Epidemiologic Survey on Alcohol and Related Conditions. J Clin Psychiatry 66:677–685, 2005

Corrigan PW, Yudofsky SC, Silver JM: Pharmacology and behavioral treatments for aggressive psychiatric inpatients. Hosp Community Psychiatry 44:125–133, 1993

Cowdry RW, Gardner DL: Pharmacotherapy of borderline personality disorder: alprazolam, carbamazepine, and tranylcypromine. Arch Gen Psychiatry 45:111–119, 1988

Crowe RR: An adoption study of antisocial personality. Arch Gen Psychiatry 31:785–791, 1974

Dahlstrom WG, Welsh GS, Dahlstrom LE: An MMPI Handbook. Minneapolis, University of Minnesota Press, 1972

Davidson KM, Tyrer P: Cognitive therapy for antisocial and borderline personality disorders: single case study series. Br J Clin Psychol 35:413–429, 1996

Davis JM, Janicak PG, Ayd FJ: Psychopharmacotherapy of the personality-disordered patient. Psychiatr Ann 25:614–620, 1995

Dinwiddie H, Reich T: Attribution of antisocial symptoms in coexistent antisocial personality disorder and substance abuse. Compr Psychiatry 34:235–242, 1993

Donovan SJ, Stewart JW, Nunes EV, et al: Divalproex treatment for youth with explosive temper and mood lability: a double-blind, placebo-controlled crossover design. Am J Psychiatry 157:818–820, 2000

D'Silva K, Duggan C, McCarthy L: Does treatment really make psychopaths worse? a review of the evidence. J Personal Disord 18:163–177, 2004

Favazza A: Bodies Under Siege: Self-Mutilation in Culture and Psychiatry. Baltimore, MD, Johns Hopkins University Press, 1987

First M, Spitzer RL, Gibbon M, et al: The Structured Clinical Interview for DSM-III-R Personality Disorders (SCID-II), I: description. J Personal Disord 9:83–91, 1995

Foley DL, Eaves LJ, Wormly JL, et al: Childhood adversity, monoamine oxidase A genotype and risk for conduct disorder. Arch Gen Psychiatry 61:738–744, 2004

Garvey MJ, Spoden F: Suicide attempts in antisocial personality disorder. Compr Psychiatry 21:146–149, 1980

Gibbons DC: Delinquent Behavior, 3rd Edition. Englewood Cliffs, NJ, Prentice Hall, 1981

Glueck S, Glueck E: Unraveling Juvenile Delinquency. Cambridge, MA, Harvard University Press, 1950

Goodwin D, Guze S: Psychiatric Diagnosis, 4th Edition. New York, Oxford University Press, 1989

Gottesman HG, Schubert DSP: Low-dose oral medroxyprogesterone acetate in the management of the paraphilias. J Clin Psychiatry 54:182–188, 1993

Goyer P, Andreasen P, Clayton A, et al: Positron emission tomography and personality disorder. Neuropsychopharmacology 10:21–28, 1994

Grant BF, Stinson FS, Dawson DA, et al: Co-occurrence of 12-month alcohol and drug use disorders and personality disorders in the United States: results from the National Epidemiologic Survey on Alcohol and Related Conditions. Arch Gen Psychiatry 61:361–368, 2004

Grilo CM, Becker DF, Fehon DC, et al: Conduct disorder, substance use disorder, and coexisting conduct and substance use disorders in adolescent inpatients. Am J Psychiatry 153:914–920, 1996

Guze S: Criminality and Psychiatric Disorders. New York, Oxford University Press, 1976

Hare RD: Twenty years of experience with the Cleckley psychopath, in Unmasking the Psychopath: Antisocial Personality and Related Syndromes. Edited by Reid WJ, Dorr D, Walker JI, et al. New York, WW Norton, 1986, pp 3–27

Hare RD: Without Conscience: The Disturbing World of Psychopaths Among Us. New York, Pocket Books, 1993

Hare RD: Psychopathy as a risk factor for violence. Psychiatr Q 70:181–197, 1999

Henn FA, Bardwell R, Jenkins R: Juvenile delinquents re-visited: adult criminal activity. Arch Gen Psychiatry 37:1160–1163, 1978

Hesselbrock V, Meyer R, Hesselbrock M: Psychopathology and addictive disorders: the specific case of antisocial personality disorder, in Addictive States. Edited by O'Brien CP, Jaffe JH. New York, Raven, 1992, pp 179–191

Jack-Roller, Snodgrass J, Geis G, et al: The Jack-Roller at Seventy: A 50-Year Follow-Up. Lexington, MA, Lexington Books, 1982

Kafka MP: Sertraline pharmacotherapy for paraphilias and paraphilia-related disorders: an open trial. Ann Clin Psychiatry 2:39–40, 1994

Kazdin AE: Treatment of antisocial behavior in children: current status and future directions. Psychol Bull 102:187–203, 1997

Kessler RC, McGonagle KA, Zhao S: Lifetime and 12-month prevalence of DSM-III-R psychiatric disorders in the United States: results from the National Comorbidity Survey. Arch Gen Psychiatry 51:8–19, 1994

Kiehl KA, Smith AM, Hare RD, et al: Limbic abnormalities in affective processing by criminal psychopaths as revealed by functional magnetic resonance imaging. Biol Psychiatry 50:677–684, 2001

Krueger RF, Hicks BM, Patrick CG, et al: Etiologic connections among substance dependence, antisocial behavior, and disinhibited personality: modeling the externalizing spectrum. J Abnorm Psychol 111:411–424, 2002

Lahey BB, Loeber R, Quay HC, et al: Validity of DSM-IV subtypes of conduct disorder based on age of onset. J Am Acad Child Adolesc Psychiatry 37:435–442, 1998

Lipsey MW: The effect of treatment on juvenile delinquents: results from a meta-analysis. Paper presented at a meeting sponsored by the National Institute of Mental Health, Bethesda, MD, October 31–November 3, 1992

Loeber R: Development and risk factors of juvenile antisocial behavior in delinquency. Clin Psychol Rev 10:1–41, 1990

Loranger AW: International Personality Disorder Examination (IPDE): DSM-IV and ICD-10 Modules. Odessa, FL, Psychological Assessment Resources, 1999

Luntz BK, Widom CS: Antisocial personality disorder in abused and neglected children grown up. Am J Psychiatry 101:670–674, 1994

McCord WM, McCord J, with Zola IK: Origins of Crime: A New Evaluation of the Cambridge-Somerville Youth Study. New York, Columbia University Press, 1959

Moffitt T: Adolescence limited and life-course persistent antisocial behavior: a developmental taxonomy. Psychol Rev 100:674–701, 1993a

Moffitt T: The neuropsychology of conduct disorder. Dev Psychopathol 5:135–151, 1993b

Neugebauer R, Hoek HW, Susser E: Prenatal exposure to wartime famine and development of antisocial personality disorder in early adulthood. JAMA 282:455–462, 1999

Nielson DA, Goldman D, Virkkunen M, et al: Suicidality and 5-hydroxyindoleacetic acid concentration associated with tryptophan hydroxylase polymorphism. Arch Gen Psychiatry 51:34–38, 1994

North C, Smith EM, Spitsnagel EL: Is antisocial personality a valid diagnosis in the homeless? Am J Psychiatry 150:578–583, 1993

Perry JL, Vaillant GE: Personality disorders, in Comprehensive Textbook of Psychiatry, Vol 2, 5th Edition. Edited by Kaplan HI, Freedman AM, Sadock BJ. Baltimore, MD, Williams & Wilkins, 1989, pp 132–135

Pfohl B, Blum N, Zimmerman M: Structured Interview for DSM-IV Personality Disorders. Washington, DC, American Psychiatric Press, 1997

Raine A, Venables PH, Williams M: Relationship between central and autonomic measures of arousal at age 15 years and criminality at age 24 years. Arch Gen Psychiatry 47:1003–1007, 1990

Raine A, Lencz T, Bihrle S, et al: Reduced prefrontal gray matter volume and reduced autonomic activity in antisocial personality disorder. Arch Gen Psychiatry 57:119–127, 2000

Regier DA, Farmer ME, Rae DS, et al: Comorbidity of mental disorders with alcohol and other drug abuse. JAMA 264:2511–2518, 1990

Reich JH, Green AI: Effect of personality disorders on outcome of treatment. J Nerv Ment Dis 179:74–82, 1991

Reti IM, Samuels JF, Eaton WW, et al: Adult antisocial personality traits are associated with experiences of low paternal care and maternal over-protection. Acta Psychiatr Scand 106:126–133, 2002

Robins LN: Deviant Children Grown Up. Baltimore, MD, Williams & Wilkins, 1966

Robins LN: The epidemiology of antisocial personality disorder, in Psychiatry, Vol 3. Edited by Michels RO, Cavenar JO. Philadelphia, PA, JB Lippincott, 1987, pp 1–14

Robins LN, Price RK: Adult disorders predicted by childhood conduct problems: results from the NIMH Epidemiologic Catchment Area project. Psychiatry 54:116–132, 1991

Robins LN, Murphy GE, Woodruff RA Jr, et al: Adult psychiatric status of black schoolboys. Arch Gen Psychiatry 24:338–345, 1971

Robins LN, Helzer JE, Weissman MM, et al: Lifetime prevalence of specific psychiatric disorders in three sites. Arch Gen Psychiatry 41:949–958, 1984

Russo MF, Beidel DC: Comorbidity of childhood anxiety and externalizing disorders. Clin Psychol Rev 14:199–221, 1994

Rutter M: Maternal Deprivation Reassessed, 2nd Edition. Harmondsworth, England, Penguin, 1982

Satterfield JH, Schell A: A prospective study of hyperactive boys with conduct problems and normal boys: adolescent and adult criminality. J Am Acad Child Adolesc Psychiatry 36:1726–1735, 1997

Scarpa A, Raine A: Psychophysiology of anger and violent behavior. Psychiatr Clin North Am 20:375–403, 1997

Shapiro S, Skinner EA, Kesler LG, et al: Utilization of health and mental health services. Arch Gen Psychiatry 14:971–978, 1984

Shaw C: The Jack-Roller: A Delinquent Boy's Own Story. Chicago, IL, University of Chicago Press, 1930

Shaw C (ed): Brothers in Crime. Chicago, IL, University of Chicago Press, 1938

Sheard MH, Morini JL, Bridges CI, et al: The effect of lithium on impulsive aggressive behavior in man. Am J Psychiatry 133:1409–1413, 1976

Slutske WS, True WR, Goldberg J, et al: A twin study of the association between pathological gambling and antisocial personality disorder. J Abnorm Psychol 110:297–308, 2001

Strasburger LH: Treatment of antisocial syndromes: the therapist's feelings, in Unmasking the Psychopath: Antisocial Personality and Related Syndromes. Edited by Reid WH, Dorr D, Walker JI, et al. New York, WW Norton, 1986, pp 191–207

Wakschlag LS, Lahey BB, Loeber R, et al: Maternal smoking during pregnancy and risk of conduct disorder in boys. Arch Gen Psychiatry 54:670–676, 1997

Walker C, Thomas J, Allen TS: Treating impulsivity, irritability, and aggression of antisocial personality disorder with quetiapine. Int J Offender Ther Comp Criminol 20:1–11, 2003

Winokur G, Crowe R: Personality disorders, in Comprehensive Textbook of Psychiatry, Vol 2. Edited by Freedman AM, Kaplan HI, Sadock BJ. Baltimore, MD, Williams & Wilkins, 1975, pp 1279–1297

Woodruff RA, Guze SB, Clayton PJ: Medical and psychiatric implications of antisocial personality (sociopathy). Dis Nerv Sys 32:712–714, 1971

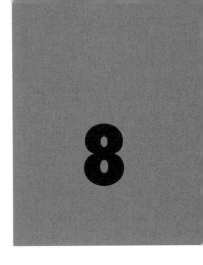

8

SEXUAL HEALTH AND PROBLEMS

Erectile Dysfunction, Premature Ejaculation, and Male Orgasmic Disorder

DAVID L. ROWLAND, PH.D.

Case Vignette

Terrence was a 44-year-old man who 2 years ago became divorced from his wife of 18 years. He and his former wife shared joint custody of their son and two daughters. The eldest child, a son age 17, lived with him. The two daughters, ages 16 and 12, lived with his former wife across town and visited Terrence every second weekend.

Since his marriage ended, Terrence had little time to pursue a new relationship, yet he fully realized that he missed the companionship of a partner. His work as a lawyer for a moderate-sized corporation kept him busy on weekdays and weekends. On those weekends when his daughters were not visiting, Terrence traveled for the company, kept the house in good shape, or simply tried to keep up with the kids' busy schedules.

Terrence's physical health was about average for his age. He was slightly overweight and out of shape because of his busy but rather sedentary lifestyle. He enjoyed a nightly drink and since his divorce had returned on and off to his old smoking habits.

Over the past 2 years, Terrence dated occasionally—mainly different women. However, unresolved issues from his first marriage generally prevented him from developing anything deeper than friendly acquaintances with these women. On two occasions, Terrence had sex with his dates, although it seemed driven more by expectation than by desire and passion. Nevertheless, Terrence's sex drive seemed adequate; he typically masturbated several times a week.

More by accident than design, Terrence recently met a woman, also divorced, on one of his recent business trips. They seemed to make an instant connection and, conveniently, she lived a 70-minute drive away. Terrence, interested in pursuing something more serious, had now been seeing her fairly regularly over the past 3 months. He felt positively toward his new partner and saw the potential for something more serious. However, when it came to sex, things were somewhat awkward and difficult. In the six times thus far, more often than not, Terrence had difficulty keeping an erection. On several occasions, his loss of erection had terminated their sexual activities; on others he had reached orgasm far too quickly for both his and his partner's satisfaction. On only one occasion had she reached orgasm. Overall, their attempts at sex had been more frustrating than satisfying, usually ending in anxiety, tension, and certainly not the sense of intimacy that each had hoped for.

Greatly distressed, fearful that his new partner saw him as a poor lover, and feeling isolated by the situation, Terrence mustered the courage to make an appointment with his physician.

The problems Terrence encountered are not uncommon in men. In this chapter, readers will gain a better understanding of men's sexual problems, including the prevalence and possible causes of these problems; options for treatment; typical treatment processes and their effectiveness; and the likelihood that sexual function will improve and result in a more sexually satisfying relationship.

Important to most men's mental health and psychological well-being is their ability to have a fulfilling sexual relationship. Not only is this a biologically and socially defining characteristic for men in our society, but recent evidence suggests that men in such relationships tend to have greater longevity and to report a higher quality of life and overall satisfaction (McCabe 1997; Palmore 1985). Men whose sexual relationships are disrupted because of their inability to respond adequately typically experience a number of psychological symptoms, including lack of confidence, anxiety, and distress.

SEXUAL DYSFUNCTION VERSUS SEXUAL DISORDER

The term *sexual disorder* refers to any sex-related problem that may or may not be clinically significant and can be of several different types.

Usually sexual disorders fall into one of three broad categories, with distinctions made among sexual dysfunctions, gender identity disorders, and atypical and paraphilia-related behaviors. *Sexual dysfunction*—a specific category of sexual disorder and the focus of this chapter—refers to the disruption or inadequacy of normal sexual responding. *Gender identity disorder* refers to cross-gender identity or the lack of assimilation of or satisfaction with the gender identity consistent with the person's biological sex or assigned gender. *Paraphilia* refers to sexual arousal and behaviors that are directed toward inappropriate objects or partners or are carried out in inappropriate situations (e.g., fetishism, pedophilia, frotteurism, voyeurism).

CHARACTERISTICS OF FUNCTIONAL SEXUAL RESPONSE AND SEXUAL HEALTH

Sexual response is complex, requiring specific preconditions, incorporating multiple behavioral responses, and including an array of psychosocial factors that relate to affective, cognitive, and relationship dimensions. Masters and Johnson (1966) characterized stages of physiological sexual response, including arousal, plateau, orgasm, and resolution. Subsequent models defined roles for sexual interest and desire within the sexual response system (Kaplan 1979). More recent refinement distinguishes between spontaneous desire and arousability, with the latter referring to sexual interest derived from a specific individual, object, or context. Other models have included separate pain-pleasure dimensions (Schover et al. 1982) and other subjective factors such as the feelings, motivations, and attitudes that surround the sexual act (Byrne and Schulte 1990). Most recently, the dyadic relationship has been emphasized, and this approach seeks to understand and treat sexual dysfunction in its relational context (Schnarch 1988, 1991).

Healthy sexual relationships are not characterized merely by the absence of dysfunctional response. Key elements of healthy sexual relationships include passion, intimacy, and commitment (Sternberg and Barnes 1988). *Passion* typically involves such characteristics as sexual feelings, physical attraction, and romantic love. *Intimacy* deals with dimensions of affection and expressiveness—the willingness to communicate and share beliefs, attitudes, and feelings. *Commitment* refers to the decision to be with one partner and to work hard to maintain the relationship. Because many sexual problems are rooted in a couple's disparate expectations and emotional struggles, including the different ways in which these elements are often experienced by each of the sexes, most sexual problems benefit from attention to general relationship factors as well as to specific sexual response issues.

DEFINITION AND PREVALENCE OF MALE SEXUAL DYSFUNCTIONS

The classification of sexual dysfunctions has evolved from the conceptual models discussed earlier and is related to the specific axes or dimensions important to functional sexual response (American Psychiatric Association 2000). These dimensions include lack of desire or interest in sex, problems with either physiological (e.g., erection) or subjective sexual arousal, and disorders of ejaculation or orgasm. Although not part of this review, problems with painful intercourse and sexual aversion also are included in the diagnostic classification system. Typically, the scope of the problem is characterized 1) as either situation (including person) specific or generalized and 2) as either lifelong or acquired (through either pathophysiological developments or sexual experiences). Several classification systems are currently in use to define sexual dysfunctions; DSM-IV-TR classifications are included in Table 8–1 (American Psychiatric Association 2000).

   Although sexual dysfunctions in men and women generally parallel one another, the incidence of the various dysfunctions differentiates the sexes, and because of differences in physiology, the dysfunctions are often manifested in different ways (Lewis et al. 2004). For example, anorgasmia and lack of sexual desire are more common among women, whereas rapid ejaculation/orgasm and physiological arousal problems (e.g., erection in men vs. lubrication in women) are more common among men (see Table 8–1 for prevalence). The dysfunctions themselves do not represent mutually exclusive categories. In fact, the interrelatedness of the components of the sexual response cycle increases the likelihood that men with one problem will exhibit another. Important to any evaluation and treatment process is distinguishing primary from secondary problems. For example, a man with significant erectile problems may eventually lose interest in sex altogether, and nearly one-third of men with premature ejaculation experience erectile difficulties.

   Sexual dysfunctions in general cause significant worry or distress to the individual. The distress may be caused not only by inadequate sexual performance but also by the impact the dysfunction has on the sexual dyad (e.g., disruption of intimacy, lack of partner satisfaction). On the other hand, some men may experience minimal distress due to their condition. For example, a man who ejaculates very rapidly may employ strategies other than coitus to ensure his partner's sexual enjoyment

TABLE 8–1. Definition and prevalence of major male sexual dysfunctions

Dysfunction/Nomenclature	Defining characteristics	DSM-IV-TR	Prevalence	Age[a]
Hypoactive sexual desire disorder Loss of libido or sexual interest	Diminished/absent interest or desire Absent sexual thoughts or fantasies Lack of responsive desire	302.71	4%–25%	++
Arousal disorder[b]	No or diminished subjective erotic feelings despite normal erection	302.70	NA	
Erectile dysfunction Impotence	Inability to attain erection Inability to maintain erection to completion of activity Coital penetration impaired ≥50%	302.72	10%–35%	+++
Premature ejaculation Rapid ejaculation Early ejaculation	Onset of orgasm and ejaculation before or shortly after penetration Ejaculation within 2 minutes or less Ejaculation occurs before desired due to lack of control	302.75	15%–30%	+
Male orgasmic disorder Ejaculatory incompetence Retarded or delayed ejaculation Inhibited ejaculation	Delayed or absent orgasm Follows normal excitement (erection) phase	302.74	5%–10%	+
Dyspareunia	Pain associated with intercourse Occurs before, during, or after intercourse	302.76	1%–5%	

[a]Indicates whether the dysfunction increases with age in a weak (+), moderate (++), or strong (+++) manner.
[b]Subjective arousal disorder does not have a dedicated classification but is increasingly recognized as a potential problem for men with orgasmic disorders; it is codable in DSM-IV-TR as "sexual disorder not otherwise specified."

and therefore may have little motivation to seek treatment. A debated question is whether such a man manifests a sexual dysfunction.

PSYCHOPHYSIOLOGY OF MALE SEXUAL FUNCTION: A BRIEF OVERVIEW

Before reviewing risk factors and treatment options, a basic familiarity with the psychophysiological processes of sexual desire, sexual arousal, and orgasm is helpful. *Libido* or *sexual interest* is a psychological construct intended to explain the likelihood or strength of a sexual response. In men, libido is usually assessed through self-reports of interest in sexual activity and a sexual partner, the presence of self-generated fantasies, and the frequency of sexual activity (coitus, masturbation). At the neural level, libido represents a state of arousability that most likely involves motivation centers in the diencephalon (e.g., medial preoptic area, paraventricular nucleus of the hypothalamus) operating in conjunction with cortical level sensory and cognitive centers responsible for processing sexually relevant information about the environment (e.g., appropriate partner, appropriate time) (Pfaus et al. 2003). Androgens, particularly testosterone, modulate sexual desire in men, priming (i.e., lowering the threshold for) neural responsivity under specific contexts or conditions and to sexually relevant stimuli.

Given the appropriate stimulus conditions, the man will respond with *sexual arousal*, a process that involves both central (brain) and genital activation. The precise brain mechanisms for arousal appear centered in the hypothalamic and limbic areas, but higher-order brain processing of contextual stimuli (sensory input), emotional state (positive or negative), and past experiences and perceived future consequences also is involved. Arousal most probably involves sympathetic activation (producing erotic feelings) integrated with the aforementioned motivational and cognitive processing centers that then regulate the descending neural impulses responsible for penile response.

Penile erection is a vascular process involving increased arterial inflow to the penis, penile engorgement with blood, and decreased venous outflow from the organ, processes that result in sufficient rigidity for sexual intercourse (Lue 1992). Whether the penis is erect or flaccid depends on the physiology of corporal cavernosal smooth muscle tone—that is, the equilibrium between proerectile and antierectile mechanisms that control, respectively, the relaxant and contractile responses of the smooth muscle cells in the penile blood vessels and cavernous tissue. Specifically, the erect penis results from *relaxation* of smooth muscle cells; the vasculature (arteries, arterioles, and capillaries) in the penis opens to allow the increased flow necessary for engorgement. The flaccid penis is characterized by *contraction* of smooth muscle cells; constricted vasculature limits the blood flow to the penis (Burnett 1999).

In response to the descending neural innervation (probably parasympathetic), a number of events occur at the target cell membrane and the intracellular level. Second messenger molecules (e.g., cyclic guanosine monophosphate [cGMP] or cyclic adenosine monophosphate [cAMP]) and ions transmit the neural signal via the action of receptor proteins at the cell membrane of the target cell (e.g., smooth muscle) or via enzyme pathways. Regarding the latter process, these enzymatic pathways (e.g., phosphodiesterase) within the muscle cell may inactivate various pathways and therefore inhibit erectile function. It is through these pathways that the pharmacotherapies for erectile dysfunction (e.g., sildenafil) operate. Such agents inhibit phosphodiesterase type 5, the enzyme that deactivates cGMP, the energy-drawing process that stimulates relaxation of corporal cavernosal tissue (and thus erection). As a result, cGMP remains active in increasing amounts to exert corporal smooth muscle relaxant effects (Boolel et al. 1996). Stated simply, these prosexual drugs for erectile dysfunction act by inhibiting the system that inhibits erection at the level of penile tissue.

Ejaculation represents the sequencing of two cerebrally controlled reflexes that typically coincide with the peak of sexual arousal (Rowland and Slob 1997). Unlike erection, which may occur in the absence of direct penile stimulation, the ejaculatory reflexes generally require penile stimulation. The first reflex—emission—is a sympathetic response that closes the bladder neck (preventing urination and retrograde ejaculation) and stimulates excretion of seminal fluid (which mixes with sperm) from the prostate into the urethral tract. This first stage of ejaculation is associated with "ejaculatory inevitability" that men experience before actual expulsion of the seminal fluid and serves as the trigger for the second reflex. The second reflex—putatively involving the parasympathetic system, the somatic motor system, or both—involves the expulsion of the seminal fluid from the urethra, achieved through the rhythmic contractions of the bulbocavernosus and ischiocavernosus muscles (associated with anal sphincter muscle contraction). The subjective (brain) perception of these contractions, mediated through sensory neurons in the region, produces the experience of orgasm, which comprises a distinct and separate loop. Thus ejaculation can and does (rarely) occur without concomitant orgasm.

The mechanism that actually triggers the entire ejaculatory process is not well understood, but the brain neurotransmitter serotonin has been strongly implicated. Accordingly, various antidepressant drugs that affect the serotonergic system (e.g., tricyclic antidepressants and selective serotonin reuptake inhibitors [SSRIs]) have been used fairly effectively to prolong intercourse in men who usually ejaculate very rapidly. Not surprisingly, because ejaculation is also mediated in part by the sympathetic nervous system, prescription and over-the-counter drugs that attenuate sympathetic response may interfere with a normal ejaculatory process.

The summary just given indicates that the basic rudiments of sexual response are complex and not fully understood. Furthermore, it underscores the many possible points at which the process could go awry. Given the high level of psychophysiological integration required for coordinated sexual response, it is not surprising that sexual response, important as it is to procreation, is sensitive to myriad physiological and psychological factors.

ETIOLOGY OF MALE SEXUAL DYSFUNCTION

The causes of sexual problems in men vary, but generally they might be attributed to one or more of three sources: physiological, psychological, and relationship. These sources constitute overlapping domains and therefore they represent convenient, rather than mutually exclusive, classifications. For example, a distressful relationship between the man and his partner may impact his psychological well-being, which in turn has the potential to influence his physiological response. Conversely, a man with a clear medical etiology responsible for diminishing erectile function may lose confidence and begin to avoid sexual intimacy, a situation that typically impacts the dyadic relationship.

The etiological factors identified herein represent *potential* causes for problems (i.e., risk factors); although these potential causes increase the likelihood of a sexual dysfunction, they do not determine it. Furthermore, it is important to recognize that the factors responsible for precipitating or predisposing a patient to a sexual problem may be quite different from those factors that eventually maintain it. For example, failure to respond with an adequate erection due to stress or medication may result in anxiety and diminished self-confidence surrounding future sexual encounters, factors that may eventually maintain the problem. Finally, there is a great deal of variation in how each of these sources (physiological, psychological, relationship) might affect any given individual, and in some instances, clear etiologies for some dysfunctions have not been fully elaborated. In the following sections, a number of common risk, predisposing, and maintaining factors for male sexual dysfunction are discussed; these factors are summarized in Table 8–2.

Pathophysiological Risk Factors

Given the priming role of testosterone in sexual arousability in men, disruption of the hypothalamic-pituitary-gonadal (HPG) axis is likely to lead to loss of libido and sexual interest. Such problems tend to be fairly uncommon and are typically accompanied by a variety of other physical or physiological problems. Although men with low or absent gonadal function (i.e., hypogonadal) may show little interest in sex, they are not necessarily impotent and may obtain erections when presented with certain kinds of psychosexual stimuli (Bancroft 1989). However, these men are less likely to seek sexual stimulation and fulfillment because of their hormone deficiency. Diseases that interfere with neural control over the HPG axis (e.g., dopamine in Parkinson's disease) or that result in high levels of prolactin may also interfere with sexual desire. In some instances, a cascading effect occurs in which decreased sexual interest results in attenuated arousal and inability to maintain an erection.

Any condition, disease, or drug that diminishes responsivity of the nervous, vascular, and smooth muscle (autonomic) systems has the potential to disrupt the "mechanics" of erection (Feldman et al. 1994). Common risk factors for erectile dysfunction directly or indirectly compromise the process of smooth muscle relaxation (and arteriole dilation) necessary for penile engorgement; thus erectile dysfunction is often associated with cardiovascular disease. Disruption of neural control due to radical prostatectomy, neuropathy, or chronic neurological diseases also accounts for erectile impairment. In some instances, the association between a specific condition (e.g., low levels of dehydroepiandrosterone sulfate) and erectile dysfunction has been documented, but the specific mechanism of action has not yet been clarified. Risk factors that affect erectile function may in some instances be additive in that the greater the number of conditions present that affect the response system (e.g., smoking plus diabetes), the greater the likelihood of impact on erectile function.

Unlike risk factors for erectile dysfunction, pathophysiological risk factors for ejaculatory disorders—premature and retarded/inhibited ejaculation—do not share easily identifiable common underlying pathways. Factors most often correlated with ejaculatory disorders are procedures, diseases, or conditions that interfere with the neural integrity in the pelvic-genital region.

TABLE 8–2. Summary of common risk, predisposing, and maintaining factors for male sexual dysfunction

Dysfunction	Pathophysiological/Biological	Psychological	Relationship
Erectile dysfunction	Tobacco use Diabetes mellitus Cardiovascular disease/hypertension Urinary tract disease Pelvic/spinal surgery or trauma Chronic neurological disease Endocrine axis disturbances Various medications	Stress/emotional Depression/anxiety Performance anxiety Psychiatric disturbances Body image Arousal disorders	Partner dysfunction Hostility/anger Lack of trust Control/dominance Partner attractiveness
Premature ejaculation	Chronic neurological disease Pelvic/spinal surgery or trauma Various medications Urinary tract disease	Anxiety (general or specific)	Partner dysfunction Hostility/anger Control/dominance
Retarded/inhibited ejaculation	Cardiovascular disease Urinary tract disease Pelvic/spinal surgery or trauma Neuropathy Various medications, alcohol	Idiosyncratic masturbation Low arousal History of sexual abuse	Partner attractiveness Partner dysfunction Lack of trust Control/dominance
Hypoactive sexual desire disorder	Endocrine disturbances Dopaminergic disturbances	Depression Psychiatric disturbances History of sexual abuse	Lack of partner History of sexual abuse Hostility/anger Lack of trust Control/dominance

Age and Medications

In as much as aging serves as a proxy for a general increase in patho-physiological conditions, it is not surprising that men age 50 years and older are much more likely to report problems with erections (Feldman et al. 1994; Lewis et al. 2004) (Table 8–1). Although age may impact ejaculatory function, the relationship between the two is not always straight-forward. An increased prevalence of premature ejaculation seen in men 50 and older probably represents the development of coexisting erectile problems in those age groups—that is, the premature ejaculation may develop in response (or be secondary) to age-related erectile dysfunction. The long-time supposition that rapid ejaculation is attenuated with age, although logically sound, has not been adequately tested in longitudinal studies, and therefore no firm conclusions can be drawn. On the other hand, given that penile sensitivity decreases substantially with age (Rowland 1998), a tendency toward increased ejaculatory latencies with aging is not implausible and may account for the slight increase in the prevalence of inhibited ejaculation in older men. Finally, as might be expected, various medications and recreational drugs may interfere with erectile and ejaculatory function, including many medications commonly used for depression, hypertension, and gastrointestinal disturbances. A comprehensive description of psychotropic agents that impact sexual function, many of which are used increasingly with age, has recently been reported by Gitlin (2003).

Psychological Risk Factors

In contrast to the pathophysiological risk factors noted earlier, the relationships among psychological risk or predisposing factors and sexual dysfunction are substantially more tenuous (although no less important) and more likely to impact the entire sexual response cycle rather than just specific components. Because psychological factors are many and varied, they have the potential to interact with sexual response through a variety of processes. For example, a major Axis I psychiatric disorder—clinical depression or schizophrenia—is likely to influence sexual response in a different manner than personality or developmental disorders. These influences may differ substantially from the way in which a lack of self-confidence stemming from anxiety about performance impacts sexual response. A number of psychological risk factors for sexual dysfunction are reviewed in the following sections.

Evaluative Factors

The overwhelming majority of erection problems—and perhaps premature ejaculation problems as well—that are psychological in nature stem from the self- and other-evaluative component of sexual response (hence the common reference to sexual "performance"). Anxiety stemming from the man's lack of confidence to perform adequately, to appear and feel attractive (body image), to satisfy his partner sexually, to experience an overall sense of self-efficacy, and—despite New Age efforts to minimize the idea—to measure up against the competition is likely to affect most men at some point in their lives (Althof et al. 2004; Zilbergeld 1993). This anxiety often generates a number of maladaptive responses, such as the man's setting unrealistic expectations or focusing attention on his own sexual response (i.e., self-monitoring) at the cost of ignoring important erotic cues from the partner. Such problems often arise from various cultural expectations and stereotypes linked to the male gender role. Although these issues tend to surface at the beginning of a new relationship, they may also emerge when the ongoing balance in a relationship is changed or disrupted. These issues may be embedded in the relationship itself (and therefore might also be viewed as "relationship" risk factors), but they may also be the consequence of factors that impact the relationship in indirect ways. Thus the man's loss of employment and his subsequent reduced self-esteem, a partner's infidelity, and the introduction of a new family member into the household (e.g., child, elderly parent) are examples that often change the ongoing sexual-dyadic relationship.

Problems Surrounding Subjective Sexual Arousal

Perhaps more a symptom than an actual risk factor, subjective sexual arousal may contribute to sexual dysfunctions. In men with erectile problems stemming from evaluative factors (such as those mentioned earlier), subjective arousal may be normal and high, but genital response may be diminished or absent. In contrast, men with inhibited or retarded ejaculation often report low levels of subjective arousal while showing strong erectile response. Similarly, men with premature ejaculation often report hyperarousability during psychosexual stimulation, and recent findings suggest that such men often underestimate their physiological and genital arousal (Rowland and Cooper 2005). Thus disorders of ejaculation represent more a problem of arousal than a problem of the ejaculatory process per se. Nonetheless, because a man's sexual arousal level is determined by multiple factors, including sexual interest, partner stimulation and attraction, context, and anticipation, sexual arousal might be a proxy measure for other psychological and relationship factors.

General Psychosocial Stressors

Significant life events that result in long-term or acute depression in men may lead to sexual dysfunction. Aging or diabetic men, for example, often show a higher incidence of depression and anxiety than do their younger or healthy counterparts, and aging or diabetic men are more likely to exhibit low sexual desire and erectile difficulties (Harland and Huws 1997; Schreiner-Engel and Schiavi 1986; Tsitouras and Alvarez 1984). However, unlike the relationship between performance anxiety and sexual dysfunction, the relationship between general psychosocial stressors and sexual dysfunction is less obvious. In addition, because nonpsychotic depression and anxiety are not easily separated from the pathophysiological effects of aging, illness, and stress, it is unclear which factors might be responsible for the sexual dysfunction: the pathophysiological condition itself or the associated psychological states of depression and anxiety. Currently, it appears safest to conclude that sexual dysfunction is compounded by the depression and anxiety in these men but is not solely the result of these disorders. Indeed, depression and anxiety associated with various life events may result from the sexual problems as well as cause them.

Developmental Factors

Early traumatic sexual experiences may impair sexual function. Although it is difficult to identify the specific events and the processes through which they operate, childhood sexual abuse consistently affects sexual interest and subsequently sexual arousal and erectile and ejaculatory function (Loeb et al. 2002). Perhaps as frequently, childhood sexual abuse is manifested in maladaptive sexual or nonsexual behaviors (e.g., paraphilias, drug use, eating disorders). Other developmental issues may play important roles in sexual problems. For example, unresolved gender identity issues and restrictive sexual attitudes or practices in the family-of-origin household may predispose individuals to sexual dysfunction. The man's ability to overcome developmental traumas is often related to therapeutic intervention and his own level of resiliency.

Personality Profiles

A number of efforts have attempted to profile the type of male personality prone to sexual dysfunction. Although results are mixed, the most consistent pattern to emerge is that men seeking help for sexual problems exhibit higher levels of depression and anxiety than do their sexually functional counterparts (Angst 1998; Costa et al. 1992). In contrasting different kinds of sexual dysfunction, Tondo et al. (1991) suggested that men with erectile problems manifest their anxiety primarily through negative self-image and low self-esteem, whereas men with premature ejaculation do so through symptoms more characteristic of hypomanic states such as agitation and mild obsession. The relationship between depression, anxiety, and sexual dysfunction appears to extend beyond erectile and ejaculatory disorders. For example, couples indicating low sexual interest (hypoactive sexual desire disorder) have a higher-than-expected propensity for past or current chronic depression, a finding that mirrors the low sexual interest in depressed populations. When depression and anxiety are excluded from the picture, no single personality profile consistently characterizes men with sexual dysfunction, although several personality characteristics appear relevant. A tendency toward greater self-consciousness and vulnerability and lower openness seems most consistently to describe dysfunctional men, characteristics that may lead to diminished appreciation of varied experiences and may act to sustain performance anxiety associated with male sexual dysfunction. Furthermore, men who score low in warmth may have difficulty with intimacy or commitment, suggesting that treatment should focus on establishing greater interpersonal intimacy.

Major Psychopathology

Chronic psychopathology has long been a suspected cause of sexual dysfunction. Both depression and schizophrenia are associated with diminished sexual desire, impairment of arousal, and loss or delay of ejaculation, and sexual dysfunction occurs in a high percentage of depressed and schizophrenic patients (estimated from 35% to 75% [Baldwin 1996; Lilleleht and Leiblum 1993]). The extent to which the psychopathology causes the dysfunction is unclear because few studies have documented sexual functioning before the onset of the mental illness or have adequately separated the influences of medication (which itself may have antisexual effects) from the effects of the mental disorder. Furthermore, the extent to which the diminished sexual response represents general malaise, social withdrawal, or inability to experience pleasure rather than a separate influence on a psychosexual process is undetermined. Although definitive studies have yet to be done, most research suggests that the primary effect on sexual dysfunction is mediated through diminished interest in sex, which in turn influences arousal, erectile, and orgasmic responses. Thus, for individuals manifesting major mental disorders, treatment typically focuses first on alleviating the psychological condition.

Relationship Risk Factors

Relationship risk factors that influence sexual function are the most difficult to isolate and describe in brief phrases. The lack of an adequate or appropriate nosology should not be interpreted as a lack of importance. Many of the dysfunction-precipitating or -maintaining factors described earlier involve a relationship component. Furthermore, because the quality of the sexual relationship often hinges on the overall quality of the marital or partner relationship, these two elements are highly interdependent (Rosen et al. 2004; Schnarch 2000).

Several specific relationship factors that have been associated with male sexual dysfunction include partner dysfunctions, partner expectations and perceived evaluation of performance, and perceived attractiveness of the partner. Within the relationship itself, the progression from a novel, partner-focused style early in the relationship to a more routinized self-gratification style, concomitantly affected by the intrusion of work and family, is often cause for emotional problems that may in part be manifested through sexual dysfunction. Cognitive-emotional issues such as lack of intimacy and trust and general anger or hostility directed toward or perceived from the partner are likely to impact sexual interactions and response. Issues of relationship control and dominance also frequently emerge as mediating factors for sexual problems. As has been noted by clinicians for years, because sexual gratification lies in the hands of the partner, the more such gratification is actively sought by one member of the dyad, the greater the control the other member exerts over that individual.

Probably more important than any single relationship factor is the overall quality of the relationship itself. Specifically, any event, factor, or situation that interferes with passion, intimacy, commitment, or communication is likely to have a disruptive effect on the sexual relationship. Thus, preceding sex therapy with couples therapy for those with significant relationship issues tends to result in better outcomes for the sex therapy, whereas couples therapy in nondistressed couples does not typically lead to improved sexual functioning (Carey 1998; Rowland et al. 1998). Conversely, sex therapy in nondistressed couples often leads to improved dyadic functioning.

ASSESSMENT OF MALE SEXUAL DYSFUNCTION

Ideally, the evaluation of a sexual problem involves a thorough analysis of the specific problem—its severity, etiology, and contributing and maintaining factors. In practice, evaluation procedures vary widely, depending on how the man enters the health care system when seeking help. In the primary care physician's office, where economic factors (third-party reimbursement) may restrict the physician's investment of time and where lack of expertise about nonmedical factors involved in sexual problems may limit the scope of the conversation, the evaluation may be cursory and superficial. In contrast, psychiatrists and behavioral or mental health clinicians, whose qualifications increase the likelihood of third-party reimbursement for examining psychological and interpersonal issues, often perform a more thorough evaluation that involves multiple sessions. Thorough evaluations typically include a complete medical and psychological history, the use of standardized assessment instruments, and a psychosexual history that includes the man's sexual partner.

Establishing the General Framework for Evaluation

The patient-directed approach to the treatment of sexual disorders has recently gained popularity within the clinical and medical community. In this approach, primary consideration is given to the specific therapeutic goals and preferences of the patient, and therefore one of the clinician's main tasks is to identify the most appropriate means to achieve those goals. Although attempts are made to identify medical disorders that interfere with sexual functioning, diagnostic procedures are generally limited because etiology often does not necessarily guide the type of treatment selected. Because patient-centered therapy focuses on a holistic approach that views patient satisfaction as a primary treatment outcome, exploration of psychological and relationship issues is needed to guide treatment. This process is consistent with the idea that the more the provider understands about potential factors responsible for the etiology and maintenance of the dysfunction, the wider the range of treatment options available becomes, and therefore the treatment can be better tailored to the specific needs of the individual. No matter what approach is taken, a critical component in the process is that the clinician works together with the patient (and his partner) in developing the treatment plan (Osborne and Rowland, in press).

Organization of the Evaluation

Reduced to its simplest elements, a sexual assessment should identify 1) the nature and severity of the sexual dysfunction; 2) the biomedical, psychological, and/or relationship factors that cause or contribute to the problem or that might diminish the effects of any particular treatment strategy; and 3) the needs and preferences of the patient and his partner regarding treatment options. The means by which each of these elements is assessed—through a face-to-face interview, a physical examination, symptom assessment scales, laboratory tests, or some combination thereof—may be influenced by multiple factors, including the specific orientation of the health care provider and the resources and time available to the patient. For the behavioral or mental health clinician who encounters a male client with sexual dysfunction, the assessment process should entail referral for a physical examination by a physician, who then can determine whether further referral to a medical specialist (e.g., urologist, endocrinologist) is warranted or may be beneficial. To optimize outcomes, medical specialists should refer any patient with a sexual dysfunction who enters the health care system through the "medical door" to a sex therapist for an assessment of general psychosocial and relationship functioning.

Process of Evaluation

Identifying the Problem and Quantifying Severity

The first step of the evaluation process requires identifying the specific problem—whether it is hypoactive sexual desire, erectile and arousal difficulty, premature ejaculation, inhibited orgasm or ejaculation, or some combination of these. Carefully worded questions related to each of these domains (Table 8–3) are usually effective in determining where the specific problem lies. Optimally, each domain question should be augmented with further questioning that affirms the presence and type of the dysfunction.

Once the problem is identified, quantification of its severity is important—for example, the frequency of occurrence of the dysfunctional response and the degree to which the response is impaired. For erectile dysfunction, such quantification may include an estimate of rigidity and the rate of successful coital attempts. For premature ejaculation, parameters such as the estimated latency to ejaculation and the ability to delay (or control) ejaculation provide measures of impairment. For inhibited ejaculation, the ratio of orgasmic to coital episodes, estimated latency to

TABLE 8–3. Typical starting questions for identifying a sexual dysfunction

Initial question	Sample elaborations
Do you…	
Have sexual interests, desire, thoughts, fantasies?	Masturbation frequency? Initiator of intercourse? Interest in or attraction to partner?
Have difficulty getting or keeping an erection?	Frequency of coital impairment? Loss of erection before ejaculating? Degree of erection (e.g., none, some)?
Ejaculate before you wish?	Ejaculate before intercourse begins? Within 1 or 2 minutes after penetration? Able to delay or postpone ejaculation? Ejaculate for fear of losing erection?
Take longer than you wish to reach orgasm?	Ever ejaculate, for example, during masturbation? Ratio of orgasms to attempts? Duration of intercourse?
Have pain during intercourse?	Before, during, or after?

Note. These prototypical items are meant only as "conversation" starters that help narrow the problem to a specific domain. A full assessment would include a complete psychosexual history and evaluation (see text and Rosen et al. 2004 for further discussion).

orgasm, and general feelings of subjective arousal during coitus (e.g., relative to masturbation) offer a rudimentary index of severity. For all dysfunctions, the level of distress, bother, or dissatisfaction regarding sexual response and function is critically important to assess. A number of standardized assessment tools are available to assist clinicians with these tasks (Rosen et al. 2004).

Identifying Etiological Factors

The second step of the evaluation process typically accounts for most of the variation across clinicians and health care providers. No matter how extensive or limited this step of the process might be, because sexual dysfunction may sometimes serve as a marker for other health problems (e.g., erectile dysfunction may signal cardiovascular disease, ejaculatory disorders may suggest prostate problems), a physical examination is always warranted.

Primary care physicians sometimes end the evaluative process at this point and move on to a discussion of treatment options. In contrast, health care specialists (e.g., urologists, sex therapists) are more likely to further assess the biological, psychological, and relationship domains of the problem, with biases toward those domains consistent with the specialist's clinical training. Although the traditional desire to differentiate psychogenic from organogenic etiologies has become less critical with the introduction of effective biomedical interventions that can alleviate specific dysfunctions of multiple origins, knowing the precise biological, psychological, or relationship components often assists in determining the most effective therapy.

Biomedical assessment. Medical assessments may be limited, moderate, or extensive. In addition to the physical examination, obtaining a family medical history and the patient's history, including the use of prescription and over-the-counter medications, nutritional supplements, and recreational substances (e.g., tobacco, alcohol, cocaine), is typical. Beyond these steps, no broad consensus exists regarding the procedures that are likely to yield information most helpful to the treatment process. For men exhibiting hypoactive sexual desire disorder, a basic endocrine analysis for testosterone and prolactin is indicated. For men with erectile dysfunction, laboratory tests for comorbidities (e.g., diabetes mellitus, hyperlipidemia, cardiovascular function) and psychiatric assessment for mood disorders can help determine whether the dysfunction is secondary to an identifiable and treatable disease or condition. More extensive evaluations assessing vascular problems, autonomic functioning, and sleep-related erections, as well as complete pituitary, gonadal, and adrenal hormone profiles, are performed less frequently nowadays (Rosen et al. 2004). For ejaculatory disorders (premature and inhibited), no specific or reliable biomedical assessments are available that provide further insight beyond information readily obtained through the medical history (e.g., pelvic trauma or neuropathy) and basic physical examination.

Psychosexual and psychological histories. In men, sexual functioning and psychological health often interact. In performing a psychosexual and general psychological evaluation, the clinician can assess whether psychological (and relationship) factors cause physiological sexual dysfunction, including whether these psychological factors sustain or exacerbate the dysfunction. Whether the clinician considers cause or effect or the mutual and reciprocal flow between the two, one of the immediate goals of psychological evaluation is to determine which factor is primary and thus where treatment should be focused.

Besides assessment for psychiatric disorders (depression, anxiety), the psychosexual history is arguably the most critical element of the overall assessment process. The sexual history may be taken verbally, may utilize a script, and/or may involve standardized assessment instruments (see Rosen et al. 2004). The evaluation should include information about current and past sexual functioning and the history (onset and duration) and specificity (e.g., with a particular partner, only during coitus and not during masturbation) of the problem. Information about the patient's understanding of and education about the problem, psychosocial factors surrounding the problem (e.g., fear of failure), specific cultural expectations, child and adolescent sexual histories and experiences, and family-of-origin attitudes and practices often reveals important factors related to the sexual problem that will suggest specific treatment strategies. Clinicians should be sensitive when exploring matters related to sexuality and try to ensure that the patient does not feel stigmatized, judged, or embarrassed.

Relationship assessment.   The potential for a relationship contribution to the problem warrants investigation. A relationship history that includes major events such as extramarital activity, divorce, separation, pregnancies, and deaths should be noted, and any current relationship concerns or distress should be discussed (see Pridal and LoPiccolo 2000). Standardized assessment instruments such as the Dyadic Adjustment Scale (Spanier 1976) and Golombok Rust Inventory of Sexual Satisfaction (Rust and Golombok 1986) may help to elicit such concerns because patients may be reluctant to appear critical of their partner's sexual, emotional, and behavioral interactions. Initially, the patient and partner may be assessed separately to avoid attributions of fault or blame, identify potential partner dysfunctions and counterproductive attitudes, and obtain each person's individual perspective (including distress) about the problem and its severity.

Defining the Desired Outcome in Terms of the Needs and Values of the Patient and Partner

In the transition between evaluation and treatment, an important preliminary step involves defining the relevant outcomes. Although the patient's and the partner's involvement is essential to this process, men sometimes focus heavily on genital issues at the cost of neglecting more subtle, but no less important, psychological and interpersonal issues. Although treatment of physical symptoms is crucial (e.g., prolongation of ejaculation latency, obtaining an erection sufficient for intercourse), most clinicians would also note that improved genital performance in the absence of improved sexual satisfaction and a better sexual relationship is not sufficient (Rowland and Burnett 2000). These latter outcomes, although not always easily quantified, typically correlate well with overall patient satisfaction with treatment (Hawton 1998).

Although these three outcomes—improved genital response, increased sexual satisfaction, and improved sexual relationship—are themselves interrelated, each may need to be addressed individually in the course of the therapeutic process. That is, in many situations, alleviation of the symptoms may improve the man's sexual satisfaction and the overall sexual relationship. In others, the change in interpersonal dynamics that results from the dysfunction (e.g., avoidance of intimacy or a partner's anger and distress) may not easily be reversed by merely "fixing" the genital dysfunction. In such cases, a number of psychological and interpersonal issues may need to be addressed if increased sexual satisfaction and an improved sexual relationship are viewed as important outcomes.

TREATMENT OF MALE SEXUAL DYSFUNCTION

In the following sections, general strategies available for the treatment of three major male sexual dysfunctions—erectile dysfunction, premature ejaculation, and male orgasmic disorder—are discussed. Some male sexual dysfunctions are not discussed in this review. Hypoactive sexual desire disorder, if not due to an endocrine deficiency that can be treated relatively easily, usually involves significant issues of anger, hostility, and control within the relationship and as such requires couples counseling. Similarly, sexual aversion disorder typically requires more extensive counseling that explores the man's relationship with his partner, his family-of-origin environment, and his developmental and sexual history.

Setting the Context

Before commencing treatment, the clinician should understand 1) the specific sexual problem; 2) the severity of the problem and the degree of functional impairment it causes; 3) at least broadly, if not in detail, the biological, psychological, and relationship factors that contribute to or maintain the problem; and 4) the specific treatment goals of the man and his partner. These four elements converge to suggest an appropriate strategy that may utilize one, some, or all of the therapeutic tools available to the health care provider. Thus, pharmacotherapy and other biomedical treatments, bibliotherapy, individual sex therapy and counseling, and couples' marital and/or sex therapy represent a range of options that may eventually constitute an effective treatment plan. Important to this approach is not only the notion that each strategy can address a specific dimension of the problem but also the idea that even when the etiology lies primarily within one domain (e.g., psychological anxiety), the use of auxiliary strategies (e.g., pharmacotherapy) may be helpful for achieving the larger goals of the patient and his partner. Finally, it is essential for both clinician and patient to recognize early in the therapeutic process the importance of and need for periodic follow-up.

Erectile Dysfunction

What once was considered the most challenging sexual problem to address through therapy and a chief cause of distress for many men—namely, erectile problems that prevent intercourse—has now become one of the most treatable sexual dysfunctions. The treatability of these erectile problems in part stems from the introduction of specific and effective medications (phosphodiesterase 5 inhibitors) that induce smooth muscle relaxation of penile vasculature, allowing engorgement of the corporal cavernosa and subsequent erection. Concurrently, recent clinical and psychophysiological research has identified situational, individual, and relationship factors that impact sexual (erectile) response in men. Based on such findings, sex therapists have developed treatment procedures that effectively assist men in overcoming erectile inhibition due to psychological and relationship issues.

Medical treatments for erectile dysfunction have been available for some time and have included surgical implants, vascular reconstruction surgery, intracavernosal injection of vasoactive agents (e.g., papaverine, prostaglandin E_1), and vacuum devices that draw blood into the penis. Although each of these treatments has assisted men in overcoming erection problems, most have been viewed as unnatural or invasive. As such, the new pharmacotherapies (sildenafil, tadalafil, vardenafil) have not only overshadowed these older medical treatments but also changed medical and cultural approaches to the treatment of erectile dysfunction. Although perhaps originally established as a treatment for erectile dysfunction of pathophysiological origin, pharmacotherapies offer a range of proven options that can be used to treat sexual problems of varied and even unidentified causes, with recent studies indicating success rates between 50% and 90% (Althof et al. 2004). Many health care providers anecdotally report that these agents are now commonly being used as performance enhancers among men who, for whatever reason, lack confidence about their erectile response.

However, having a fully functional penis is of limited value in the context of a dysfunctional relationship or one that has been stressed by a major sexual dysfunction. For this reason, it is perhaps not surprising that the adherence rate for medications for erectile dysfunction approaches only 50%. The emotional and interpersonal issues that interact with the erectile problem (lack of understanding and communication about sexual issues, blame, distrust, guilt, emotional distance, reduced self-confidence and self-esteem, and anxiety) have not undergone major change. Yet as the treatment of erectile dysfunction further shifts from the urologist's or sex therapist's office to the office of the primary care physician, attention to relevant psychological and relationship factors may be further neglected. This situation may be exacerbated by the man's resistance to recognize and deal with important emotional and relationship issues. Thus the burden falls increasingly on sex therapists and counselors to devise effective, affordable treatments that can be readily and effectively integrated with the use of the new pharmacotherapies. Even before the advent of medications for erectile dysfunction, therapies combining medical with psychological treatment—extending from simple education to more extensive counseling—have been known to result in greater adherence and overall satisfaction for the couple.

Before the onset of psychotherapy for erectile dysfunction, the therapist should consider whether the partner should be included, whether couples therapy should precede sex therapy, and whether augmentation with available medical treatments should be undertaken. Regarding this last point, Althof (2000) recommended medical augmentation when the man with erectile dysfunction has had a lifelong problem, low self-confidence, significant medical etiology, or a history of unremediated problems despite prior sex therapy. Many therapists agree that preliminary treatment with medication helps to quickly reestablish a man's self-confidence and reduce his anxiety, thus increasing his willingness or ability to address other psychological and relationship issues.

The components of sex therapy strategies for erectile dysfunction have evolved since the 1970s and include a variety of elements. Approaches typically include sex education and dyadic communication as core elements of the therapy. Systematic desensitization and anxiety reduction involve the learning of new and productive behaviors and the elimination of anxiety—a state incompatible with the erectogenic process—to improve the erectile response. Therapeutic procedures such as sensate focus, relaxation exercises, and other behavioral exercises are typically used to facilitate this process. Concomitantly, the highly internalized performance demands of men with erectile dysfunction may be modified through the use of cognitive restructuring. This process enables the patient to set expectations that are more realistic and less culturally derived, develop positive sexual imagery that strengthens self-confidence, and expand the sexual repertoire to include varied and gradational kinds of stimulation beyond intercourse. Although it is unclear which particular component of these therapeutic processes imparts the greatest benefit, cumulative effects probably accrue whereby the inclusion of more strategies results in better outcomes. Furthermore, when larger relationship issues emerge as contributing or maintaining factors for erectile dysfunction, augmentation of sex therapy with general couples therapy becomes critically important.

Satisfaction rates from sex therapy for erectile dysfunction are high, typically in the range of 50%–70%, and remain so 12 months or more posttreatment. Key elements for long-term success and satisfaction include relapse prevention strategies and periodic follow-up or "booster" sessions. The inclusion of medications in erectile dysfunction psychotherapy treatment protocols is likely to further improve satisfaction and success rates. Combined treatment strategies also offer the advantage of decreasing the number of sessions required for successful outcomes, thereby making core elements of sex therapy accessible to greater numbers of couples.

Premature Ejaculation

Premature ejaculation is characterized by a short latency to ejaculation (usually 2 minutes or less) before or after penetration. This short latency is due to the inability to control or delay the ejaculatory response. The off-label use of moderate doses of tricyclic and SSRI antidepressants and stimulus-reduction creams has proven effective, with results indicating prolongation of intercourse anywhere from about 1 to 5 minutes (Waldinger 2002). Unlike existing medications that require daily dosing or administration 3–6 hours before anticipated intercourse, new medications that may be taken shortly before intercourse, with effects continuing up to several hours thereafter, are probably not far away. All these medications presumably work by inhibiting serotonin transporters within the central nervous system to delay ejaculation. The disadvantages of medications for premature ejaculation include the symptomatic approach to treatment—that is, relapse occurs in the absence of drug use because men do not develop better control over their ejaculatory response—and, as with any drug, unwanted side effects may occur, although most drugs are well tolerated.

Cognitive-behavioral factors are involved in premature ejaculation, and health care providers should be aware of and sensitive to such factors in the treatment of premature ejaculation. Although cognitive-behavioral therapy for premature ejaculation has been criticized by some as lacking long-term efficacy, long-term success rates for premature ejaculation treatment have not been adequately investigated, and the reasons for purported failures remain largely unknown. For example, it is not known whether relapse occurs because cognitive-behavioral techniques become less effective with continued use or because couples merely cease using them once the novelty has worn off. Furthermore, cognitive-behavioral techniques enjoy the advantages of being highly specific to the problem, neither harmful nor painful, and well tolerated. Once learned and incorporated into lovemaking, these techniques become personally integrated such that men with premature ejaculation will have access to the tools that enable them to control their ejaculatory response. On the negative side, cognitive-behavioral techniques typically require significant cooperation of the partner; entail greater effort, expense, and time on the part of the patient; and have less support in terms of efficacy (Rowland et al. 1998).

The severity of premature ejaculation may suggest varied treatment approaches that combine medications and stimulus-reduction creams (applied to the penis) with either brief or extended cognitive-behavioral counseling. As with erectile dysfunction, pharmacological strategies can assist the man in improving self-confidence and self-efficacy and afford him the opportunity to develop and use cognitive-behavioral strategies as his response latency approximates a more typical pattern. These strategies may be acquired through bibliotherapy, but the patient and his partner can also benefit from a counselor who can educate them about the sexual response cycle, facilitate communication about sexual issues, and give permission regarding an expanded repertoire of behaviors for greater sexual satisfaction. For example, the clinician might encourage the couple to enjoy a second intercourse after one involving a short ejaculation latency, to take advantage of the decreased sexual arousal most men experience during the refractory period. Alternatively, the couple could be encouraged to vary their intercourse-related behaviors to attenuate the patient's level of sexual arousal for the purpose of keeping it below the level of ejaculatory inevitability.

Standard behavioral strategies for the treatment of premature ejaculation include the frenulum squeeze and start-pause techniques introduced by Masters and Johnson (1970) and Kaplan (1979). In addition, the couple could be encouraged to experiment with the partner (e.g., female) in superior or lateral positions, because these typically provide men with a greater sense of ejaculatory control. Couples could also be advised to engage in mutual masturbation and then oral sex before coitus (depending on the acceptability of the sexual behaviors to the couple). Other suggestions include slowing down during intercourse, breathing deeply, having shallower penile penetration, or moving the pelvis in circular motion. Excellent resources for both men (Zilbergeld 1993) and women (Heiman and LoPiccolo 1988) are available to assist couples.

Relevant cognitive strategies include increasing the man's 1) attention to his somatic sensations so that he might better monitor his level of physical arousal and detect pre-ejaculatory sensations and 2) use of sensate focus, which permits enjoyment of physical sensations without necessarily generating sexual arousal (Carey 1998). This latter procedure de-emphasizes the focus on intercourse and orgasm within the sexual relationship and may help reduce the man's performance anxiety, which, because it presumably operates through sympathetic pathways, may serve to prime the ejaculatory response prematurely. As the man and his partner gain a greater sense of self-efficacy, reliance on medications can be reduced.

Important to any treatment plan is the substitution of counterproductive behaviors and beliefs with positive therapeutic strategies. Strong emphases on latency to ejaculation or using distracting stimuli (at the cost of ignoring relevant body cues) can increase premature ejaculation symptoms. Deliberate strategies to prevent relapse of premature ejaculation involve 1) predicting the likelihood of occasional "setbacks" and preparing couples appropriately and 2) using increased spacing between sessions as progress is noted (McCarthy 1993). Depending on the level of premature ejaculation severity, the goals mentioned earlier may be achieved in several sessions or, if significant relationship issues and partner dysfunction exist, 10–20 sessions may be required. By itself cognitive-behavioral treatment has a fairly high initial success rate, although for reasons as yet undetermined, this success rate falls to 50% or less by a year posttreatment. When therapy is combined with medications the long-term success rates are likely to increase, assuming couples continue to practice their newly acquired strategies and adhere to treatment procedures.

Male Orgasmic Disorder

Male orgasmic disorder (MOD) is the DSM-IV-TR terminology for absent, inhibited, or delayed/retarded ejaculation—a condition in which the man does not reach orgasm (because he does not ejaculate) or reaches it only after prolonged stimulation. Many instances of delayed or inhibited ejaculation can be traced to a pathophysiological event (pelvic surgery) or condition (e.g., prostatitis, degenerative neural diseases, medications). However, in men for whom a medical etiology cannot be thus traced, MOD represents one of the more challenging male sexual disorders for the clinician. Unlike premature ejaculation and erectile dysfunction, MOD has no widely accepted drugs approved for treatment in humans (although some off-label agents have been used with mild success) and no obvious or common psychological or relationship etiologies to account for the majority of cases. It also is not clear when a man actually meets the criteria for this dysfunction, because operationalized criteria for the disorder currently do not exist. Given that most sexually functional men ejaculate within about 7–10 minutes after intromission, a clinician might assume that men with latencies beyond 20 or 30 minutes or men who simply cease sexual activity due to exhaustion or irritation qualify for this diagnosis. Such symptoms, together with the fact that a man and/or his partner decide to seek help for the problem, are usually sufficient for an MOD diagnosis.

Important to the treatment plan for MOD is an understanding of the kinds of problems, behaviors, or contexts sometimes associated with the disorder. It is particularly useful to know whether the problem occurs under any circumstance (including masturbation) or only during intercourse. Men who are anorgasmic during masturbation as well as intercourse are often more difficult to treat, although they may still benefit from exploration and analysis of the predisposing risk or maintaining factors that follow. Men with MOD usually have no difficulty attaining or keeping their erections—in fact, they often are able to maintain erections for prolonged periods of time. Despite their good erections, these men often report low levels of subjective sexual arousal as compared with sexually functional men (Rowland et al. 2004). Men with MOD sometimes indicate greater arousal and enjoyment from masturbation than from intercourse. This autosexual orientation may involve an idiosyncratic and vigorous masturbation style—carried out with high frequency—with which the vagina is unable to compete. Apfelbaum (2000) labels this as a desire disorder specific to partnered sex. These men may experience a mismatch between the sexual fantasies used during masturbation and the behaviors and appearance of their partners, thereby attenuating their levels of arousal during intercourse. Particularly relevant as men and their partners age, both penile sensitivity and vaginal tautness decrease, thus exacerbating any preexisting tendencies for this dysfunction. Other factors may contribute, including specific religious beliefs or taboos against masturbation or a fear of pregnancy, and such information should be obtained as part of the psychosexual history.

Treatment strategies for MOD have typically been based on the kinds of problems identified earlier, and most approaches require cooperation of the sexual partner. Masters and Johnson (1970) advocated masturbation with the assistance of the partner, who simulates the patient's techniques (sometimes forceful and aggressive and involving the use of vibrators) to the point of ejaculatory inevitability, at which point the couple switches to intercourse. Aligned with this particular approach but generally more fruitful in generating a satisfying outcome for the couple is that of masturbatory retraining, where the man uses self-stimulation techniques more consistent with the stimulation experienced during intercourse (Perelman 2004). In conjunction with this approach, sexual fantasies can be realigned (i.e., stimulus fading) so that ideations during masturbation better match those that might occur during intercourse with the partner. The attractiveness and proceptive or arousing behaviors of the partner might also be increased. Other therapists such as Apfelbaum (2000) have emphasized the need to remove the "demand" (and thus anxiety-producing) characteristics of the situation, noting that men with MOD may be overconscientious about pleasing their partner. The anxiety for the man with MOD is not about having an orgasm (a psychodynamic perspective) but about not having one. This ejaculatory performance anxiety interferes with the erotic sensations of genital stimulation, resulting in levels of sexual excitement and arousal that are insufficient for climax (although more than adequate to maintain the man's erections). Treatment strategies based on this view include validation of (although not necessarily encouragement of) the man's autosexual orientation, removal of stigmas suggesting hostility or withholding toward the partner, and anxiety reduction. In this respect, the treatment emphasizes normalizing the anorgasmic response and exploring factors that facilitate the man's arousal (similar to treatment of anorgasmia in women) rather than assigning responsibility or fault. Usually, after end points such as these are achieved, the likelihood of becoming orgasmic greatly increases.

Although pharmacological agents are not a common approach to the treatment of inhibited or retarded ejaculation, several agents have been used to facilitate orgasm in patients taking SSRI antidepressants, the latter drugs known to delay or completely inhibit ejaculatory response. Specifically, the antiserotonergic agent cyproheptadine and the dopamine agonist amantadine have been used with moderate success in this population of patients (McMahon et al. 2004). The lack of large-scale, well-controlled studies involving these and other agents that facilitate ejaculation in men with noniatrogenic MOD suggests the need for further study to investigate these agents' efficacies and tolerabilities. A lack of efficacy of pharmacotherapies in men with MOD may result in part from the potentially strong psychological and relationship contributions to this dysfunction. As research continues to uncover greater understanding of the ejaculatory process, the likelihood of identifying proejaculatory agents increases. As with both premature ejaculation and erectile dysfunction, if and when safe and effective pharmacological treatment becomes available for MOD, treatment for this dysfunction will likely undergo a major paradigm shift.

Despite the lack of an easily identified etiology for MOD, reported success rates have been high, approximating 70%–80%. Confidence in such reports, however, is limited by the few studies that have been conducted, their uncontrolled designs (including lack of placebo groups), the lack of standardized treatment formulations, and heterogeneous samples that included men with varying biological and psychological etiologies.

CONCLUSION

Since the 1980s, the understanding of the biological, psychological, and relationship factors involved in sexual response and dysfunction has increased substantially. With this progress have come integrated assessment and treatment strategies that make amelioration of male sexual dysfunctions more likely than ever. Important to the ongoing understanding and treatment of male sexual dysfunction is recognition of not only the complex interplay among relationship, psychological, and physiological systems required for adequate sexual response but also the important role that a fulfilling sexual relationship has on men's psychological well-being and quality of life.

KEY POINTS

- Sexual dysfunctions in men—that is, the inability to perform adequately—are subcategorized into problems of sexual desire or interest, problems of arousal (either genital response or feelings of sexual excitement), and problems of ejaculation (either earlier or later than the man or his partner desires—or not ejaculating at all).

- Diagnosis of sexual dysfunction is typically aimed at understanding the nature of the problem, determining problem severity and the functional impairment it causes, identifying possible etiologies, and collaborating with the man and his partner to identify specific treatment goals.

- Although some aspects of men's sexual dysfunctions are not yet fully understood, the wide range of available treatment strategies holds significant promise for reinstatement of adequate sexual functioning in the majority of men.

PRACTICE GUIDELINES

1. Sexual health and satisfaction are usually embedded in a relationship with a partner and involve elements of passion, intimacy, caring, commitment, and communication. Clinicians treating men with sexual dysfunctions should evaluate and target relationship elements that might be contributing to the sexual dysfunction.

2. Sexual response is multidimensional and incorporates physiological, psychological, and relationship components. Sexual dysfunctions may stem from problems in one or more of these areas. Treatment for men with sexual dysfunctions should target these domains.

3. Treatment of sexual dysfunction may involve pharmacotherapy, psychotherapy, or a combination of both. The extent to which the sexual problem has affected the man and his relationship with his partner should help guide the treatment strategy.

REFERENCES

Althof SE: Erectile dysfunction: psychotherapy with men and couples, in Principles and Practice of Sex Therapy, 3rd Edition. Edited by Leiblum SR, Rosen RC. New York, Guilford, 2000, pp 242–275

Althof SE, Leiblum SR, Chevert-Measson M, et al: Psychological and interpersonal dimensions of sexual function and dysfunction, in Sexual Medicine: Sexual Dysfunctions in Men and Women. Edited by Lue TF, Basson R, Rosen R, et al. Paris, International Consultation on Sexual Dysfunctions, 2004, pp 73–116

American Psychiatric Association: Diagnostic and Statistical Manual of Mental Disorders, 4th Edition, Text Revision. Washington, DC, American Psychiatric Association, 2000

Angst J: Sexual problems in healthy and depressed persons. Int Clin Psychopharmacol 13 (suppl 6):S1–S4, 1998

Apfelbaum B: Retarded ejaculation: a much misunderstood syndrome, in Principles and Practice of Sex Therapy, 3rd Edition. Edited by Leiblum SR, Rosen RC. New York, Guilford, 2000, pp 205–241

Baldwin DS: Depression and sexual function. J Psychopharmacol 10(suppl):30–34, 1996

Bancroft J: Human Sexuality and Its Problems. Edinburgh, Scotland, Churchill Livingstone, 1989

Boolell M, Allen MJ, Ballard SA, et al: Sildenafil: an orally active type 5 cyclic GMP-specific phosphodiesterase inhibitor for the treatment of penile erectile dysfunction. Int J Impot Res 8:47–52, 1996

Burnett AL: Neurophysiology of erectile function and dysfunction, in The Handbook of Sexual Dysfunction. Edited by Hellstrom WJG. San Francisco, CA, American Society of Andrology, 1999, pp 12–17

Byrne D, Schulte L: Personality dispositions as mediators of sexual response. Annu Rev Sex Res 1:93–117, 1990

Carey MP: Cognitive-behavioral treatment of sexual dysfunction, in International Handbook of Cognitive and Behavioural Treatments for Psychological Disorders. Edited by Caballo VE. Oxford, England, Pergamon, 1998, pp 251–280

Costa PT Jr, Fagan P, Piedmont RL, et al: The five-factor model of personality and sexual functioning in outpatient men and women. Psychiatr Med 10:199–215, 1992

Feldman HA, Goldstein I, Hatzichristou DG, et al: Impotence and its medical and psychosocial correlates: results of the Massachusetts Male Aging Study. J Urol 151:54–61, 1994

Gitlin M: Sexual dysfunction with psychotropic drugs. Expert Opin Pharmacother 4:2259–2269, 2003

Harland R, Huws R: Sexual problems in diabetes and the role of psychological intervention. Sex Marital Ther 12:147–157, 1997

Hawton K: Integration of treatments for male erectile dysfunction. Lancet 351:7–8, 1998

Heiman JR, LoPiccolo J: Becoming Orgasmic: A Sexual and Personal Growth Program for Women, Revised Edition. New York, Prentice Hall, 1988

Kaplan HS: Disorders of Sexual Desire and Other New Concepts and Techniques in Sex Therapy. New York, Brunner/Mazel, 1979, pp 3–40

Lewis RW, Fugl-Meyer KS, Bosch R, et al: Definitions, classification, and epidemiology of sexual dysfunction, in Sexual Medicine: Sexual Dysfunctions in Men and Women. Edited by Lue TF, Basson R, Rosen R, et al. Paris, France, International Consultation on Sexual Dysfunctions, 2004, pp 37–72

Lilleleht E, Leiblum SR: Schizophrenia and sexuality: a critical review of the literature. Annu Rev Sex Res 4:247–276, 1993

Loeb TB, Williams JK, Carmona JV, et al: Child sexual abuse: associations with the sexual functioning of adolescents and adults. Annu Rev Sex Res 13:307–345, 2002

Lue TF: Physiology of erection and pathophysiology of impotence, in Campbell's Urology. Edited by Walsh PC, Retik AB, Stamey TA, et al. Philadelphia, PA, WB Saunders, 1992, pp 709–728

Masters WH, Johnson VE: Human Sexual Response. Boston, MA, Little, Brown, 1966

Masters WH, Johnson VE: Human Sexual Inadequacy. Boston, MA, Little, Brown, 1970

McCabe MP: Intimacy and quality of life among sexually dysfunctional men and women. J Sex Marital Ther 23:276–290, 1997

McCarthy BW: Relapse prevention strategies and techniques in sex therapy. J Sex Marital Ther 19:142–146, 1993

McMahon C, Abdo C, Incrocci L, et al: Disorders of orgasm and ejaculation in men. J Sex Med 1:58–65, 2004

Osborne C, Rowland DL: Evaluation of psychological functioning in men with sexual dysfunctions, in Pathophysiology and Treatment of Male Sexual and Reproductive Dysfunction. Edited by Kandeel F. New York, Marcel Dekker, in press

Palmore EB: How to live longer and like it. J Appl Gerontol 4:1–8, 1985

Perelman MA: Retarded ejaculation. Current Sexual Health Reports 1:95–101, 2004

Pfaus JG, Kippin TE, Coria-Avila G: What can animal models tell us about human sexual response? Annu Rev Sex Res 14:1–63, 2003

Pridal CG, LoPiccolo J: Multielement treatment of desire disorders: integration of cognitive, behavioral, and systemic therapy, in Principles and Practice of Sex Therapy, 3rd Edition. Edited by Leiblum SR, Rosen RC. New York, Guilford, 2000, pp 205–241

Rosen R, Hatzichristou D, Broderick G, et al: Clinical evaluation and symptom scales: sexual dysfunction assessment in men, in Sexual Medicine: Sexual Dysfunctions in Men and Women. Edited by Lue TF, Basson R, Rosen R, et al. Paris, France, International Consultation on Sexual Dysfunctions, 2004, pp 173–220

Rowland DL: Penile sensitivity in men: an overview of recent findings. Urology 52:1101–1105, 1998

Rowland DL, Burnett A: Pharmacotherapy in the treatment of male sexual dysfunction. J Sex Res 37:226–243, 2000

Rowland DL, Cooper SE: Behavioral and psychologic models in ejaculatory function research. Current Sexual Health Reports 2:29–34, 2005

Rowland DL, Slob AK: Premature ejaculation: psychophysiological considerations in theory, research, and treatment. Annu Rev Sex Res 8:224–253, 1997

Rowland DL, Cooper SE, Slob AK: Treatment of premature ejaculation: psychological and biological strategies. Drugs Today 34:879–899, 1998

Rowland DL, Keeney C, Slob AK: Sexual response in men with inhibited or retarded ejaculation. J Sex Med 16:270–274, 2004

Rust J, Golombok S: The Golombok Rust Inventory of Sexual Satisfaction. Odessa, FL, Psychological Assessment Resources, 1986

Schnarch DM: Talking to patients about sex, part II. Med Aspects Hum Sex 22:97–106, 1988

Schnarch DM: Constructing the Sexual Crucible: An Integration of Sexual and Marital Therapy. New York, WW Norton, 1991

Schnarch DM: Desire problems: a systemic perspective. in Principles and Practice of Sex Therapy, 3rd Edition. Edited by Leiblum SR, Rosen RC. New York, Guilford, 2000, pp 17–56

Schover LR, Friedman JM, Weiler SJ, et al: Multiaxial problem-oriented system for sexual dysfunctions: an alternative to DSM-III. Arch Gen Psychiatry 39:614–619, 1982

Schreiner-Engel P, Schiavi RC: Lifetime psychopathology in individuals with low sexual desire. J Nerv Ment Dis 174:646–651, 1986

Spanier GB: Measuring dyadic adjustment: new scales for assessing the quality of marriage and similar dyads. J Marriage Fam 38:15–28, 1976

Sternberg RJ, Barnes M: The Psychology of Love. New Haven, CT, Yale University Press, 1988

Tondo L, Cantone M, Carta M, et al: An MMPI evaluation of male sexual dysfunction. J Clin Psychol 47:391–396, 1991

Tsitouras PD, Alvarez RR: Etiology and management of sexual dysfunction in elderly men. Psychiatr Med 2:43–55, 1984

Waldinger M: The neurobiological approach to premature ejaculation. J Urol 168:2359–2367, 2002

Zilbergeld B: The New Male Sexuality. New York, Bantam Books, 1993

9

IMPULSE CONTROL DISORDERS

JON E. GRANT, M.D., M.P.H., J.D.
MARC N. POTENZA, M.D., PH.D.

Case Vignette 1

Justin, a 45-year-old man, started gambling with college roommates at age 18. He began playing poker with friends for money, and by age 28 he was gambling alone at casinos. Justin reported that his urges to gamble were often triggered by advertisements for the local casino and fantasies of winning large amounts of money.

For the past 4 years, Justin had played blackjack approximately three evenings each week. Always intending on staying only 2 or 3 hours at the casino, Justin would often play blackjack for 8–10 hours each evening. In addition, he began gambling with larger amounts of money. He was a successful self-employed businessman, but his work suffered as a result of his gambling. Over time, he became too tired from staying late at the casino, the quality of his work deteriorated, and he lost business.

Justin's marriage was also affected because he often missed events at home, choosing instead to go to the casino. In addition, Justin began lying to his wife about his whereabouts. This deception led to guilt and marital strain. With fear of impending divorce and loss of his business, Justin sought help for gambling.

Case Vignette 2

Kevin, a 37-year-old married man who owned his own business, reported that although he was happy in his marriage, he felt strong urges to have sex with strange women. "I'm not really after the thrill. I have these urges when I feel tense or anxious. The urges are uncontrollable." Kevin detailed a 14-year history of multiple sexual affairs (exceeding 300 sexual partners), each one followed by feelings of remorse and guilt. On average, Kevin was having extramarital sexual relations at least once every 2 or 3 weeks. In addition, Kevin reported that the preoccupation with having sex "consumed" him daily. He described thoughts of sex that totaled more than 6 hours each day, multiple episodes of masturbation each day, and hours spent on the Internet viewing pornography. Kevin reported that these sexual behaviors interfered with his work and that he found his "lack of control" distressing.

Kevin's compulsive sexual behavior started at age 16. Getting married did not dampen the urges: "Even when I see that my behavior is destroying my life, my self-respect, and my marriage, I continue doing it." Kevin reported symptoms consistent with depression that started only after many years of compulsive sexual behavior. He denied symptoms of mania or substance use disorders. He had no history of sexual or physical abuse. Kevin sought psychiatric treatment after contracting a sexually transmitted disease and being referred by his internist.

Disorders characterized by an impaired ability to resist impulses to engage in ultimately self-destructive behaviors (or ones with deleterious long-term consequences) have been categorized in DSM-IV-TR as impulse control disorders (ICDs) not elsewhere classified (American Psychiatric Association 2000). These disorders, which currently include pathological gambling, kleptomania, intermittent explosive disorder (IED), pyromania, trichotillomania, and ICD not otherwise specified, have historically received little clinical and research attention. In addition, diagnostic criteria for compulsive sexual behavior (CSB) and compulsive buying have been proposed, because preliminary data suggest that these behaviors may be linked to ICDs currently operationalized in DSM (Black et al. 1997a; McElroy et al. 1994).

Data suggest that ICDs are relatively common (Grant et al. 2005; Shaffer et al. 1999), carry significant morbidity and mortality, and may be effectively treated with behavior and pharmacological therapies (Grant and Potenza 2004). Although the ICDs often share similarities in phenomenology, family history, comorbidity, neurobiology, and response to treatment interventions, certain ICDs appear more commonly in men (pathological gambling, CSB) whereas others are seen more frequently in women (kleptomania, trichotillomania, compulsive buying). In addition, the clinical presentation of ICDs often differs in men, and interventions, both psychological and pharmacological, should be tailored for issues unique to men. In this chapter, we review findings concerning how ICDs manifest in men within a clinical context (pyromania is not included because studies of individuals with rigorously diagnosed pyromania are lacking) and discuss how treatment of ICDs may be uniquely tailored for men as compared with women.

ADOLESCENT MALE DEVELOPMENT AND PREDISPOSITION TOWARD IMPULSE CONTROL DISORDERS

ICDs tend to start during adolescence and can be conceptualized as belonging to a larger constellation of behavioral addictions. Data support a relationship between behavioral and drug addictions in both adults and adolescents. For example, high rates of both problem gambling and substance use disorders have been reported during adolescence (Chambers and Potenza 2003; Wagner and Anthony 2002), and gambling, substance use, and other risky behaviors frequently co-occur in adolescents (Proimos et al. 1998; Romer 2003). More specifically, this co-occurrence of risky behaviors appears particularly strong in adolescent males. Arguably the most consistent and robust findings across youth gambling studies indicate that boys are more involved in gambling than girls and have higher rates of problem gambling than girls (e.g., Gupta and Derevensky 1998; Stinchfield 2001; Wallisch 1993; Wynne Resources 1996). Similarly, adolescent males have a greater likelihood of developing a substance use disorder than do adolescent females (Chambers et al. 2003).

A growing body of literature suggests the importance of environmental and genetic influences on brain function that lead to vulnerability to and expression of addictive disorders (Shah et al. 2005; Slutske et al. 2000; Tsuang et al. 2001). Both environmental and genetic factors are important influences on brain function and thus can contribute to addiction vulnerability in adolescence.

Motivated behavior involves integrating information about a person's internal state (e.g., hunger, sexual desire, pain), environmental factors (e.g., resource or reproductive opportunities, the presence of danger), and personal experiences (e.g., recollections of events deemed similar in nature). Specific brain regions provide the primary motivational system with this information. For example, the hypothalamic and septal nuclei provide information about nutrient ingestion, aggression, and reproductive drive; the amygdala provides affective information; and the hippocampus provides contextual memory data. Although numerous neurotransmitters are involved in processing this information, including glutamate and γ-aminobutyric acid (GABA), the neurotransmitters that are arguably the best characterized and that influence motivated behavior are dopamine and serotonin.

Dopamine release into the nucleus accumbens has been associated with a wide array of experiences, including those that are rewarding and reinforcing, novel, and aversive or stressful (Chambers et al. 2003). Dopamine release into the nucleus accumbens seems maximal when reward probability is most uncertain, suggesting that dopamine plays a central role in guiding behavior during risk-taking situations (Fiorillo et al. 2003). Importantly, the structure and function of dopamine neuronal projections to the nucleus accumbens, in conjunction with glutamatergic afferent and intrinsic GABAergic activities, change after experiences influencing function of the nucleus accumbens. That is, in reward-related learning, future behavior is determined in part according to past reward-related experiences via neuroplastic changes involving the nucleus accumbens. In this manner, dopamine function within the nucleus accumbens may serve to narrow motivational repertoires over time.

Adolescence is a time of remarkable changes in brain structure and function, and developmental changes within primary motivational pathways may lead to increased novelty seeking and risk taking (Chambers et al. 2003). Adolescence may reflect a state of heightened dopaminergic activity. In a related context, animals show heightened behavioral responses (e.g., increased motoric activity and novelty seeking) following exposure to pro-dopaminergic drugs. Therefore, vulnerability to addictive behaviors, particularly during adolescence, might be increased by a heightened dopaminergic state. Furthermore, the relationship between dopamine and novelty-seeking behaviors may have a stronger genetic association in adolescent males (Laucht et al. 2005).

Diminished inhibitory mechanisms could also underlie risk-taking behaviors. Among the most well-studied inhibitory pathways is that involving serotonin function within the prefrontal cortex (Chambers et al. 2003). Decreased measures of serotonin have long been associated with a variety of adult risk-taking behaviors, including alcoholism, fire setting, and pathological gambling (Potenza and Hollander 2002). Although the precise mechanism has not been fully determined, serotonin projections from the raphe nuclei to motivational circuitry, including the ventral tegmental area, nucleus accumbens, prefrontal cortex, amygdala, and hippocampus, appear involved (Chambers et al. 2003). For example, blunted serotonergic responses in the ventromedial prefrontal cortex have been observed in individuals with impulsive aggression (New et al. 2002), and this region has been implicated in disadvantageous decision making, as has been observed in adults with gambling or substance use disorders (Bechara 2003).

PATHOLOGICAL GAMBLING

A recent meta-analysis of the available literature concluded that 2.2 million adults in North America (1.6%) are pathological gamblers, with an additional 5.3 million adults (3.9%) at risk for the disorder (Shaffer et al. 1999). In epidemiological studies, men represent approximately 68% of the pathological gamblers in the United States (Cunningham-Williams et al. 1998; Shaffer et al. 1999; Volberg 1994). Nationally based studies in other countries confirm the overrepresentation of men among those with pathological gambling (Abbott et al. 2004; Gotestam and Johansson 2003; Legarda et al. 1992; Wong and So 2003).

Clinical Characteristics

As in the case of Justin, pathological gambling usually begins in childhood or adolescence, with males tending to start at an earlier age than females (Chambers and Potenza 2003; Grant and Kim 2001b). High rates of pathological gambling in adolescents and young adults suggest a similar natural history to that observed in individuals with substance use disorders (Chambers and Potenza 2003). In fact, male gender appears to be a risk factor for developing a gambling addiction in adolescence (Pietrzak et al. 2003). Male pathological gamblers are more likely to be young, single, and living alone without children compared with their female counterparts (Crisp et al. 2004). In addition, males tend to incur larger gambling debts than women. Financial and marital problems are common (Grant and Kim 2001b), as are illegal behaviors such as stealing, embezzlement, and writing bad checks (Grant and Kim 2001b; Potenza et al. 2000).

One of the most replicated findings with respect to differences between male and female pathological gamblers has been that the course of illness seems to be different for men. The interval between the age of starting to gamble and of developing a problem with gambling seems to be longer for men (Grant and Kim 2001b; Ibanez et al. 2003; Ladd and Petry 2002; Martins et al. 2002; Potenza et al. 2001; Tavares et al. 2001). These findings suggest a "telescoping" progression of the disorder in women as compared with men, although gender differences in patterns of treatment seeking may also contribute to these findings. A slower development of addiction in males has been documented in other addictive disorders such as alcohol use disorders and opiate dependence (Anglin et al. 1987; Piazza et al. 1989).

Strategic forms of gambling, such as sports and card gambling, are more prevalent in male pathological gamblers, whereas nonstrategic forms of gambling, such as using slot machines and playing bingo, are more prevalent in females (Potenza et al. 2001). A man's choice of strategic gambling may be more action oriented (e.g., sports gambling or blackjack; Potenza et al. 2001) and may reflect a higher level of sensation seeking among male pathological gamblers (Vitaro et al. 1997).

Male gamblers report that advertisements are a common trigger of their urges to gamble, whereas females are more likely to report that feeling bored or lonely may trigger their urges to gamble (Grant and Kim 2001b; Ladd and Petry 2002). Men are more likely to report urges to gamble unrelated to their emotional state (Grant and Kim 2002b; Ladd and Petry 2002; Potenza et al. 2001). Social situations may explain why affective state is a less prominent trigger for males, and some research suggests that the home environment may be more stable and supportive for male pathological gamblers (Ladd and Petry 2002).

Co-occurring Disorders

Studies have consistently reported that subjects with pathological gambling have high rates of lifetime mood (60%–76%; Linden et al. 1986; McCormick et al. 1984; Roy et al. 1988), anxiety (16%–40%; Crockford and el-Guebaly 1998; Ibanez et al. 2001), and substance use (33%–63%; Black and Moyer 1998; Grant et al. 2002) disorders. In terms of gender differences in comorbidity, one study found that male pathological gamblers were more likely to have a current alcohol use disorder but less likely to have a comorbid mood disorder (Ibanez et al. 2001). Some evidence suggests that men with gambling problems are less likely to have symptoms of depression (Getty et al. 2000) and less likely to attempt suicide (Martins et al. 2004). However, a large community sample of male twins found high rates of depression when sociodemographic and other co-occurring disorders were controlled and that the co-occurrence between pathological gambling and major depression was largely determined by genetic factors (Potenza et al. 2005). Males with pathological gambling are also more likely to engage in risky sexual behavior (Martins et al. 2004), have CSB, and have comorbid intermittent explosive disorder (Black and Moyer 1998).

Other aspects of comorbidity have been found less consistently in the literature. For example, one study found that men with gambling problems were less likely than women with gambling problems to report anxiety due to their gambling (Potenza et al. 2001). Differences in scores on the Hamilton Anxiety Scale, however, have not been found between genders in adults with pathological gambling (Grant et al. 2003). Also, among people with pathological gambling, men do not report different rates of categorical anxiety disorders than women (Ibanez et al. 2003). Rates of personality disorders also do not differ between genders, although there is some indication that antisocial traits may be higher among men with pathological gambling (Ibanez et al. 2003).

Although the number of categorical personality disorders does not appear to differ between male and female pathological gamblers (Ibanez et al. 2003), gender may still influence the personality characteristics of pathological gamblers. The extent to which male and female gamblers differ with respect to personality traits, however, remains unclear. One study found that men with pathological gambling reported greater sensation seeking (Ibanez et al. 2003). Additional studies are needed to define more precisely the gender differences in personality characteristics between men and women with pathological gambling.

Treatment

Pharmacotherapy

Various classes of medication have been studied in the treatment of pathological gambling. Studies using selective serotonin reuptake inhibitors (SSRIs; e.g., paroxetine, fluvoxamine), lithium, and opioid antagonists have all demonstrated efficacy in double-blind studies of pathological gambling (Grant and Potenza 2004). Of the 10 double-blind studies (Blanco et al. 2002; Grant et al. 2003, 2006; Haller and Hinterhuber 1994; Hollander et al. 1992, 2000, 2005; Kim et al. 2001, 2002; Saiz-Ruiz et al. 2005) and 7 open-label or single-blind studies (Black 2004; Grant and Potenza 2006; Hollander et al. 1998; Kim and Grant 2001a; Pallanti et al. 2002a, 2002b; Zimmerman et al. 2002) in the published literature, 6 assessed whether men responded differently to treatment. In trials of nefazodone, paroxetine, naltrexone, and nalmefene, there were no gender differences associated with response to medication (Grant et al. 2003, 2006; Kim et al. 2001; Pallanti et al. 2002a, 2002b). In 1 trial of fluvoxamine, however, young male pathological gamblers appeared to respond preferentially to the medication (Blanco et al. 2002). However, the reported gender difference in treatment response should be viewed cautiously given the small number of subjects and particularly the small group of men completing treatment in the study.

Psychotherapy

Multiple behavioral treatments have been investigated, with promising preliminary results (Hodgins and Petry 2004). Cognitive therapy, which focuses on changing the patient's beliefs regarding perceived control over randomly determined events, has demonstrated success in small, randomized trials (Hodgins and Petry 2004). Cognitive-behavioral therapy has also been used effectively to treat pathological gambling (Hodgins and Petry 2004). Brief interventions in the form of motivational interventions and self-directed workbooks have resulted in significant reductions in gambling behavior (Hodgins et al. 2001). Aversion therapy and imaginal desensitization have also resulted in improvement for pathological gamblers (McConaghy et al. 1983, 1991). Gamblers Anonymous and self-exclusion programs may also aid in reducing gambling behavior. Of the various psychosocial interventions, however, none has assessed whether men respond differently than women. The relatively small samples studied in reports published to date have limited power in detecting gender-related differences in treatment response. It is anticipated that future studies involving larger samples will provide additional insight into optimal treatments for men with pathological gambling.

A better understanding of gender differences in treatment response may help in developing more prevention and treatment strategies. For example, given the reported gender differences in triggers to gambling, an appropriate treatment for men might target visual processing of salient gambling cues. In addition, cognitive-behavioral therapy directed at sensation-seeking behaviors may be a more appropriate treatment for men. Alcohol use disorders in male pathological gamblers may require more intense treatment because these patients are likely to have more functional impairment and a poorer prognosis than are those with either condition alone. Finally, because men are less likely to seek treatment for mental health issues (see Chapter 17, "Overcoming Stigma and Barriers to Mental Health Treatment"), brief interventions may prove particularly useful for men with pathological gambling.

COMPULSIVE SEXUAL BEHAVIOR

CSB is characterized by inappropriate or excessive sexual behaviors or thoughts that lead to subjective distress or impaired functioning (Black et al. 1997a). Although not currently included in DSM-IV-TR, CSB may be relatively common. No epidemiological studies have been performed, but the prevalence of CSB in adults is estimated to range from 3% to 6% (Coleman 1992). A recent study of patients admitted to a psychiatric hospital found that 4.4% had current CSB (Grant et al. 2005). The disorder is believed to predominately affect men. In the three large case series that have been published to date, men accounted for 77 of 87 subjects (88.5%; Black et al. 1997a; Kafka and Prentky 1994; Raymond et al. 2003). CSB may be underreported in women because women tend to focus on romantic or emotional aspects of sexual behavior whereas males appear to focus on physical aspects.

Clinical Characteristics

CSB can involve a wide range of sexual behaviors, often including a mixture of paraphilic and nonparaphilic behaviors (Coleman 1992; Kafka and Prentky 1994). Nonparaphilic CSB involves conventional sexual behaviors (e.g., masturbation, promiscuity, pornography, fixation on an unobtainable partner) that have become excessive or uncontrolled. Many people with CSB may also satisfy criteria for one of the paraphilias, such as exhibitionism, voyeurism, sexual masochism and sadism, or transvestic fetishism.

Sexual behavior in CSB may be intermittent or continuous. Although the compulsive sexual acts are gratifying, albeit briefly, the behavior is followed by remorse or guilt (Barth and Kinder 1987). The behavior is often driven by either pleasure seeking or anxiety reduction (Coleman 1992). As seen in the case of Kevin described earlier, individuals often report a feeling of being "out of control" with their sexual behavior and fear losing their jobs, friends, or family (Quadland 1985). One study that compared 28 men and 8 women with CSB found that the men had significantly more sexual partners (Black et al. 1997a). Although no other gender differences have been reported, the sample of women with CSB described in the literature is relatively small. Thus few empirical data are available to describe how clinical features of CSB might differ based on gender.

Co-occurring Disorders

Comorbidity in CSB is high, with individuals frequently meeting criteria for mood, anxiety (social phobia), and substance use disorders (Black et al. 1997a; Kafka and Prentky 1994; Raymond et al. 2003). One study of 36 subjects found that other ICDs were also frequent in this population: compulsive buying (14%), kleptomania (14%), pathological gambling (11%), and pyromania (8%) (Black et al. 1997a). Cluster B personality disorders are also commonly seen in individuals with CSB (44%; Black et al. 1997a).

Treatment

Little published treatment research exists for nonparaphilic CSB. Case series and open-label trials, all treating only men with CSB, suggest that various medications may be efficacious. Fluoxetine demonstrated efficacy in reducing sexual urges and behavior in 10 men with nonparaphilic sexual addiction (Kafka and Prentky 1992). A smaller case series of 5 men with CSB treated with fluoxetine, however, did not produce similarly robust effects (Stein et al. 1992). A retrospective study looking at 14 men receiving nefazodone (mean dosage, 200 mg/day) reported that 55% of the men improved, with 45% achieving remission of CSB symptoms (Coleman et al. 2000). Other medications with possible efficacy in treating CSB in men include imipramine, lithium, buspirone, naltrexone, and naltrexone augmentation of an antidepressant (Grant and Kim 2001a; Potenza and Hollander 2002; Raymond et al. 2002). Hormonal treatments, including antiandrogens, estrogens, and gonadotropin-releasing hormone analogues, have also been reported to be helpful in men with CSB (Potenza and Hollander 2002).

Psychotherapy is commonly recommended, and a variety of behavioral techniques have been employed such as imaginal desensitization, aversion therapy, group therapy, and psychodynamic therapies (Carnes 1983; Goodman 1993). A randomized trial found that imaginal desensitization was more effective at 1-year follow-up than covert sensitization in 20 men with CSB (McConaghy et al. 1985).

INTERMITTENT EXPLOSIVE DISORDER

IED was first established as a psychiatric diagnosis in ICD-9-CM (World Health Organization 1978) and later included in DSM-III in 1980 (American Psychiatric Association 1980). IED is defined by recurrent significant outbursts of aggression, often leading to assaultive acts against people or property, that are disproportionate to outside stressors and not better explained by another psychiatric diagnosis (American Psychiatric Association 2000). Although IED was once considered relatively uncommon, recent research suggests that IED may in fact be quite prevalent. One study found that 6.3% of a community sample had lifetime IED, with 2.4% reporting symptoms consistent with IED in the previous month (Coccaro et al. 2004). A study of 1,300 psychiatric outpatients found that 3.1% had current IED (Posternak and Zimmerman 2002). In addition, a study of psychiatric inpatients found that 6.4% and 6.9% had current and lifetime IED, respectively (Grant et al. 2005).

Clinical Characteristics

Early reports suggest that most individuals with IED are male (74% of one sample) (McElroy et al. 1998), but recent research suggests that IED may be more common in females than previously thought (Coccaro et al. 2004). There is no evidence yet, however, that the disorder presents differently in women. IED symptoms tend to start in adolescence and appear to be chronic (Coccaro et al. 2004; McElroy et al. 1998). Although individuals with IED report that their anger outbursts provide relief from tension or may in fact be pleasurable, they also regard the behavior as distressing and problematic (McElroy et al. 1998). Outbursts are generally short-lived (usually less than 30 minutes in duration) and frequent (multiple times per month) (McElroy et al. 1998). Legal and occupational difficulties due to IED symptoms are common (McElroy et al. 1998).

Co-occurring Disorders

Studies of comorbidity in IED have found elevated rates of mood disorders, substance use disorders, ICDs, and anxiety disorders (Coccaro et al. 2004; McElroy et al. 1998; Olvera 2002). Many individuals with IED report that their aggressive outbursts are secondary to changes in mood (McElroy et al. 1998). Although some studies suggest that IED and personality disorders frequently co-occur (Galovski et al. 2002), the rates of borderline personality and antisocial personality disorders appear to be low (Coccaro et al. 2004).

Treatment

Although pharmacotherapies have long been studied in the treatment of aggression, impulsivity, and violent behavior, research specific to IED is limited. One double-blind study of 116 subjects with IED found that divalproex had no significant influence on aggression (Hollander et al. 2003). An open-label study of citalopram in subjects with either Cluster B personality disorder or IED ($N=8$) who displayed impulsive aggression found some benefit in the decrease of aggression and irritability (Reist et al. 2003). In case series, various other medications have shown promise. In one report, 5 of 10 subjects with IED had a favorable response to antidepressant monotherapy (venlafaxine or sertraline) and 7 of 10 subjects responded to either lithium or valproate (McElroy et al. 1998). A case series of 3 subjects reported response to sertraline (50–100 mg/day; Feder 1999). Other reports have suggested that propranolol (Jenkins and Maruta 1987) and clozapine (Kant et al. 2004) may provide benefit for IED.

In terms of psychotherapy for IED, there is some indication that insight-oriented psychotherapy and behavior therapy may be beneficial, but a small number of subjects ($N=4$) with IED reported no benefit from group, couples, or family therapy (McElroy et al. 1998).

The treatment research to date has enrolled primarily men with IED. No clear treatment for IED emerges from the available data, nor are there empirical data for gender differences in treatment responses.

PROBLEMATIC INTERNET USE

Problematic Internet use, also called compulsive computer use (Black et al. 1999; Potenza and Hollander 2002), is characterized by either irresistible preoccupations with use of the Internet or excessive use of the Internet for longer periods of time than planned (Shapira et al. 2003). The use or the preoccupation leads to clinically significant distress or impaired functioning (Shapira et al. 2003). Although problematic Internet use has been frequently discussed in the medical literature over the past several years, there have been no epidemiological studies of the disorder (Goldsmith and Shapira 2005). Clinical samples, however, suggest that the disorder may be somewhat more prevalent in men (Black et al. 1999; Shapira et al. 2000.

Clinical Characteristics

Early evidence suggests that the majority of people with problematic Internet use have some college education and are employed (Black et al. 1999; Shapira et al. 2000). Individuals with this disorder have reported a mean of 27 hours per week spent on the Internet for "nonessential" purposes (Black et al. 1999). Consequently, these individuals tend to report significant social impairment, financial difficulties, and vocational impairment (Shapira et al. 2000). Individuals with problematic Internet use report that the behavior allows for a distraction from other concerns, helps them feel more social, and relieves anxiety (Black et al. 1999). Preliminary studies suggest that clinical characteristics are largely similar in men and women.

Co-occurring Disorders

Co-occurring disorders are common in individuals with problematic Internet use. Lifetime mood (33%–85%), substance use (38%–70%), and impulse control (30%–38%) disorders appear to be the most common (Black et al. 1999; Shapira et al. 2000). Personality disorders also appear to be common (52%; Black et al. 1999).

Treatment

Individuals with problematic Internet use have reported favorable responses to paroxetine, mirtazapine, bupropion, lithium, and gabapentin as monotherapies (Shapira et al. 2000). A combination pharmacotherapy of mood stabilizer and antipsychotic drugs has also been reported as beneficial in individual cases (Shapira et al. 2000). There are, however, no published systematic studies evaluating pharmacotherapy in the treatment of problematic Internet use. Similarly, no systematic studies evaluating psychotherapy for this disorder have been published to date (Goldsmith and Shapira 2005).

KLEPTOMANIA

Kleptomania ("stealing madness") was formally designated a psychiatric disorder in DSM-III, and the core features are 1) a recurrent failure to resist an impulse to steal unneeded objects; 2) an increasing sense of tension before committing the theft; 3) an experience of pleasure, gratification, or release at the time of committing the theft; and 4) the stealing is not performed due to anger, vengeance, or psychotic symptoms (American Psychiatric Association 2000).

No national epidemiological studies of kleptomania have been performed. Prevalence studies of kleptomania in clinical samples suggest that the disorder is not uncommon. Studies have reported rates of kleptomania of 3.7% among depressed patients ($N=107$; Lejoyeux et al. 2002), 3.8% among patients with alcohol dependence ($N=79$; Lejoyeux et al. 1999), 2.1%–5% among patients with pathological gambling (Grant and Kim 2003), and 24% among patients with bulimia (Hudson et al. 1983). A recent study of psychiatric inpatients with multiple disorders ($N=204$) revealed that 7.8% ($n=16$) endorsed current kleptomania and 9.3% ($n=19$) met lifetime criteria (Grant et al. 2006). Studies using clinical samples have consistently reported that the majority (approximately two-thirds) of kleptomania patients are women (Grant and Kim 2002a; McElroy et al. 1991; Presta et al. 2002; Sarasalo et al. 1996).

Clinical Characteristics

Kleptomania usually appears first during late adolescence or early adulthood (McElroy et al. 1991). One study found that men with kleptomania are more likely to have a history of birth trauma (Presta et al. 2002). The course of illness for both men and women with kleptomania is generally chronic, with waxing and waning of symptoms. Individuals with kleptomania try unsuccessfully to stop. In one study, all participants reported increased urges to steal when trying to stop (Grant and Kim 2002a). The diminished ability to stop often leads to feelings of shame and guilt, reported in most subjects (77.3%; Grant and Kim 2002a). Of married subjects, fewer than half had disclosed their behavior to their spouses because of shame and guilt (Grant and Kim 2002a). Studies have found that men and women with kleptomania do not appear to differ on measures of impulsivity (Bayle et al. 2003; Grant and Kim 2002a).

Although people with kleptomania often steal various items from multiple places, most individuals steal from stores. In one study, 68.2% of patients reported that the value of stolen items had increased over time (Grant and Kim 2002a). Patients may keep, hoard, discard, gift, or return stolen items (McElroy et al. 1991). Many (64%–87%) have been apprehended at some time due to their behavior (McElroy et al. 1991), and 15%–23% report having been jailed (Grant and Kim 2002a). Although most patients who are apprehended report that their urges to steal diminish after the apprehension, symptom remission generally lasts only for a few days or weeks (McElroy et al. 1991).

Co-occurring Disorders

High rates of co-occurring psychiatric disorders have been found in individuals with kleptomania. Rates of lifetime co-occurring affective disorders range from 59% (Grant and Kim 2002a) to 100% (McElroy et al. 1991). The rate of co-occurring bipolar disorder has been reported as ranging from 9% (Grant and Kim 2002a) to 60% (McElroy et al. 1991). Studies have also found high lifetime rates of co-occurring anxiety disorders (60%–80%; McElroy et al. 1991, 1992), ICDs (20%–46%; Grant 2003), substance use disorders (23%–50%; Grant and Kim 2002a; McElroy et al. 1991), and eating disorders (60%; McElroy et al. 1991). Men with kleptomania appear less likely to have a co-occurring eating disorder or bipolar disorder (Presta et al. 2002), but they appear to have higher rates of co-occurring paraphilias (McElroy et al. 1991).

Treatment

Rigorous studies examining treatment response in kleptomania are few. Various medications have been studied in case reports or case series, and several medications have suggestive efficacies: fluoxetine, nortriptyline, trazodone, clonazepam, valproate, lithium, fluvoxamine, paroxetine, and topiramate (Grant and Potenza 2004; McElroy et al. 1991). The only formal trial of medication for kleptomania involved 10 subjects (3 men) in a 12-week, open-label study of naltrexone. At a mean dosage of 145 mg/day, medication resulted in a significant decline in the intensity of urges to steal, thoughts of stealing, and stealing behavior (Grant and Kim 2002c). The response to medication was similar for men and women.

Although multiple types of psychotherapies have been described in the treatment of kleptomania, no controlled trials exist in the literature. Forms of psychotherapy described in case reports as demonstrating success include psychoanalytic, insight-oriented, and behavioral psychotherapy (Goldman 1991; McElroy et al. 1991). Because no controlled trials of therapy for kleptomania have been published, the differential efficacies of these interventions in men and women with kleptomania have not been adequately evaluated.

TRICHOTILLOMANIA

Hair pulling is a grooming behavior that has often been reported to frequently occur in milder forms. Especially in childhood and early adolescence, episodes of recurrent hair pulling are common and are often accompanied by spontaneous remissions (Christenson and Mansueto 1999). Pathological hair pulling—trichotillomania—has been defined as repetitive, intentionally performed pulling that causes noticeable hair loss and results in clinically significant distress or functional impairment (American Psychiatric Association 2000).

The prevalence of trichotillomania is difficult to estimate in the absence of a consensually agreed-upon definition of the problem (e.g., 17%–23% of people with clinically meaningful hair pulling fail to meet DSM criteria requiring either tension immediately before pulling or pleasure, gratification, or relief when pulling) (Christenson et al. 1991a). However, current research suggests that the severe, debilitating form of hair pulling is fairly frequent, with estimated prevalence rates of 1%–3% (Christenson et al. 1991b).

Clinical Characteristics

Although hair pulling can begin at any age, the mean age at onset for trichotillomania is approximately 13 years (Christenson and Mansueto 1999; Schlosser et al. 1994a; Swedo and Leonard 1992). Although no prospective study has documented associated events at the onset of trichotillomania, the genesis of hair pulling has been associated with scalp disease and stressful life events (Christenson and Mansueto 1999). Hair pulling is subject to great fluctuations in severity, with worsening of symptoms often related to stress.

Trichotillomania has traditionally been thought of as a disorder predominantly affecting females (Cohen et al. 1995; Graber and Arndt 1993; Swedo and Leonard 1992). In children with trichotillomania, however, boys are found in numbers nearly equal to girls (Tay et al. 2004). A question exists whether trichotillomania is less common in men or whether men with trichotillomania avoid seeking professional help (see Chapter 17, "Overcoming Stigma and Barriers to Mental Health Treatment") or blame hair loss on male pattern baldness (Christenson et al. 1994b). Another theory posits that men may pull hair primarily from the beard and mustache and shaving may serve as a means by which men treat themselves (Christenson and Mansueto 1999). When men do have trichotillomania, however, the age at onset, severity, and related clinical features of the disorder appear similar to those found in women (Christenson et al. 1994b; Cohen et al. 1995).

Co-occurring Disorders

Individuals with trichotillomania report frequent co-occurring psychiatric disorders. Frequently co-occurring depression (39%–65%), generalized anxiety disorder (27%–32%), and substance abuse (15%–20%) have been reported (Christenson and Mansueto 1999; Swedo and Leonard 1992). Rates of obsessive-compulsive disorder (13%–23%) appear higher than found in the general population (1%–3%) (Cohen et al. 1995; Swedo and Leonard 1992). In addition, trichotillomania frequently co-occurs with nail biting and skin picking (Bohne et al. 2005). Co-occurring psychiatric disorders do not appear to differ for men with trichotillomania, although the numbers of subjects limit definitive statements on this issue.

Treatment

Medical and nonmedical treatments may be effective in the treatment of trichotillomania.

Antidepressant medications with serotonergic properties (e.g., clomipramine and other serotonin reuptake inhibitors) are in many cases effective in reducing hair pulling (O'Sullivan et al. 1999). As in the treatment of obsessive-compulsive disorder, D_2 dopamine receptor antagonists seem to be especially useful as augmenting agents with serotonin reuptake inhibitors (Stein and Hollander 1992). Lithium and the opiate antagonist naltrexone have also been reported to be helpful in some cases (O'Sullivan et al. 1999). Medications, however, are not effective with all patients, and drugs may lose their efficacy over time. Although the number of men enrolled in pharmacotherapy trials has been limited, men appear to respond as well as women to these interventions.

Men with trichotillomania appear to respond to behavioral treatment. Habit-reversal training is considered the first-line intervention for these problems (Azrin and Nunn 1973; Ninan et al. 2000b; Twohig et al. 2003). The intervention is a multicomponent treatment package that entails, among other techniques, self-monitoring of urges and behavior, incompatible-response training, and coping skills training. Awareness of habit occurrence and training in the use of alternative coping responses are viewed as critical treatment steps. Relaxation techniques and stimulus control procedures have also been successfully integrated into treatment (Barrios 1977).

COMPULSIVE BUYING

Originally termed "oniomania" by Kraepelin and Bleuler, compulsive buying has been described for more than 100 years (Christenson et al. 1994a). Although compulsive buying is not specifically recognized in DSM-IV-TR, the following diagnostic criteria have been proposed: 1) maladaptive preoccupation with or engagement in buying (evidenced by frequent preoccupation with or irresistible impulses to buy; frequent buying of items that are not needed or not affordable; or shopping for longer periods of time than intended); 2) preoccupations with buying or the buying itself leads to significant distress or impairment; and 3) the buying does not occur exclusively during hypomanic or manic episodes (McElroy et al. 1994).

Clinical Characteristics

The onset of compulsive buying generally occurs during late adolescence or early adulthood, although the full disorder may take several years to develop (Christenson et al. 1994a). Compulsive buying shows a female preponderance ranging from 80% to 92% in clinical samples (Christenson et al. 1994a; McElroy et al. 1994; Schlosser et al. 1994b) and is characterized by repetitive urges to shop that are most often unprovoked but may be triggered by being in stores. These urges may worsen during times of stress, emotional difficulties, or boredom. Urges are generally intrusive, and most patients attempt to resist them, although usually unsuccessfully. Buying often results in large debts, marital or family disruption, and legal consequences (Christenson et al. 1994a). The behavior is pleasurable and momentarily relieves the urges to shop, but guilt, shame, and embarrassment generally follow compulsive buying episodes.

A positive interaction with salespeople is often described as a motivating factor in compulsive buying. The items bought vary considerably and can include clothing, jewelry, books, and auto parts. Men often buy electronic or mechanical items. Most items are not used or removed from the packaging, and many are given away, returned, or hoarded (Christenson et al. 1994a).

Co-occurring Disorders

Rates of co-occurring mood disorders range from 28% to 95% (Christenson et al. 1994a; McElroy et al. 1994; Schlosser et al. 1994b), with the mood disorder often preceding the compulsive buying by at least 1 year (Christenson et al. 1994a). Lifetime histories of anxiety (41%–80%), substance use (30%–46%), eating (17%–35%), and impulse control (21%–40%) disorders are common (Christenson et al. 1994a; McElroy et al. 1994; Schlosser et al. 1994b).

Treatment

The effectiveness of pharmacotherapies in treating compulsive buying is beginning to be systematically investigated. Case reports and open-label studies have suggested that the following agents may be beneficial: nortriptyline, fluoxetine, bupropion, lithium, clomipramine, naltrexone, fluvoxamine, citalopram, and valproate (Black et al. 1997b; Koran et al. 2002; McElroy et al. 1994). Although a double-blind study using citalopram suggested the possible efficacy of SSRIs in treating the disorder (Koran et al. 2003), two double-blind fluvoxamine studies failed to show a difference between medication and placebo (Black et al. 2000; Ninan et al. 2000a).

There are no formal studies of psychotherapy for compulsive buying. Several case reports suggest possible effective psychotherapeutic interventions might include exposure and response prevention and supportive or insight-oriented psychotherapy (McElroy et al. 1994).

CONCLUSION

ICDs represent a clinically relevant group of disorders that appear relatively common and frequently go unrecognized. Treatments for these disorders are poorly understood given a paucity of controlled trials for behavioral and pharmacological interventions. When large samples of individuals with ICDs have been studied, gender-related differences have typically been identified. Future research into how men with ICDs differ from similarly diagnosed women should help advance prevention and treatment strategies for both men and women with these disorders.

KEY POINTS

- Certain ICDs—pathological gambling, CSB, IED—occur more commonly in men than in women.

- ICDs frequently co-occur with other psychiatric disorders, and general gender differences in patterns of psychopathology (in men, higher rates of externalizing disorders such as alcohol dependence and lower rates of internalizing disorders such as major depression) appear to transcend ICDs.

- Men with ICDs appear to respond as well as do women to both psychosocial and pharmacological treatments.

PRACTICE GUIDELINES

1. Screen men for ICDs, particularly those men who present with mental health concerns such as substance use and mood disorders.

2. Assess multiple domains of social and functional impairment in men with ICDs.

3. Consider both pharmacological and behavioral treatment interventions.

REFERENCES

Abbott MW, Volberg RA, Ronnberg S: Comparing the New Zealand and Swedish national surveys of gambling and problem gambling. J Gambl Stud 20:237–258, 2004

American Psychiatric Association: Diagnostic and Statistical Manual of Mental Disorders, 3rd Edition. Washington, DC, American Psychiatric Association, 1980

American Psychiatric Association: Diagnostic and Statistical Manual of Mental Disorders, 4th Edition, Text Revision. Washington, DC, American Psychiatric Association, 2000

Anglin MD, Hser YI, Booth MW: Sex differences in addict careers. Am J Drug Alcohol Abuse 13:253–280, 1987

Azrin NH, Nunn RG: Habit reversal: a method of eliminating nervous habits and tics. Behav Res Ther 11:619–628, 1973

Barrios BA: Cue-controlled relaxation in reduction of chronic nervous habits. Psychol Rep 41:703–706, 1977

Barth RJ, Kinder BN: The mislabeling of sexual impulsivity. J Sex Marital Ther 13:15–23, 1987

Bayle FC, Caci H, Millet B, et al: Psychopathology and comorbidity of psychiatric disorders in patients with kleptomania. Am J Psychiatry 160:1509–1513, 2003

Bechara A: Risky business: emotion, decision-making, and addiction. J Gambl Stud 19:23–51, 2003

Black DW: An open-label trial of bupropion in the treatment of pathologic gambling. J Clin Psychopharmacol 24:108–110, 2004

Black DW, Moyer T: Clinical features and psychiatric comorbidity of subjects with pathological gambling behavior. Psychiatr Serv 49:1434–1439, 1998

Black DW, Kehrberg LLD, Flumerfelt DL, et al: Characteristics of 36 subjects reporting compulsive sexual behavior. Am J Psychiatry 154:243–249, 1997a

Black DW, Monahan P, Gabel J: Fluvoxamine in the treatment of compulsive buying. J Clin Psychiatry 58:159–163, 1997b

Black DW, Belsare G, Schlosser S: Clinical features, psychiatric comorbidity, and health-related quality of life in persons reporting compulsive computer use behavior. J Clin Psychiatry 60:839–844, 1999

Black DW, Gabel J, Hansen J, et al: A double-blind comparison of fluvoxamine versus placebo in the treatment of compulsive buying disorder. Ann Clin Psychiatry 12:205–211, 2000

Blanco C, Petkova E, Ibanez A, et al: A pilot placebo-controlled study of fluvoxamine for pathological gambling. Ann Clin Psychiatry 14:9–15, 2002

Bohne A, Wilhelm S, Keuthen N: Pathologic hair pulling, skin picking, and nail biting. Ann Clin Psychiatry 17:227–232, 2005

Carnes P: Out of the Shadows: Understanding Sexual Addiction. Minneapolis, MN, CompCare, 1983

Chambers RA, Potenza MN: Neurodevelopment, impulsivity, and adolescent gambling. J Gambl Stud 19:53–84, 2003

Chambers RA, Taylor JR, Potenza MN: Developmental neurocircuitry of motivation in adolescence: a critical period of addiction vulnerability. Am J Psychiatry 160:1041–1052, 2003

Christenson GA, Mansueto CS: Trichotillomania: descriptive characteristics and phenomenology, in Trichotillomania. Edited by Stein DJ, Christenson GA, Hollander E. Washington, DC, American Psychiatric Press, 1999, pp 1–42

Christenson GA, Mackenzie TB, Mitchell JE: Characteristics of 60 adult chronic hair pullers. Am J Psychiatry 148:365–370, 1991a

Christenson GA, Pyle RL, Mitchell JE: Estimated lifetime prevalence of trichotillomania in college students. J Clin Psychiatry 52:415–417, 1991b

Christenson GA, Faber RJ, de Zwaan M, et al: Compulsive buying: descriptive characteristics and psychiatric comorbidity. J Clin Psychiatry 55:5–11, 1994a

Christenson GA, Mackenzie TB, Mitchell JE: Adult men and women with trichotillomania: a comparison of male and female characteristics. Psychosomatics 35:142–149, 1994b

Coccaro EF, Schmidt CA, Samuels JF, et al: Lifetime and 1-month prevalence rates of intermittent explosive disorder in a community sample. J Clin Psychiatry 65:820–824, 2004

Cohen LJ, Stein DJ, Simeon D, et al: Clinical profile, comorbidity, and treatment history in 123 hair pullers: a survey study. J Clin Psychiatry 56:319–326, 1995

Coleman E: Is your patient suffering from compulsive sexual behavior? Psychiatr Ann 22:320–325, 1992

Coleman E, Gratzer T, Nesvacil L, et al: Nefazodone and the treatment of nonparaphilic compulsive sexual behavior: a retrospective study. J Clin Psychiatry 61:282–284, 2000

Crisp BR, Thomas SA, Jackson AC, et al: Not the same: a comparison of female and male clients seeking treatment from problem gambling counseling services. J Gambl Stud 20:283–299, 2004

Crockford DN, el-Guebaly N: Psychiatric comorbidity in pathological gambling: a critical review. Can J Psychiatry 43:43–50, 1998

Cunningham-Williams RM, Cottler LB, Compton WM 3rd, et al: Taking chances: problem gamblers and mental health disorders. Results from the St. Louis Epidemiologic Catchment Area Study. Am J Public Health 88:1093–1096, 1998

Feder R: Treatment of intermittent explosive disorder with sertraline in 3 patients (letter). J Clin Psychiatry 60:195–196, 1999

Fiorillo CD, Tobler PN, Schultz W: Discrete coding of reward probability and uncertainty by dopamine neurons. Science 299:1898–1902, 2003

Galovski T, Blanchard EB, Veazey C: Intermittent explosive disorder and other psychiatric comorbidity among court-referred and self-referred aggressive drivers. Behav Res Ther 40:641–651, 2002

Getty HA, Watson J, Frisch GR: A comparison of depression and styles of coping in male and female GA members and controls. J Gambl Stud 16:377–391, 2000

Goldman M: Kleptomania: making sense of the nonsensical. Am J Psychiatry 148:986–996, 1991

Goldsmith TD, Shapira NA: Problematic Internet use, in Clinical Manual of Impulse Control Disorders. Edited by Hollander E, Stein DJ. Washington, DC, American Psychiatric Publishing, 2005, pp 291–308

Goodman A: What's in a name? terminology for designating a syndrome of driven sexual behavior. Sexual Addiction and Compulsivity 8:191–213, 1993

Gotestam KG, Johansson A: Characteristics of gambling and problem gambling in the Norwegian context: a DSM-IV–based telephone interview study. Addict Behav 28:189–197, 2003

Graber J, Arndt WB: Trichotillomania. Compr Psychiatry 34:340–346, 1993

Grant JE: Family history and psychiatric comorbidity in persons with kleptomania. Compr Psychiatry 44:437–441, 2003

Grant JE, Kim SW: A case of kleptomania and compulsive sexual behavior treated with naltrexone. Ann Clin Psychiatry 13:229–231, 2001a

Grant JE, Kim SW: Demographic and clinical features of 131 adult pathological gamblers. J Clin Psychiatry 62:957–962, 2001b

Grant JE, Kim SW: Clinical characteristics and associated psychopathology of 22 patients with kleptomania. Compr Psychiatry 43:378–384, 2002a

Grant JE, Kim SW: Gender differences in pathological gamblers seeking medication treatment. Compr Psychiatry 43:56–62, 2002b

Grant JE, Kim SW: An open label study of naltrexone in the treatment of kleptomania. J Clin Psychiatry 63:349–356, 2002c

Grant JE, Kim SW: Comorbidity of impulse control disorders in pathological gamblers. Acta Psychiatr Scand 108:207–213, 2003

Grant JE, Potenza MN: Impulse control disorders: clinical characteristics and pharmacological management. Ann Clin Psychiatry 16:27–34, 2004

Grant JE, Potenza MN: Escitalopram in the treatment of pathological gambling with co-occurring anxiety: an open-label study with double-blind discontinuation. Int Clin Psychopharmacol 21:203–209, 2006

Grant JE, Kushner MG, Kim SW: Pathological gambling and alcohol use disorder. Alcohol Res Health 26:143–150, 2002

Grant JE, Kim SW, Potenza MN, et al: Paroxetine treatment of pathological gambling: a multi-center randomized controlled trial. Int Clin Psychopharmacol 18:243–249, 2003

Grant JE, Levine L, Kim D, et al: Impulse control disorders in adult psychiatric inpatients. Am J Psychiatry 162:2184–2188, 2005

Grant JE, Potenza MN, Hollander E, et al: A multicenter investigation of the opioid antagonist nalmefene in the treatment of pathological gambling. Am J Psychiatry 163:303–312, 2006

Gupta R, Derevensky JL: Adolescent gambling behavior: a prevalence study and examination of the correlates associated with problem gambling. J Gambl Stud 14:319–345, 1998

Haller R, Hinterhuber H: Treatment of pathological gambling with carbamazepine (letter). Pharmacopsychiatry 27:129, 1994

Hodgins DC, Petry NM: Cognitive and behavioral treatments, in Pathological Gambling: A Clinical Guide to Treatment. Edited by Grant JE, Potenza MN. Washington, DC, American Psychiatric Publishing, 2004, pp 169–187

Hodgins DC, Currie SR, el-Guebaly N: Motivational enhancement and self-help treatments for problem gambling. J Consult Clin Psychol 69:50–57, 2001

Hollander E, Frenkel M, DeCaria C, et al: Treatment of pathological gambling with clomipramine (letter). Am J Psychiatry 149:710–711, 1992

Hollander E, DeCaria CM, Mari E, et al: Short-term, single-blind fluvoxamine treatment of pathological gambling. Am J Psychiatry 155:1781–1783, 1998

Hollander E, DeCaria CM, Finkell JN, et al: A randomized double-blind fluvoxamine/placebo crossover trial in pathologic gambling. Biol Psychiatry 47: 813–817, 2000

Hollander E, Tracy KA, Swann AC, et al: Divalproex in the treatment of impulsive aggression: efficacy in cluster B personality disorders. Neuropsychopharmacology 28:1186–1197, 2003

Hollander E, Pallanti S, Allen A, et al: Does sustained-release lithium reduce impulsive gambling and affective instability versus placebo in pathological gamblers with bipolar spectrum disorders? Am J Psychiatry 162:137–145, 2005

Hudson JI, Pope HG Jr, Jonas JM, et al: Phenomenologic relationship of eating disorders to major affective disorder. Psychiatry Res 9:345–354, 1983

Ibanez A, Blanco C, Donahue E, et al: Psychiatric comorbidity in pathological gamblers seeking treatment. Am J Psychiatry 158:1733–1735, 2001

Ibanez A, Blanco C, Moreryra P, et al: Gender differences in pathological gambling. J Clin Psychiatry 64:295–301, 2003

Jenkins SC, Maruta T: Therapeutic use of propranolol for intermittent explosive disorder. Mayo Clin Proc 62:204–214, 1987

Kafka MP, Prentky R: Fluoxetine treatment of nonparaphilic sexual addictions and paraphilias in men. J Clin Psychiatry 53:351–358, 1992

Kafka MP, Prentky R: Preliminary observations of DSM-III-R Axis I comorbidity in men with paraphilias and paraphilia-related disorders. J Clin Psychiatry 55:481–487, 1994

Kant R, Chalansani R, Chengappa KN, et al: The off-label use of clozapine in adolescents with bipolar disorder, intermittent explosive disorder, or posttraumatic stress disorder. J Child Adolesc Psychopharmacol 14:57–63, 2004

Kim SW, Grant JE: An open naltrexone treatment study of pathological gambling disorder. Int Clin Psychopharmacol 16:285–289, 2001a

Kim SW, Grant JE: Personality dimensions in pathological gambling disorder and obsessive-compulsive disorder. Psychiatry Res 104:205–212, 2001b

Kim SW, Grant JE, Adson DE, et al: Double-blind naltrexone and placebo comparison study in the treatment of pathological gambling. Biol Psychiatry 49:914–921, 2001

Kim SW, Grant JE, Adson DE, et al: A double-blind, placebo-controlled study of the efficacy and safety of paroxetine in the treatment of pathological gambling disorder. J Clin Psychiatry 63:501–507, 2002

Koran LM, Bullock KD, Hartston HJ, et al: Citalopram treatment of compulsive shopping: an open-label study. J Clin Psychiatry 63:704–708, 2002

Koran LM, Chuong HW, Bullock KD, et al: Citalopram for compulsive shopping disorder: an open-label study followed by double-blind discontinuation. J Clin Psychiatry 64:793–798, 2003

Ladd GT, Petry NM: Gender differences among pathological gamblers seeking treatment. Exp Clin Psychopharmacol 10:302–309, 2002

Laucht M, Becker K, El-Faddagh M, et al: Association of the DRD4 exon III polymorphism with smoking in fifteen-year-olds: a mediating role for novelty seeking? J Am Acad Child Adolesc Psychiatry 44:477–484, 2005

Legarda JJ, Babio R, Abreu JM: Prevalence estimates of pathological gambling in Seville (Spain). Br J Addict 87:767–770, 1992

Lejoyeux M, Feuche N, Loi S, et al: Study of impulse control disorders among alcohol-dependent patients. J Clin Psychiatry 60:302–305, 1999

Lejoyeux M, Arbaretaz M, McLoughlin M, et al: Impulse control disorders and depression. J Nerv Ment Dis 190:310–314, 2002

Linden RD, Pope HG Jr, Jonas JM: Pathological gambling and major affective disorder: preliminary findings. J Clin Psychiatry 47:201–203, 1986

Martins SS, Lobo DSS, Tavares H, et al: Pathological gambling in women: a review. Rev Hosp Clin Fac Med Sao Paulo 57:235–242, 2002

Martins SS, Tavares H, da Silva Lobo DS, et al: Pathological gambling, gender, and risk-taking behaviors. Addict Behav 29:1231–1235, 2004

McConaghy N, Armstrong MS, Blaszczynski A, et al: Controlled comparison of aversive therapy and imaginal desensitization in compulsive gambling. Br J Psychiatry 142:366–372, 1983

McConaghy N, Armstrong MS, Blaszczynski A: Expectancy, covert sensitization and imaginal desensitization in compulsive sexuality. Acta Psychiatr Scand 72:176–187, 1985

McConaghy N, Blaszczynski A, Frankova A: Comparison of imaginal desensitisation with other behavioural treatments of pathological gambling: a two to nine year follow-up. Br J Psychiatry 159:390–393, 1991

McCormick RA, Russo AM, Ramirez LF, et al: Affective disorders among pathological gamblers seeking treatment. Am J Psychiatry 41:215–218, 1984

McElroy SL, Pope HG Jr, Hudson JI, et al: Kleptomania: a report of 20 cases. Am J Psychiatry 148:652–657, 1991

McElroy SL, Hudson JI, Pope HG Jr, et al: The DSM-III-R impulse control disorders not elsewhere classified: clinical characteristics and relationship to other psychiatric disorders. Am J Psychiatry 149:318–327, 1992

McElroy SL, Keck PE Jr, Pope HG Jr, et al: Compulsive buying: a report of 20 cases. J Clin Psychiatry 55:242–248, 1994

McElroy SL, Soutullo CA, Beckman DA, et al: DSM-IV intermittent explosive disorder: a report of 27 cases. J Clin Psychiatry 59:203–210, 1998

New AS, Hazlett EA, Buchsbaum MS, et al: Blunted prefrontal cortical [18]fluorodeoxyglucose positron emission tomography response to meta-chlorophenylpiperazine in impulsive aggression. Arch Gen Psychiatry 59:621–629, 2002

Ninan PT, McElroy SL, Kane CP, et al: Placebo-controlled study of fluvoxamine in the treatment of patients with compulsive buying. J Clin Psychopharmacol 20:362–366, 2000a

Ninan PT, Rothbaum BO, Marsteller FA, et al: A placebo-controlled trial of cognitive-behavioral therapy and clomipramine in trichotillomania. J Clin Psychiatry 61:47–50, 2000b

Olvera RL: Intermittent explosive disorder: epidemiology, diagnosis and management. CNS Drugs 16:517–526, 2002

O'Sullivan RL, Christenson GA, Stein DJ: Pharmacotherapy of trichotillomania, in Trichotillomania. Edited by Stein DJ, Christenson GA, Hollander E. Washington, DC, American Psychiatric Press, 1999, pp 93–123

Pallanti S, Quercioli L, Sood E, et al: Lithium and valproate treatment of pathological gambling: a randomized single-blind study. J Clin Psychiatry 63:559–564, 2002a

Pallanti S, Rossi NB, Sood E, et al: Nefazodone treatment of pathological gambling: a prospective open-label controlled trial. J Clin Psychiatry 63:1034–1039, 2002b

Piazza NJ, Vrbka JL, Yeager RD: Telescoping of alcoholism in women alcoholics. Int J Addict 24:19–28, 1989

Pietrzak RH, Ladd GT, Petry NM: Disordered gambling in adolescents: epidemiology, diagnosis, and treatment. Paediatr Drugs 5:583–595, 2003

Posternak MA, Zimmerman M: Anger and aggression in psychiatric outpatients. J Clin Psychiatry 63:665–672, 2002

Potenza MN, Hollander E: Pathological gambling and impulse control disorders, in Neuropsychopharmacology: The 5th Generation of Progress. Edited by Coyle JT, Nemeroff C, Charney D, et al. Baltimore, MD, Lippincott Williams & Wilkins, 2002, pp 1725–1741

Potenza MN, Steinberg MA, McLaughlin SD, et al: Illegal behaviors in problem gambling: analysis of data from a gambling helpline. J Am Acad Psychiatry Law 28:389–403, 2000

Potenza MN, Steinberg MA, McLaughlin SD, et al: Gender-related differences in the characteristics of problem gamblers using a gambling helpline. Am J Psychiatry 158:1500–1505, 2001

Potenza MN, Xian H, Shah K, et al: Shared genetic contributions to pathological gambling and major depression in men. Arch Gen Psychiatry 62:1015–1021, 2005

Presta S, Marazziti D, Dell'Osso L, et al: Kleptomania: clinical features and comorbidity in an Italian sample. Compr Psychiatry 43:7–12, 2002

Proimos J, DuRant RH, Pierce JD, et al: Gambling and other risk behaviors among 8th- to 12th-grade students. Pediatrics 102:e23, 1998

Quadland MC: Compulsive sexual behavior: definition of a problem and an approach to treatment. J Sex Marital Ther 11:121–132, 1985

Raymond NC, Grant JE, Kim SW, et al: Treatment of compulsive sexual behavior with naltrexone and serotonin reuptake inhibitors. Int Clin Psychopharmacol 17:201–205, 2002

Raymond NC, Coleman E, Miner MH: Psychiatric comorbidity and compulsive/impulsive traits in compulsive sexual behavior. Compr Psychiatry 44:370–380, 2003

Reist C, Nakamura K, Sagart E, et al: Impulsive aggressive behavior: open-label treatment with citalopram. J Clin Psychiatry 64:81–85, 2003

Romer D (ed): Reducing Adolescent Risk: Toward an Integrated Approach. Thousand Oaks, CA, Sage, 2003

Roy A, Ardinoff B, Roehrich L, et al: Pathological gambling: a psychobiological study. Arch Gen Psychiatry 45:369–373, 1988

Saiz-Ruiz J, Blanco C, Ibanez A, et al: Sertraline treatment of pathological gambling: a pilot study. J Clin Psychiatry 66:28–33, 2005

Sarasalo E, Bergman B, Toth J: Personality traits and psychiatric and somatic morbidity among kleptomaniacs. Acta Psychiatr Scand 94:358–364, 1996

Schlosser S, Black DW, Blum N, et al: The demography, phenomenology, and family history of 22 persons with compulsive hair pulling. Ann Clin Psychiatry 6:147–152, 1994a

Schlosser S, Black DW, Repertinger S, et al: Compulsive buying: demography, phenomenology, and comorbidity in 46 subjects. Gen Hosp Psychiatry 16:205–212, 1994b

Shaffer HJ, Hall MN, Vander Bilt J: Estimating the prevalence of disordered gambling behavior in the United States and Canada: a research synthesis. Am J Public Health 89:1369–1376, 1999

Shah KR, Eisen SA, Xian H, et al: Genetic studies of pathological gambling: a review of methodology and analyses of data from the Vietnam Era Twin (VET) Registry. J Gambl Stud 21:179–203, 2005

Shapira NA, Goldsmith TD, Keck PE Jr, et al: Psychiatric features of individuals with problematic internet use. J Affect Disord 57:267–272, 2000

Shapira NA, Lessig MC, Goldsmith TD, et al: Problematic internet use: proposed classification and diagnostic criteria. Depress Anxiety 17:207–216, 2003

Slutske WS, Eisen S, True WR, et al: Common genetic vulnerability for pathological gambling and alcohol dependence in men. Arch Gen Psychiatry 57:666–673, 2000

Stein DJ, Hollander E: Low-dose pimozide augmentation of serotonin reuptake blockers in the treatment of trichotillomania. J Clin Psychiatry 53:123–126, 1992

Stein DJ, Hollander E, Anthony DT, et al: Serotonergic medications for sexual obsessions, sexual addictions, and paraphilias. J Clin Psychiatry 53:267–271, 1992

Stinchfield R: A comparison of gambling among Minnesota public school students in 1992, 1995 and 1998. J Gambl Stud 17:273–296, 2001

Swedo SE, Leonard HL: Trichotillomania: an obsessive compulsive spectrum disorder? Psychiatr Clin North Am 15:777–790, 1992

Tavares H, Zilberman ML, Beites FJ, et al: Gender differences in gambling progression. J Gambl Stud 17:151–159, 2001

Tay YK, Levy ML, Metry DW: Trichotillomania in childhood: case series and review. Pediatrics 113:e494–e498, 2004

Tsuang MT, Bar JL, Harley RM, et al: The Harvard Twin Study of Substance Abuse: what we have learned. Harv Rev Psychiatry 9:267–279, 2001

Twohig MP, Woods DW, Marcks BA, et al: Evaluating the efficacy of habit reversal: comparison with a placebo control. J Clin Psychiatry 64:40–48, 2003

Vitaro F, Arseneault L, Tremblay RE: Dispositional predictors of problem gambling in male adolescents. Am J Psychiatry 154:1769–1770, 1997

Volberg RA: The prevalence and demographics of pathological gamblers: implications for public health. Am J Public Health 84:237–240, 1994

Wagner FA, Anthony JC: From first drug use to drug dependence: developmental periods of risk for dependence upon marijuana, cocaine, and alcohol. Neuropsychopharmacology 26:479–488, 2002

Wallisch L: Gambling in Texas: 1992 Texas survey of adolescent gambling behavior. Austin, Texas Commission on Alcohol and Drug Abuse, 1993

Wong IL, So EM: Prevalence estimates of problem and pathological gambling in Hong Kong. Am J Psychiatry 160:1353–1354, 2003

World Health Organization: International Classification of Diseases, 9th Revision, Clinical Modification. Ann Arbor, MI, Commission on Professional and Hospital Activities, 1978

Wynne Resources: Adolescent Gambling and Problem Gambling in Alberta. Edmonton, AB, Canada, Alberta Alcohol and Drug Abuse Commission, 1996

Zimmerman M, Breen RB, Posternak MA: An open-label study of citalopram in the treatment of pathological gambling. J Clin Psychiatry 63:44–48, 2002

10

POSTTRAUMATIC STRESS DISORDER

DOLORES VOJVODA, M.D.
STEVEN SOUTHWICK, M.D.

Case Vignette

At age 18, Owen enlisted in the army hoping to become a career soldier. After basic and specialized training he was sent to Vietnam in 1969 as a gunman on a helicopter. He flew numerous missions, which were almost always dangerous. While retrieving the wounded and the dead from deep inside enemy territory, he often came under enemy fire. The crew of his helicopter developed a close relationship, depending on each other for survival. During one of the missions the helicopter was hit, caught fire, and crashed into the jungle. Owen was injured but escaped the burning helicopter. He helped pull several soldiers from the blazing debris but in the process saw some of his friends burn to death.

After his return to the United States, Owen had a hard time adjusting to civilian life. He frequently encountered antiwar sentiment, and his family did not understand the experiences he had been through. He felt emotionally numb and distant from his wife and parents, unable to relate to the routine events of everyday life. The helicopter crash constantly replayed in his mind, and he could not sleep for more than an hour without bolting out of bed to check for the enemy. Even with a loaded gun under his pillow, he did not feel safe. Owen would get irritated by small things. This reaction surprised his family, who knew him as a soft-spoken person.

For years after returning from Vietnam, Owen worked at an aircraft manufacturing plant. Unfortunately, the frequent sound and sight of helicopters served as painful and vivid reminders of his Vietnam traumas. In order to deal with his constant vigilance, irritability, and insomnia, he started to drink excessively. Although drinking helped him to sleep, it only aggravated his irritability. Owen and his wife had two children in quick succession, but Owen participated little in their upbringing. He was unable to deal with the everyday stresses of family life and would often isolate himself in the cellar. With the passage of time, his posttraumatic symptoms failed to improve. His days consisted of going to work and then drinking heavily at night so that he could pass out and get a few hours of sleep. At night while in bed, he would often smell burning flesh, and memories of the helicopter crash would overwhelm him. When he was able to sleep, he frequently dreamed about the crash and sometimes thrashed about and unintentionally struck his wife, who was sleeping next to him. At other times, he would dream he was under enemy fire and would reach under his pillow for his gun. Eventually his wife removed the ammunition from his gun but could not convince Owen to remove the gun from their bedroom. He found a partial solution for the olfactory flashbacks: he started applying Vicks VapoRub under his nose immediately before he went to bed, and this tactic helped reduce some of the vivid memories. However, nightmares continued unchanged. At one point he heard a rumor that Vicks VapoRub production was going to be discontinued, so he wrote to the company. The company reassured him that they planned to continue making the product and sent him a large case of it.

Owen did not seek treatment for nearly 20 years. He finally saw a psychiatrist for his alcoholism and his inability to function at work or at home. By that time, his wife had left him twice for several months at a time. She finally gave him an ultimatum: "Get better or I am leaving for good." Initially he presented for treatment of the alcoholism, but it quickly became clear to his psychiatrist that Owen was also tormented by symptoms of posttraumatic stress disorder (PTSD). A slow recovery process began and involved several years and multiple inpatient hospitalizations for Owen to achieve full sobriety. Through the use of several modalities of psychotherapy and with medications, Owen experienced a reduction in his symptoms. His insomnia decreased so that he was able to sleep for several hours at night, and he experienced fewer nightmares. Profound feelings of guilt related to the helicopter crash diminished, and he was gradually able to talk about his experiences. As his depression resolved, Owen started enjoying activities with his family. He became more active in raising his children, and his relationship with his wife improved. However, some symptoms did not resolve. Owen still liked to be alone and felt uncomfortable in large gatherings. He had very few social contacts and continued to apply Vicks VapoRub under his nose every night. Although Owen continued to experience PTSD symptoms, the reduction in their intensity allowed him to rejoin his family and devote his energy to supporting his wife and children.

HISTORICAL BACKGROUND

The negative impact of exposure to traumatic events has been recognized and described for centuries. In 1952, DSM-I (American Psychiatric Association 1952) included the diagnosis "gross stress reaction" in an attempt to classify psychologically distraught survivors of trauma. According to DSM-I, this reaction developed after an exposure to "severe physical demands or extreme emotional stress, such as in combat or in civilian catastrophe" (p. 40). However, DSM-I did not identify the symptom criteria needed to diagnose gross stress reaction. It was not until 1980, with the publication of DSM-III, that the diagnosis of PTSD was introduced and the three clusters of PTSD symptoms (reexperiencing, avoidance, and hyperarousal) were identified (American Psychiatric Association 1980).

PREVALENCE AND TYPES OF TRAUMA IN MEN

Traumatic events are highly prevalent in the general population. Three well-conducted epidemiological studies provide estimates of prevalence and types of trauma experienced by adult residents of the United States. In the National Comorbidity Survey (NCS), 2,800 men and 3,000 women ages 15–54 were asked about 12 specific types of trauma (Kessler et al. 1995), and 61% of men and 51% of women reported at least one traumatic event during their lifetime. Of those who had been traumatized, most (56.4% of men vs. 48.7% of women) had experienced more than one trauma. More men than women reported having been involved in a life-threatening accident (25.0% vs. 13.8%); having experienced a fire, flood, or natural disaster (18.9% vs. 15.2%); or having witnessed someone being badly injured or killed (35.6% vs. 15.2%). Men were also more likely to have been physically attacked (11.1% vs. 6.9%); been threatened with a weapon (19.0% vs. 6.8%); or experienced combat (6.4% vs. 0.0%). Women, on the other hand, reported greater rates of rape (9.2% of women vs. 0.7% of men); sexual molestation (12.3% vs. 2.8%); and childhood physical abuse (4.8% vs. 3.2%) than did men.

In the 1996 Detroit Area Survey of Trauma, in which 2,180 adults ages 18–45 were interviewed, Breslau's expanded inventory of qualifying traumatic events detected an even higher (90%) prevalence of lifetime exposure to trauma (Breslau et al. 1998). Men experienced an average of 5.3 distinct traumatic events as compared with 4.3 in women. The nature of traumatic events in men compared with women was consistent with Kessler's study.

Finally, in a study of 1,000 adults ages 18–90, Norris (1992) reported a 74% overall lifetime prevalence rate for exposure to trauma in men and a 65% rate in women. Consistent with the other two studies, more men had experienced physical assault, motor vehicle accidents, and combat, whereas more women had experienced sexual assault or molestation. These data consistently indicate that the rates of trauma are high in the United States and that men tend to experience a greater number of lifetime traumas than do women.

STRESSOR CRITERION

The first issue in diagnosing PTSD involves determining whether the individual has been exposed to a traumatic event. The definition of a *qualifying traumatic event* has evolved since its introduction into the psychiatric nosology: in DSM-III, a qualifying traumatic stressor was identified as an event that would cause "significant symptoms of distress in almost everyone" (p. 238), whereas in DSM-III-R it was described as being "outside the range of usual human experience" (American Psychiatric Association 1987, p. 250). The DSM-IV-TR definition of a qualifying traumatic stressor is divided into two criteria (American Psychiatric Association 2000). The first, Criterion A1, requires that "the person experienced, witnessed, or was confronted with an event…that involved actual or threatened death or serious injury, or a threat to the physical integrity of self or others" (p. 467). Criterion A2 requires that "the person's response involved intense fear, helplessness, or horror" (p. 467). This two-part definition is a significant departure from previous DSM editions because it stresses the importance of the subjective experience of the trauma and acknowledges that similar events evoke varying responses from different people. The subjective experience of a trauma is believed to be a key factor in determining whether a person develops PTSD and might explain why some individuals, even after exposure to severely traumatic events, do not develop symptoms of PTSD (Breslau et al. 1991; Davidson et al. 1991). For example, it is possible that some individuals experience a traumatic event without feeling loss of control but instead master the event and, as a result, feel invigorated and triumphant rather than victimized and vulnerable (Harvey and Yehuda 1999).

It is not known whether women have a greater vulnerability to the PTSD effects of trauma than men. Vulnerability might be influenced by differences in the memory and appraisal of the trauma. For example, men rated motor vehicle accidents less frightening than did women (Ehlers et al. 1998) and described childhood sexual assault as more neutral or positive and less negative than did females (Rind et al. 1998). It is also possible that fewer men than women respond to the same type of trauma with intense fear, helplessness, and horror—and that some men thus fail to meet Criterion A2—despite the fact that they develop symptoms of PTSD.

TRAUMATIC STRESS RESPONSE SYMPTOMS

The same pattern of symptoms emerges following a variety of traumas, such as natural disasters (McFarlane 1988), accidents (Schottenfeld and Cullen 1986), and combat (Foa 1997). Immediately following a traumatic event, most people feel distressed and have frequent and intense intrusive thoughts about the trauma. With time, the intensity of the memories decreases and less frequently preoccupies the survivor. In a substantial number of individuals, however, traumatic stress can continue to have profound and chronic effects on psychological, biological, social, and spiritual life (van der Kolk and McFarlane 1996). The specific types of responses that mark PTSD are discussed below:

- *Reexperiencing*. Reexperiencing symptoms manifest in the form of repeated traumatic memories, flashbacks, and nightmares. Traumatic memories and flashbacks may recur spontaneously or be triggered by trauma-related stimuli. Traumatic memories are typically unwanted and intrude against the person's will. Intrusive memories can remain painful, arousing, and vivid for decades. Survivors often report that, despite the passage of time, memories and images of trauma feel "as if they happened just yesterday." Flashbacks, in which the survivor acts or feels as though the traumatic event is recurring in the present, are less common than intrusive memories but tend to be extremely upsetting. Trauma-related nightmares can last for a lifetime, as documented by World War II and Holocaust survivors, and these nightmares can markedly disrupt a person's life (Kuch and Cox 1992). Trauma survivors with PTSD often report sleep deprivation, daytime fatigue, and irritability. Some even dread going to sleep for fear of having another trauma-related nightmare. The reexperiencing symptoms and internal and external cues that symbolize or resemble an aspect of the traumatic event often cause intense psychological distress and physiological arousal.

- *Avoidance*. Individuals with PTSD avoid situations, people, and conversations that are reminiscent of the traumatic event or that cause excessive arousal. As a result, they gradually live increasingly restricted lives. Symptoms of avoidance and emotional numbing sometimes dominate the clinical picture, especially in a more chronic form of PTSD (van der Kolk and McFarlane 1996). Many trauma survivors with PTSD feel detached from others and unable to form close relationships. They tend to avoid loving relationships, particularly if they have witnessed or have been involved in the traumatic death of others. Some researchers believe that these individuals are afraid to lose another person. Clinicians also have suggested that for individuals with PTSD, feeling emotionally numb is preferable to feeling the grief and torment that accompany past or potential future tragedies or deaths. Many trauma survivors with PTSD also seem unable to derive a sense of pleasure from most activities and live with a sense of a foreshortened future. Avoidance and the tendency to retreat from life often severely influence their psychosocial functioning.

- *Hyperarousal.* PTSD is in large part a disorder of arousal. Increased arousal is characterized by disturbance of sleep, difficulties with concentration and memory, irritability, hypervigilance, and exaggerated startle response. It is as though the survivor is reacting to a current danger, even when no real danger is present. Individuals sleep "with one eye open," startle to common everyday noises, and remain vigilant and on guard. The hypervigilant trauma survivor tends to have difficulty in busy places and in crowds, positions himself or herself in a manner that allows for monitoring of the environment (e.g., sitting with his or her back to the wall), does not like surprises, and sees potential danger in many situations. Often survivors will compulsively check their environment to ensure safety (e.g., multiple locks and alarms at home). Persistent irritability and anger tend to accompany hypervigilance and can become the symptoms that cause the greatest disruption in social, occupational, and family functioning.

The manifestation of core PTSD symptoms does not differ between genders. However, men more often exhibit aggression or violent impulses, whereas women are more likely to be withdrawn and dysthymic (Jannoff-Buman and Frieze 1987). These differences are evident in traumatized children, with boys demonstrating higher rates of externalizing disorders (e.g., oppositional defiant disorder) compared with girls (Ackerman et al. 1998). There is also evidence that women report a greater number of reexperiencing symptoms than do men (Zlotnick et al. 2001).

PREVALENCE OF POSTTRAUMATIC STRESS DISORDER

The earliest community prevalence estimates of PTSD were generated from the Epidemiologic Catchment Area study. Lifetime prevalence estimates of 1.0% in St. Louis (Helzer et al. 1987) and 1.3% in North Carolina (Davidson et al. 1991) were observed. Later studies found higher rates of PTSD in the general population. In the NCS (Kessler et al. 1995), the estimated lifetime prevalence of PTSD was 5.0% for men and 10.4% for women. In this study, 8.2% of men exposed to trauma developed PTSD as opposed to 20.4% of exposed women. Similarly, Norris (1992) reported that 6% of men and 9% of women met criteria for lifetime PTSD. Finally, the National Vietnam Veterans Readjustment Study (Kulka et al. 1990) found that 30% of 3.1 million Vietnam veterans developed PTSD at some time after the war, and 15% had PTSD 15 years after the war.

RISK FACTORS FOR DEVELOPMENT OF POSTTRAUMATIC STRESS DISORDER

The most frequently occurring traumas, such as witnessing someone being injured or killed, life-threatening accidents, or natural disasters, result in PTSD in less than 10% of victims (Kessler et al. 1999). Traumas such as rape, child abuse, or combat are more likely to result in PTSD (Kessler et al. 1995). Rape is the most likely cause of PTSD in both men and women (Kessler et al. 1995). The national U.S. study of rape prevalence and PTSD (Kilpatrick et al. 1992) found that 31% of rape victims developed PTSD sometime after the event. These data are consistent with the lifetime prevalence of 32% observed in a national survey of women (Resnick et al. 1993). In the NCS (Kessler et al. 1995), of those persons who had been raped, the rate of lifetime PTSD was 65% for men and 46% for women. In the National Vietnam Veterans Readjustment Study (Kulka et al. 1990), the lifetime prevalence of combat-related PTSD was 30% in male veterans. Hyer et al. (1996) diagnosed PTSD in 39% of 125 World War II and Korean War veterans. Disasters are likely to cause lifetime PTSD in 13% of cases (McFarlane and Papay 1992). Motor vehicle crashes result in a 23% rate of lifetime PTSD (Norris 1992). Several other factors play a role in how people respond to trauma.

In a meta-analysis of risk factors for PTSD in adults, a consistent pattern was observed for women to be at higher risk than men for developing civilian trauma–related PTSD (Brewin et al. 2000). Data indicate that the risk associated with female gender begins in childhood and continues throughout middle adulthood (Breslau et al. 1997). Other risk factors include social, educational, and intellectual disadvantage; childhood abuse; and family psychiatric history (Bremner et al. 1993; Davidson et al. 1991). Resick (2001a) suggested that early traumatic childhood experiences, as well as poor modeling by parents, may influence a person's ability to cope with stressors later in life. The presence of preexisting mental health problems is one of the most powerful variables influencing the risk for PTSD (Kulka et al. 1990; Ruch and Leon 1983); McFarlane (1989) found that the presence of preexisting illnesses better predicted posttraumatic symptoms than the degree of exposure to trauma.

In general, women are twice as likely as men to develop PTSD after a trauma. However, male victims of rape are an exception to this pattern. NCS data indicate that men have an increased likelihood of developing PTSD associated with rape (65% in men vs. 46% in women; Kessler et al. 1995). This pattern is especially strong in survivors of adult sexual assault. Adult male sexual victims are more likely to have been assaulted by multiple perpetrators and to have been beaten during the assault (Kaufman et al. 1980). The masculine gender role may additionally contribute to the feelings of helplessness, vulnerability, and incompetence in men who are raped (Eagly 1987). These factors may contribute to the high PTSD rates among sexually abused men (Tolin and Foa 2002).

COURSE OF ILLNESS

After a traumatic event, most people will develop some trauma-related symptoms that may include a range of emotional, cognitive, physical, and behavioral responses. PTSD symptom rates have been reported to be as high as 94% in rape victims 1 week after the trauma (Foa et al. 1991). However, most people will recover from the effects of the trauma. Kessler et al. (1995) found that 60% of victims recovered from early PTSD, and most recovered within 1 year of the traumatic event (gender and type-of-trauma differences were not reported). Similar recovery or remission rates were found in the National Vietnam Veterans Readjustment Study, in which the difference between lifetime and current (15 years after the trauma) combat-related PTSD rates in men were 30% and 15.2%, respectively. Predicting PTSD from early symptoms is difficult, and it is often challenging for clinicians to identify who is most likely to remain symptomatic. Known predictors include early presence of dissociative symptoms, depression, and elevated autonomic (e.g., heart rate) responses to the traumatic event (McFarlane 1999). Early identification and treatment are important because delayed treatment predicts poor response to treatment (Foa 1997; Kessler et al. 1995) and is a risk factor for chronicity in both men and women.

A small subgroup of patients will have delayed-onset PTSD (onset 6 months or longer after the trauma), and most will have a variable course of illness. Individuals who are doing well at one time may find that stressors (often unrelated to the trauma) reactivate their symptoms (Schnurr et al. 2002). In veterans, reactivation of symptoms is often precipitated by anniversary reactions (Morgan et al. 1999).

CO-OCCURRING DISORDERS

In PTSD, the rates of psychiatric co-occurrence are very high. Kessler et al. (1995) found that 88% of men and 79% of women diagnosed with PTSD also met criteria for one or more co-occurring psychiatric disorders. For men, the most commonly co-occurring disorders include alcohol use disorder (52%), major depressive disorder (48%), conduct disorder (43%), drug use disorder (35%), and phobias (28%–31%). Personality disorders are also common in people with PTSD. The National Vietnam Veterans Readjustment Study (Kulka et al. 1990) reported a rate of 31% of antisocial personality disorder among veterans with PTSD. NCS data indicate antisocial personality disorder in 43% of men and 15% of women with PTSD (Kessler et al. 1995). Other personality disorders (borderline, obsessive-compulsive, avoidant, and paranoid personality disorders) were reported to be more prevalent than antisocial personality in a sample of male Vietnam combat veterans (Southwick et al. 1993b). Several factors, including pretrauma features of borderline personality disorder, trauma exposure, and PTSD symptoms, contribute to development of borderline personality disorder symptoms in traumatized male and female veterans (Axelrod et al. 2005).

Relatively few people have only PTSD. Most people with PTSD have one or more additional psychiatric disorders. Clinicians should consider co-occurring disorders when developing treatment plans for patients with PTSD.

Substance Use and Symptoms of Posttraumatic Stress Disorder

Trauma survivors with both PTSD and substance use problems constitute more than half of the individuals (52%) diagnosed with PTSD (Kessler et al. 1995). High rates of co-occurrence between PTSD and substance use disorders suggest that these disorders are functionally related to one other (Jacobsen et al. 2001). Most published data support a model in which substance use follows or parallels traumatic exposure and the development of PTSD (Keane et al. 1988). In a longitudinal study of traumatized civilians, Chilcoat and Breslau (1998) found increased risk for development of a substance use disorder specifically in patients with PTSD but not in trauma-exposed subjects who did not develop PTSD. Individuals with PTSD may use substances to self-medicate or temporarily quiet symptoms related to central nervous system overactivation, such as hyperarousal, irritability, and insomnia. Consistent with this notion, male combat veterans report that central nervous system depressants (e.g., alcohol, cannabis, opioids, and benzodiazepines) acutely improve PTSD symptoms (Bremner et al. 1996).

Complex Posttraumatic Stress Disorder

Herman (1992) suggested that many PTSD patients with comorbid personality disorders would be better understood and served by a more comprehensive diagnosis called *complex posttraumatic stress disorder*. Herman (1992) proposed that when men and women experience prolonged or repeated trauma, usually sexual or physical abuse starting in childhood, the traumatic effects can be so wide-ranging that the person appears to have a personality disorder. Herman argued that the diagnostic criteria for "simple" PTSD do not capture the full range of symptoms (e.g., impaired affect modulation; self-destructive and impulsive behavior; somatic complaints; feelings of ineffectiveness, shame, despair, or hopelessness; feeling permanently damaged) that these individuals experience. The symptoms of complex PTSD are listed in DSM-IV-TR as associated features of PTSD.

BIOLOGY OF POSTTRAUMATIC STRESS DISORDER

PTSD is associated with multiple neurobiological alterations or abnormalities. Trauma survivors with PTSD, as a group, have shown exaggerated reactivity of the sympathetic nervous system in response to current stressors when compared with healthy control subjects (Southwick et al. 1999). When compared with control subjects, subjects with PTSD have exaggerated increases in heart rate, blood pressure, norepinephrine, and epinephrine in response to traumatic reminders administered in the laboratory; elevated 24-hour urine excretion of norepinephrine and epinephrine; elevated 24-hour plasma norepinephrine; reduced platelet α_2-adrenergic receptor number; increased subjective, behavioral, physiological, and biochemical (increased plasma methoxyhydroxyphenylglycol) responses to intravenous yohimbine (an α_2-adrenoreceptor antagonist); blunted response to clonidine; and altered yohimbine-induced cerebral blood flow (Bremner et al. 1997; Friedman et al. 1995;

Perry et al. 1987; Southwick et al. 1993a; Yehuda and McFarlane 1997). Norepinephrine is important in orienting behaviors, selective attention, vigilance, and the encoding and consolidation of emotional memories (Southwick et al. 1997, 1999). Dysregulation of noradrenergic systems in PTSD may contribute to symptoms of reexperiencing and hyperarousal (Southwick et al. 1997). Potential gender differences in the magnitude of changes in the noradrenergic system have not been well researched. In a study of healthy subjects, men were found to have greater urinary norepinephrine and epinephrine responses to mental stress compared with premenopausal women (Frankenhaeuser et al. 1978).

Abnormalities in hypothalamic-pituitary-adrenal (HPA) axis functioning among trauma survivors with PTSD have been reported. Studies have described alterations in 24-hour urine excretion, 24-hour plasma cortisol levels, lymphocyte glucocorticoid receptor number, cortisol response to dexamethasone, adrenocorticotropic hormone (ACTH) response to corticotropin-releasing factor (CRF), and β-endorphin and ACTH response to metyrapone, as well as adrenal androgen abnormalities (Rasmusson et al. 2004; Yehuda et al. 2004). Elevated resting cerebrospinal fluid levels of CRF have been reported in two studies of male combat veterans with chronic PTSD (Baker et al. 1999; Bremner et al. 1997). Unfortunately, there is a lack of studies examining gender differences in HPA axis function in PTSD.

Neurocognitive and brain imaging studies comparing individuals with PTSD and individuals without psychiatric disorders have reported that subjects with PTSD show biased attention to negative and potentially dangerous information, reductions in hippocampal volume and function, exaggerated amygdalar responses to stressful cues, and stress-induced reduction in prefrontal cortical metabolism (Bremner et al. 1995).

Overall, data support multiple neurobiological models related to PTSD, including stress sensitization, enhanced encoding and consolidation of emotional memory, fear conditioning, and possible structural and functional abnormalities in neurobiological systems involved in response to fear. In general, there are no known gender differences regarding most biological factors of PTSD. However, neuroendocrine responses to fear and trauma may well differ between men and women, and research has suggested that women may be at greater risk for developing PTSD because of greater variability in hormonal responses to stress (Rasmusson and Friedman 2002).

ASSESSMENT AND TREATMENT

Assessment

Owen's case illustrates the complexity of symptoms clinicians often encounter when treating men with PTSD. A careful assessment of trauma symptoms is important in determining the most appropriate treatment. The clinician should be guided by the temporal presentation of PTSD symptoms (acute, chronic, delayed), their severity, the degree of functional impairment, and the presence of co-occurring psychiatric illnesses. Gender differences in response to treatment have not been studied systematically. Thus the extent to which gender predicts or influences treatment outcome is not well understood (Foa et al. 2000). Nonetheless, men with PTSD often present differently from women with the disorder (e.g., in patterns of co-occurring disorders), and clinicians should be cognizant of these differences and their potential impact on treatment.

Pharmacological Treatments

Pharmacotherapy is an important component of treating PTSD. Patients exhibit abnormalities in several neurobiological systems, and medications that target these symptoms often generate clinical improvement. Additionally, PTSD frequently co-occurs with other psychiatric disorders (e.g., depression and other anxiety disorders) that frequently respond to medication treatment.

When choosing a medication for treatment of PTSD, the clinician should

- choose a medication whose actions might target the biological abnormalities associated with PTSD;
- select a drug based on proven efficacy against a targeted symptom, cluster of symptoms, or co-occurring disorder;
- monitor the effect of medication and readjust the dosage to optimize therapeutic effect and minimize side effects; and
- augment treatment with an additional drug or switch to a different medication if the patient remains symptomatic after an adequate therapeutic trial (Friedman et al. 2000).

Although many patients will experience a reduction in their symptoms with currently available medications, most will need psychotherapy to achieve a more complete improvement of PTSD symptoms (Friedman et al. 2000).

Selective Serotonin Reuptake Inhibitors

Multiple studies have implicated serotonin abnormalities in PTSD patients (Friedman and Southwick 1995; Southwick et al. 2005). In addition, serotonin has also been associated with illnesses that are frequently comorbid with PTSD (e.g., depression, anxiety, impulsivity, substance abuse). Several selective serotonin reuptake inhibitors (SSRIs) have been studied in the treatment of PTSD: sertraline (Brady et al. 2000; Davidson et al. 2001), paroxetine (Marshall et al. 2001), fluoxetine (Connor et al. 1999; Martenyi et al. 2002; van der Kolk et al. 1994), and fluvoxamine (Marmar et al. 1996). These studies have each found global improvements and reductions in all three PTSD clusters of symptoms: reexperiencing, arousal, and avoidance (including numbing). The SSRIs also have been effective in treating symptoms associated with PTSD such as impulsivity, depression, suicidal thoughts, obsessive thinking, and substance abuse. Currently, the only two medications approved by the U.S. Food and Drug Administration for the treatment of PTSD are sertraline and paroxetine.

A gender-specific analysis of data from a placebo-controlled sertraline study in the treatment of PTSD found that following a 12-week trial, women responded more robustly to sertraline than did men (Brady and Farfel 1999), both in PTSD and in depressive symptomatology. However, after subjects completed the third, 28-week, double-blind, placebo-controlled maintenance phase of this study (which enrolled subjects who had completed the original 12-week, placebo-controlled phase and the 24-week, open-label continuation phase), no difference was found in the prophylactic benefit of sertraline on recurrence of PTSD between men and women (Davidson et al. 2001). One possible explanation for this finding is that men may need longer antidepressant trials before full benefit of the medication is exhibited. A large paroxetine study (Marshall et al. 2001), however, showed equal effectiveness on PTSD symptoms in men and women.

Monoamine Oxidase Inhibitors

A comprehensive review of monoamine oxidase inhibitor (MAOI) trials (Southwick et al. 1994) found moderate to good global improvement in patients with PTSD, especially in reexperiencing symptoms and insomnia. No improvement was found in avoidant or hyperarousal symptoms. Most studies included both men and women. A study by Kosten et al. (1991) compared phenelzine, imipramine, and placebo in a group of male combat veterans, and phenelzine was superior to imipramine in the degree and range of improvement. The use of MAOIs has been traditionally limited because of potential side effects, particularly in patients who continue to use substances of abuse.

Tricyclic Antidepressants

The most frequently studied tricyclic antidepressants (TCAs) for the treatment of PTSD have been imipramine, amitriptyline, and desipramine (Davidson et al. 1990; Kosten et al. 1991; Reist et al. 1989). Although these antidepressants are effective for treatment of depression and anxiety, they show mixed and generally modest improvement of PTSD symptoms. The TCAs appear to reduce reexperiencing and avoidance symptoms but do so less efficiently than SSRIs or MAOIs. Many patients do not tolerate TCAs. In men, imipramine and amitriptyline have shown positive results in treatment of PTSD, whereas desipramine has had negative results (Reist et al. 1989).

Antiadrenergic Agents

Clonidine, guanfacine, and propranolol reduce reexperiencing and hyperarousal symptoms in PTSD patients (Horrigan 1996; Kolb et al. 1984; Pitman et al. 2002). A pilot study by Pitman et al. (2002) found that propranolol may prevent subsequent PTSD when administered after acute trauma. However, randomized clinical trials are needed to investigate the efficacy of these medications.

Benzodiazepines

Although the efficacies and tolerabilities of benzodiazepines in the treatment of PTSD have not been well established, these agents are frequently prescribed for reduction of anxiety and treatment of insomnia in PTSD patients. However, data suggest that benzodiazepines do not improve the three PTSD symptom clusters (Braun et al. 1990; Friedman et al. 2000). Moreover, prescribing these medications for PTSD patients carries risks of tolerance, dependence, and serious withdrawal symptoms; the high rates of co-occurring substance use disorders in PTSD patients, particularly men, further limit the utility of benzodiazepines.

Antipsychotics

Antipsychotic medications should be reserved for patients with PTSD who are not responding to other medications and those patients who exhibit psychotic symptoms (Friedman et al. 2000). Case reports involving treatment with risperidone and quetiapine (Leyba and Wampler 1998; Sattar et al. 2002) and preliminary controlled trials of risperidone in male combat veterans (Bartzokis et al. 2005; Hamner et al. 2003) suggest that these medications might be effective in reducing symptoms from the reexperiencing and the hyperarousal clusters. However, further research is needed to empirically validate the efficacies and tolerabilities of these drugs.

Psychological Treatments

Exposure-based treatments were first used for treatment of phobias and obsessive-compulsive disorder and later successfully applied for treatment of PTSD.

In *systematic desensitization*, the therapist and patient generate a hierarchy of fear cues related to the traumatic event (Wolpe 1958). The patient is trained in relaxation skills and is then exposed to fear cues in imagination, along a graded hierarchy.

Another exposure technique, called *flooding*, or *direct therapeutic exposure*, involves the patient's confrontation of conditioned feared cues, at first in imagination and then in vivo. The specific exposure protocol for PTSD, called prolonged exposure, focuses on remembering the traumatic event in detail (Foa et al. 1991). Prolonged exposure combines repeated detailed recall of the traumatic event with behavioral exposures outside of the therapist's office. The treatment protocol usually consists of nine sessions, which include relaxation training, imaginal exposures to the trauma, and in vivo exposures to trauma-related cues. During initial exposure sessions, anxiety is expected to be high. With repeated exposures in the therapeutic setting, anxiety diminishes (Resick 2001b). In a study comparing male combat veteran groups receiving nonspecific PTSD treatment with those receiving exposure therapy, the exposure group showed a greater reduction in PTSD symptoms (Cooper and Clum 1989).

Cognitive-Behavioral Therapies

Stress inoculation training is the cognitive-behavioral package developed for treatment of anxiety (Meichenbaum 1974). In the 1980s, this training became the first treatment approach for posttraumatic stress-related symptoms (Kilpatrick et al. 1982). The goal of the therapy is to help patients understand and manage their trauma-related fear reactions, with a resultant decrease in avoidance behaviors. The protocol ranges from 8 to 20 sessions and is composed of three phases: education, skill building, and application. In the education phase, patients are taught to identify their different models of response (emotions, behaviors, physical reactions, and thoughts) and are given an overview of treatment. In the skill-building phase, patients are first taught muscle relaxation and then learn cognitive techniques that include thought stopping, covert rehearsal, problem solving, and guided self-dialogue. In the third phase, patients are taught to apply these skills in situations that provoke anxiety.

Cognitive processing therapy was developed by Resick and Schnicke (1992). Initially it was used to treat victims of sexual trauma, but more recently it has been found effective for both PTSD and trauma-induced depression. The treatment consists of two integrated components: cognitive therapy and exposure therapy. Cognitive processing therapy is manual-driven and organized in 12 sessions. Initially, the focus of therapy is on assimilated distorted beliefs (e.g., denial). The therapy then shifts to overgeneralized beliefs that patients hold about themselves and the world. Once distorted beliefs are corrected, patients begin the exposure component of treatment and write detailed accounts of their traumas, which they then read to themselves and to the therapist. Patients are encouraged to experience their emotions and identify areas of conflicting beliefs and distorted logic.

Comparisons of the effectiveness of the cognitive and exposure-based treatments have not shown significant differences (Marks et al. 1998; Tarrier et al. 1999). A controlled study of cognitive processing therapy involving 171 subjects found that this treatment approach successfully reversed PTSD in 80% of subjects and was as efficacious as prolonged exposure therapy (Resick et al. 2002).

Eye Movement Desensitization and Reprocessing

Eye movement desensitization and reprocessing (EMDR) combines components of exposure and cognitive therapy with lateral eye movements (Shapiro 1995). Patients recall aspects of the traumatic event while visually following back-and-forth hand movements by the therapist. Although studies suggest effectiveness of this treatment for PTSD (Wilson et al. 1995), the value of lateral eye movements has not been established nor is it likely to be essential (Renfrey and Spates 1994). A treatment study by Devilly and Spence (1999) compared EMDR with cognitive-behavioral therapy and found the latter to be superior.

CONCLUSION

Exposure to traumatic events is common. Although men are exposed to a greater number of traumas than are women, they are less likely to develop PTSD. This difference in vulnerability might be influenced by the differences in the appraisal and memory of the traumatic event between men and women. Features of PTSD differ between men and women. Men show increased sensitivity to certain types of trauma (i.e., adult sexual trauma) and differences in symptoms of PTSD and response to treatment for the disorder. In the immediate aftermath of a trauma, most individuals will develop some trauma-related symptoms, but with time those symptoms will remit for most trauma survivors. A significant number of individuals will, however, develop PTSD, a disorder that often causes a major disruption in functioning. During the course of PTSD, men are more likely to exhibit aggression and violent impulses, and women are more likely to be withdrawn and dysthymic. Up to 88% of men with PTSD are diagnosed with one or more comorbid psychiatric disorders, most commonly with alcohol use disorder, major depression, or disorders of conduct.

Early identification and treatment of PTSD are important because they result in higher rates of recovery. Currently available treatments involve psychopharmacological treatments and psychotherapeutic approaches. Although multiple treatment studies of SSRIs show evidence of significant improvement in all three PTSD symptom clusters for both men and women, some data indicate that men may need longer antidepressant trials to achieve full treatment benefit. Trials of other antidepressants indicate less robust treatment response for both genders. Early trials with adrenergic antagonists and antipsychotic drugs are promising, but further research is needed in order to establish efficacy of those medications. The most effective psychotherapeutic treatments involve exposure-based treatments and cognitive processing therapy, both of which appear effective for men and women. Further exploration of the etiology of PTSD phenomena in men and women will help guide development of better treatments and improve long-term outcome of this illness for both gender groups.

KEY POINTS

- PTSD occurs commonly in men who seek treatment, particularly in men who have experienced combat and sexual abuse traumas.
- PTSD in men frequently co-occurs with other psychiatric disorders, such as substance use disorders, depression, and antisocial personality disorder.
- Men with PTSD appear to respond well to both psychosocial and pharmacological treatments.

PRACTICE GUIDELINES

1. Screen men for PTSD, particularly those presenting with substance use and mood disorders.

2. Consider early pharmacological and behavioral treatment interventions to prevent chronicity of symptoms.

3. Treat co-occurring disorders when present in conjunction with PTSD.

REFERENCES

Ackerman PT, Newton JE, McPherson WB, et al: Prevalence of post traumatic stress disorder and other psychiatric diagnoses in three groups of abused children (sexual, physical, and both). Child Abuse Negl 22:759–774, 1998

American Psychiatric Association: Diagnostic and Statistical Manual: Mental Disorders. Washington, DC, American Psychiatric Association, 1952

American Psychiatric Association: Diagnostic and Statistical Manual of Mental Disorders, 3rd Edition. Washington, DC, American Psychiatric Association, 1980

American Psychiatric Association: Diagnostic and Statistical Manual of Mental Disorders, 3rd Edition, Revised. Washington, DC, American Psychiatric Association, 1987

American Psychiatric Association: Diagnostic and Statistical Manual of Mental Disorders, 4th Edition, Text Revision. Washington, DC, American Psychiatric Association, 2000

Axelrod SR, Morgan CA 3rd, Southwick SM: Symptoms of posttraumatic stress disorder and borderline personality disorder in veterans of Operation Desert Storm. Am J Psychiatry 162:270–275, 2005

Baker DG, West SA, Nicholson WE, et al: Serial CSF corticotropin-releasing hormone levels and adrenocortical activity in combat veterans with posttraumatic stress disorder. Am J Psychiatry 156:585–588, 1999

Bartzokis G, Lu PH, Turner J, et al: Adjunctive risperidone in the treatment of chronic combat-related posttraumatic stress disorder. Biol Psychiatry 57:474–479, 2005

Brady KT, Farfel G: Effects of sertraline and placebo in women with PTSD. Paper presented at the annual meeting of the International Society for Traumatic Stress Studies, Miami, FL, November 1999

Brady K, Pearlstein T, Asnis GM, et al: Efficacy and safety of sertraline treatment of posttraumatic stress disorder: a randomized controlled trial. JAMA 283:1837–1844, 2000

Braun P, Greenberg D, Dasberg H, et al: Core symptoms of posttraumatic stress disorder unimproved by alprazolam treatment. J Clin Psychiatry 51:236–238, 1990

Bremner JD, Southwick SM, Johnson DR, et al: Childhood physical abuse and combat-related posttraumatic stress disorder in Vietnam veterans. Am J Psychiatry 150:235–239, 1993

Bremner JD, Randall P, Scott TM, et al: MRI-based measurement of hippocampal volume in patients with combat-related posttraumatic stress disorder. Am J Psychiatry 152:973–981, 1995

Bremner JD, Southwick SM, Darnell A, et al: Chronic PTSD in Vietnam combat veterans: course of illness and substance abuse. Am J Psychiatry 153:369–375, 1996

Bremner JD, Licinio J, Darnell A, et al: Elevated CSF corticotropin-releasing factor concentrations in posttraumatic stress disorder. Am J Psychiatry 154:624–629, 1997

Breslau N, Davis GC, Andreski P, et al: Traumatic events and posttraumatic stress disorder in an urban population of young adults. Arch Gen Psychiatry 48:216–222, 1991

Breslau N, Davis GC, Andreski P, et al: Sex differences in posttraumatic stress disorder. Arch Gen Psychiatry 54:1044–1048, 1997

Breslau N, Kessler RC, Chilcoat HD, et al: Trauma and posttraumatic stress disorder in the community: the 1996 Detroit Area Survey of Trauma. Arch Gen Psychiatry 55:626–632, 1998

Brewin CR, Andrews B, Valentine JD: Meta-analysis of risk factors for posttraumatic stress disorder in trauma-exposed adults. J Consult Clin Psychol 68:748–766, 2000

Chilcoat HD, Breslau N: Posttraumatic stress disorder and drug disorders: testing causal pathways. Arch Gen Psychiatry 55:913–917, 1998

Connor KM, Sutherland SM, Tupler LA, et al: Fluoxetine in posttraumatic stress disorder: randomised, double-blind study. Br J Psychiatry 175:17–22, 1999

Cooper NA, Clum GA: Imaginal flooding as a supplementary treatment for PTSD in combat veterans: a controlled study. Behav Ther 20:381–391, 1989

Davidson J, Kudler H, Smith R, et al: Treatment of posttraumatic stress disorder with amitriptyline and placebo. Arch Gen Psychiatry 47:259–266, 1990

Davidson JR, Hughes D, Blazer DG, et al: Posttraumatic stress disorder in the community: an epidemiological study. Psychol Med 21:713–721, 1991

Davidson J, Pearlstein T, Londborg P, et al: Efficacy of sertraline in preventing relapse of posttraumatic stress disorder: results of a 28-week double-blind, placebo-controlled study. Am J Psychiatry 158:1974–1981, 2001

Devilly GJ, Spence SH: The relative efficacy and treatment distress of EMDR and a cognitive-behavior trauma treatment protocol in the amelioration of posttraumatic stress disorder. J Anxiety Disord 13:131–157, 1999

Eagly A: Sex Differences in Social Behavior: A Social Role Interpretation. Hillsdale, NJ, Erlbaum, 1987

Ehlers A, Mayou RA, Bryant B: Psychological predictors of chronic posttraumatic stress disorder after motor vehicle accidents. J Abnorm Psychol 107:508–519, 1998

Foa EB: Psychological processes related to recovery from a trauma and an effective treatment for PTSD. Ann N Y Acad Sci 821:410–424, 1997

Foa EB, Rothbaum BO, Riggs DS, et al: Treatment of posttraumatic stress disorder in rape victims: a comparison between cognitive-behavioral procedures and counseling. J Consult Clin Psychol 59:715–723, 1991

Foa EB, Keane TM, Friedman MJ: Introduction, in Effective Treatments for PTSD. Edited by Foa EB, Keane TM, Friedman MJ. New York, Guilford, 2000, pp 1–17

Frankenhaeuser M, von Wright MR, Collins A, et al: Sex differences in psychoneuroendocrine reactions to examination stress. Psychosom Med 40:334–343, 1978

Friedman MJ, Southwick SM: Towards pharmacotherapy for PTSD, in Neurobiological and Clinical Consequences of Stress: From Normal Adaptation to Posttraumatic Stress Disorder. Edited by Friedman MJ, Charney DS, Deutch A. Philadelphia, PA, Lippincott-Raven, 1995, pp 465–481

Friedman MJ, Charney DS, Deutch A: Neurobiological and Clinical Consequences of Stress: From Normal Adaptation to Posttraumatic Stress Disorder. Philadelphia, PA, Lippincott-Raven, 1995

Friedman MJ, Davidson JRT, Mellman TA: Pharmacotherapy, in Effective Treatments for PTSD. Edited by Foa EB, Keane TM, Friedman MJ. New York, Guilford, 2000, pp 84–105

Hamner MB, Faldowski RA, Ulmer HG, et al: Adjunctive risperidone treatment in posttraumatic stress disorder: a preliminary controlled trial of effects on comorbid psychotic symptoms. Int Clin Psychopharmacol 18:1–8, 2003

Harvey PD, Yehuda R: Strategies to study risk for the development of PTSD, in Risk Factors for Posttraumatic Stress Disorder. Edited by Yehuda R. Washington, DC, American Psychiatric Press, 1999, pp 1–22

Helzer JE, Robins LN, McEvoy L: Posttraumatic stress disorder in the general population: findings of the Epidemiologic Catchment Area survey. N Engl J Med 317:1630–1634, 1987

Herman JL: Complex PTSD: a syndrome in survivors of prolonged and repeated trauma. J Trauma Stress 5:377–391, 1992

Horrigan JP: Guanfacine for PTSD nightmares (letter). J Am Acad Child Adolesc Psychiatry 35:975–976, 1996

Hyer L, Summers MN, Boyd S, et al: Assessment of older combat veterans with the Clinician-Administered PTSD Scale. J Trauma Stress 9:587–593, 1996

Jacobsen LK, Southwick SM, Kosten TR: Substance use disorders in patients with posttraumatic stress disorder: a review of the literature. Am J Psychiatry 158:1184–1190, 2001

Jannoff-Buman R, Frieze IH: The role of gender in reactions to criminal victimization, in Gender and Stress. Edited by Barnett RC, Biener L. New York, Free Press, 1987, pp 159–184

Kaufman A, Divasto P, Jackson R, et al: Male rape victims: noninstitutionalized assault. Am J Psychiatry 137:221–223, 1980

Keane TM, Gerardi RJ, Lyons JA, et al: The interrelationship of substance abuse and posttraumatic stress disorder: epidemiological and clinical considerations. Recent Dev Alcohol 6:27–48, 1988

Kessler RC, Sonnega A, Bromet E, et al: Posttraumatic stress disorder in the National Comorbidity Survey. Arch Gen Psychiatry 52:1048–1060, 1995

Kessler RC, Sonnega A, Bromet E: Epidemiological risk factors for trauma and PTSD, in Risk Factors for Posttraumatic Stress Disorder. Edited by Yehuda R. Washington, DC, American Psychiatric Press, 1999, pp 23–59

Kilpatrick DG, Veronen LJ, Resick PA: Psychological sequelae to rape: assessment and treatment strategies, in Behavioral Medicine: Assessment and Treatment Strategies. Edited by Dolays RL, Meredith RL, Ciminero AR. New York, Plenum, 1982, pp 473–497

Kilpatrick DG, Edmunds CN, Seymour AK: Rape in America: A Report to the Nation. Arlington, VA, National Victim Center, 1992

Kolb LC, Burris BC, Griffiths S: Propranolol and clonidine in the treatment of the chronic posttraumatic stress disorders of war, in Posttraumatic Stress Disorder: Psychological and Biological Sequelae. Edited by van der Kolk BA. Washington, DC, American Psychiatric Press, 1984, pp 98–105

Kosten TR, Frank JB, Dan E, et al: Pharmacotherapy for posttraumatic stress disorder using phenelzine or imipramine. J Nerv Ment Dis 179:366–370, 1991

Kuch K, Cox BJ: Symptoms of PTSD in 124 survivors of the Holocaust. Am J Psychiatry 149:337–340, 1992

Kulka RA, Schlenger WE, Fairbank JA: Trauma and the Vietnam War generation. New York, Brunner/Mazel, 1990

Leyba CM, Wampler TP: Risperidone in PTSD. Psychiatr Serv 49:245–246, 1998

Marks I, Lovell K, Noshirvani H, et al: Treatment of posttraumatic stress disorder by exposure and/or cognitive restructuring: a controlled study. Arch Gen Psychiatry 55:317–325, 1998

Marmar CR, Schoenfeld F, Weiss DS, et al: Open trial of fluvoxamine treatment for combat-related posttraumatic stress disorder. J Clin Psychiatry 57(suppl): 66–70, 1996

Marshall RD, Beebe KL, Oldham M, et al: Efficacy and safety of paroxetine treatment for chronic PTSD: a fixed-dose, placebo controlled study. Am J Psychiatry 158:1982–1988, 2001

Martenyi F, Brown EB, Zhang H, et al: Fluoxetine versus placebo in posttraumatic stress disorder. J Clin Psychiatry 63:199–206, 2002

McFarlane AC: The phenomenology of posttraumatic stress disorders following a natural disaster. J Nerv Ment Dis 176:22–29, 1988

McFarlane AC: The aetiology of posttraumatic morbidity: predisposing, precipitating and perpetuating factors. Br J Psychiatry 154:221–228, 1989

McFarlane AC: Risk factors for the acute biological and psychological response to trauma, in Risk Factors for Posttraumatic Stress Disorder. Edited by Yehuda R. Washington, DC, American Psychiatric Press, 1999, pp 163–190

McFarlane AC, Papay P: Multiple diagnoses in posttraumatic stress disorder in the victims of a natural disaster. J Nerv Ment Dis 180:498–504, 1992

Meichenbaum D: Cognitive Behavioral Modification. Morristown, NJ, General Learning Press, 1974

Morgan CA 3rd, Hill S, Fox P, et al: Anniversary reactions in Gulf War veterans: a follow-up inquiry 6 years after the war. Am J Psychiatry 156:1075–1079, 1999

Norris FH: Epidemiology of trauma: frequency and impact of different potentially traumatic events on different demographic groups. J Consult Clin Psychol 60:409–418, 1992

Perry BD, Giller EL Jr, Southwick SM: Altered platelet alpha 2–adrenergic binding sites in posttraumatic stress disorder. Am J Psychiatry 144:1511–1512, 1987

Pitman RK, Sanders KM, Zusman RM, et al: Pilot study of secondary prevention of posttraumatic stress disorder with propranolol. Biol Psychiatry 51:189–192, 2002

Rasmusson A, Friedman MJ: Gender issues in the neurobiology of PTSD, in Gender and PTSD. Edited by Kimerling R, Ouimette P, Wolfe J. New York, Guilford, 2002, pp 43–75

Rasmusson AM, Vasek J, Lipschitz DS, et al: An increased capacity for adrenal DHEA release is associated with decreased avoidance and negative mood symptoms in women with PTSD. Neuropsychopharmacology 29:1546–1557, 2004

Reist C, Kauffmann CD, Haier RJ, et al: A controlled trial of desipramine in 18 men with posttraumatic stress disorder. Am J Psychiatry 146:513–516, 1989

Renfrey G, Spates CR: Eye movement desensitization: a partial dismantling study. J Behav Ther Exp Psychiatry 25:231–239, 1994

Resick PA: Psychological risk factors: pre-trauma and peri-trauma influences, in Stress and Trauma. Hove, East Sussex, United Kingdom, Psychology Press, 2001a, pp 95–115

Resick PA: Treatment of traumatic stress reactions, in Stress and Trauma. Hove, East Sussex, United Kingdom, Psychology Press, 2001b, pp 141–166

Resick PA, Schnicke MK: Cognitive processing therapy for sexual assault victims. J Consult Clin Psychol 60:748–756, 1992

Resick PA, Nishith P, Weaver TL, et al: A comparison of cognitive-processing therapy with prolonged exposure and a waiting condition for the treatment of chronic posttraumatic stress disorder in female rape victims. J Consult Clin Psychol 70:867–879, 2002

Resnick HS, Kilpatrick DG, Dansky BS, et al: Prevalence of civilian trauma and posttraumatic stress disorder in a representative national sample of women. J Consult Clin Psychol 61:984–991, 1993

Rind B, Tromovitch P, Bauserman R: A meta-analytic examination of assumed properties of child sexual abuse using college samples. Psychol Bull 124: 22–53, 1998

Ruch LO, Leon JJ: Sexual assault trauma and trauma change. Women Health 8:5–21, 1983

Sattar SP, Ucci B, Grant K, et al: Quetiapine therapy for posttraumatic stress disorder. Ann Pharmacother 36:1875–1878, 2002

Schnurr PP, Friedman MJ, Bernardy NC: Research on posttraumatic stress disorder: epidemiology, pathophysiology, and assessment. J Clin Psychol 58:877–889, 2002

Schottenfeld RS, Cullen MR: Recognition of occupation-induced posttraumatic stress disorders. J Occup Med 28:365–369, 1986

Shapiro F: Eye Movement Desensitization and Reprocessing: Basic Principles, Protocols and Procedures. New York, Guilford, 1995

Southwick SM, Krystal JH, Morgan CA, et al: Abnormal noradrenergic function in posttraumatic stress disorder. Arch Gen Psychiatry 50:266–274, 1993a

Southwick SM, Yehuda R, Giller EL Jr: Personality disorders in treatment-seeking combat veterans with posttraumatic stress disorder. Am J Psychiatry 150:1020–1023, 1993b

Southwick SM, Yehuda R, Giller EL Jr: Use of tricyclics and monoamine oxidase inhibitors in the treatment of PTSD: a quantitative review, in Catecholamine Function in Posttraumatic Stress Disorder: Emerging Concepts. Edited by Murburg MM. Washington, DC, American Psychiatric Press, 1994, pp 293–305

Southwick SM, Krystal JH, Bremner JD, et al: Noradrenergic and serotonergic function in posttraumatic stress disorder. Arch Gen Psychiatry 54:749–758, 1997

Southwick SM, Bremner JD, Rasmusson A, et al: Role of norepinephrine in the pathophysiology and treatment of posttraumatic stress disorder. Biol Psychiatry 46:1192–1204, 1999

Southwick SM, Rasmusson A, Barron J: Neurobiological and neurocognitive alterations in PTSD: a focus on norepinephrine, serotonin and the HPA axis, in Neuropsychology of PTSD: Biological, Cognitive and Clinical Perspectives. Edited by Vasterling JJ, Brewin CR. New York, Guilford, 2005, pp 27–58

Tarrier N, Pilgrim H, Sommerfield C, et al: A randomized trial of cognitive therapy and imaginal exposure in the treatment of chronic posttraumatic stress disorder. J Consult Clin Psychol 67:13–18, 1999

Tolin DF, Foa EB: Gender and PTSD: A Cognitive Model. Edited by Kimerling R, Ouimette P, Wolfe J. New York, Guilford, 2002, pp 76–97

van der Kolk BA, McFarlane AC: The black hole of trauma, in Traumatic Stress. Edited by van der Kolk BA, McFarlane AC, Weisaeth L. New York, Guilford, 1996, pp 3–23

van der Kolk BA, Dreyfuss D, Michaels M, et al: Fluoxetine in posttraumatic stress disorder. J Clin Psychiatry 55:517–522, 1994

Wilson SA, Becker LA, Tinker RH: Eye movement desensitization and reprocessing (EMDR) treatment for psychologically traumatized individuals. J Consult Clin Psychol 63:928–937, 1995

Wolpe J: Psychotherapy by Reciprocal Inhibition. Stanford, CA, Stanford University Press, 1958

Yehuda R, McFarlane AC (eds): Psychobiology of Posttraumatic Stress Disorder (Annals of the New York Academy of Sciences, Vol 821). New York, New York Academy of Sciences, 1997

Yehuda R, Golier JA, Halligan SL, et al: The ACTH response to dexamethasone in PTSD. Am J Psychiatry 161:1397–1403, 2004

Zlotnick C, Zimmerman M, Wolfsdorf BA, et al: Gender differences in patients with posttraumatic stress disorder in a general psychiatric practice. Am J Psychiatry 158:1923–1925, 2001

PART III

SOCIOCULTURAL ISSUES
FOR MEN

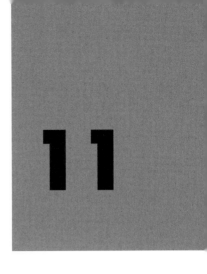

FATHERING AND THE MENTAL HEALTH OF MEN

THOMAS J. MCMAHON, PH.D.
AARON Z. SPECTOR, M.S.N., A.P.N.

Case Vignette 1

Robert was a 37-year-old carpenter of Puerto Rican heritage who was receiving methadone maintenance treatment for a 13-year history of opioid dependence when he enrolled in a research project focusing on the development of a parent intervention for men enrolled in drug abuse treatment. When he began the research project, Robert reported that he had been released from prison approximately 10 months earlier after completing a 9-year sentence for possession of narcotics with intent to sell. Although he had expected to live with his wife and 12-year-old son when released, he had learned that his wife had filed for divorce the day he was released and that she was now pursuing a relationship with another man. After relapsing almost immediately after his return to the community, Robert had enrolled in methadone maintenance treatment, secured a job, and begun a relationship with another woman. After writing to his son consistently while incarcerated, Robert had been visiting his son several times weekly, and as the divorce proceedings began, Robert's wife unexpectedly agreed to have the son live with Robert and his new girlfriend.

As he began the research project, Robert reported feeling very guilty about having relapsed while his wife was pregnant with his son. He also

259

reported missing his son intensely while incarcerated, and he reported that, while away, he had decided that if given a second chance, he would be a better father for his son than his absent, frequently incarcerated, alcoholic father had been for him. During his first psychotherapy session, Robert complained that he wanted to help his son avoid the mistakes he had made during his adolescence but did not know how to do so. He also expressed a desire to secure a stable, well-paying job to better support his family, and although he acknowledged that playing the trumpet in after-hours clubs as a member of a popular salsa band had contributed to his abuse of heroin, he expressed a desire to help his son learn to play the saxophone in a school band like he had done when he was the same age.

While doing a genogram, Robert also reluctantly acknowledged that he had a 17-year-old son with a third woman. He recently had been able to locate this son through extended family. Unsure of how to reestablish contact with the boy because the boy's mother would not speak with him, Robert had been walking through the neighborhood where the son lived, hoping to see him outside the local high school.

Case Vignette 2

Max was a 42-year-old computer programmer of Irish heritage who came reluctantly to marital counseling after his 40-year-old wife discovered he had been involved in a sexual liaison with another woman. When seen alone during the couple's initial evaluation, Max reported that he had become increasingly depressed and angry over several months' time after his wife had a miscarriage. After several years of unsuccessful infertility treatments, the couple had decided to make one last effort to have a child, and Max had been hopeful that he and his wife would finally be able to have a son. When a new treatment had produced a viable pregnancy involving a male fetus, the couple had been ecstatic. However, when the pregnancy had ended after 11 weeks, Max and his wife had become very despondent, and they had gradually withdrawn from one another. Believing that talking about his feelings would just upset his wife even further, Max had not shared his profound sense of loss with her or anyone else. Instead, he had focused his time and energy on a special project at work that he thought might earn him a new position as the leader of a special programming team being created at the financial institution where he worked.

As his wife had grown more depressed, Max had noted that her female friends and family seemed to join forces to support her. Several months after the miscarriage, his wife's closest friends had decided that she needed a 2-week winter vacation on a Caribbean island to improve her spirits. Although he thought it might have been better if they had gone away alone as a couple, Max had agreed that his wife should go on a vacation without him, after an initial discussion about the possibility of adopting a child had ended in an intense argument. About the same time, Max had been missing his deceased father, who had been a secondary school teacher and his high school baseball coach. By his report, no one had noticed when, having given up hope that he and his wife would ever have a child, Max had given an old baseball glove he had been saving for his unborn son to a nephew who had registered to play Little League baseball.

Feeling isolated and neglected while his wife was away with her sister and friends, Max accepted an invitation to have dinner with a female coworker after they had been working late. According to Max, he had been surprised when the dinner date ended with a night of sexual relations in the woman's apartment. Angry, depressed, and confused when he came for his initial consultation, Max was not sure how his wife had learned of his transgression; he was not sure how he felt about what had happened with the other woman; and given what the couple had been through, he was not sure he wanted to continue the marriage. He was, however, very clear that he still hoped to someday be a father.

Since the 1980s, a number of social forces have converged in this culture to make fatherhood one of the more prominent public policy issues of the new millennium. From a policy perspective, fathers moved to the forefront in 1995 when President Clinton directed all federal agencies to review existing policies, programs, and initiatives to ensure that they supported men as much as possible in their role as fathers. Shortly thereafter, the U.S. Department of Health and Human Services began its fatherhood initiative, and most states have since developed programs to prevent unplanned pregnancy, enhance financial support of children, and promote positive father–child relationships (for reviews, see Bernard and Knitzer 1999; Cabrera and Peters 2000; Mincy and Pouncy 2002).

Ironically, in the context of increased attention to fatherhood as a social issue, links between fatherhood and the mental health of men are rarely acknowledged in the conceptualization of public policy, service delivery, or research focusing on the nature of family process (McMahon and Rounsaville 2002). Amid calls for creative intervention to increase the presence of men in the lives of children, relatively little is known about links between fathering and men's mental health. Given the focus of this volume, two related questions are critical for professionals who work with men throughout the health care system: 1) How do psychiatric, personality, and substance use disorders contribute to the compromise of fathering? and 2) How do family transitions involving parenting issues affect the psychosocial adjustment of men?

Although the literature is evolving on the impact that positive and negative fathering can have on the psychosocial adjustment of children under a variety of circumstances, this discussion focuses on the importance of fathering in the lives of men. Moreover, although negative consequences in the reciprocal influence of mental health on fathering and fathering on mental health are explored, the discussion—as suggested by several scholars (e.g., Hawkins and Dollahite 1997; Parke and Brott 1999)—moves beyond a deficit perspective on men's parenting. The chapter acknowledges ways in which fathering promotes the mental health of men and in which men with behavioral health problems struggle to parent children in a socially responsible manner. Throughout the discussion, the primary goal is to highlight ways that the expanding literature on fathering and men's mental health should be used to inform assessment and intervention pursued by professionals who treat fathers throughout the health care system.

FATHERHOOD AND THE PSYCHOSOCIAL DEVELOPMENT OF MEN: A DEVELOPMENTAL-ECOLOGICAL PERSPECTIVE

Research indicates that undoubtedly fatherhood has a significant impact on most men (Palkovitz 2002). With growing awareness of the multidimensional nature of adult development, scholars have begun to consider fathering as a developmental pathway that men choose. Beginning early in childhood, men, like women, develop psychological representations of themselves as human beings with the capacity to create and parent children, and most men begin to think of themselves as parents long before puberty (Marsiglio and Hutchinson 2002). Moreover, although men become biological fathers under a wide range of circumstances, decisions to parent children, rather than simply conceive them, evolve out of a complex psychosocial process that has important implications for fathers, mothers, and children (Palkovitz 2002).

Although an important developmental issue in the lives of men, fathering also occurs in a social context. Many scholars believe it is useful to think of fathering as a developmental process that unfolds in a social ecology, and there is accumulating evidence that men's parenting is influenced by a broad range of intertwined social, interpersonal, and psychological factors (Parke 2002; J.H. Pleck and Masciadrelli 2003). Researchers repeatedly recognize that fathering occurs in a historical context broadly influenced by cultural, political, and economic changes (for a discussion see E.H. Pleck 2003). Researchers also recognize that the extent to which men choose to parent children is broadly influenced by gender-role norms, marital status, and patterns of employment (for reviews see Parke 2002; J.H. Pleck and Masciadrelli 2003). Moreover, research indicates that regardless of ethnic heritage, socioeconomic status, or marital status, the quality of men's relationships with the mothers of their children is probably the single most important influence on men's parenting behavior (Parke 2002).

PSYCHIATRIC DIFFICULTIES AND COMPROMISE OF FATHERING

As responsible fatherhood has become a prominent social issue, researchers have begun to examine the attitudes toward parenting and parenting behavior within special populations of fathers, particularly disenfranchised populations of fathers living outside traditional two-parent family structures. Recognizing that psychopathology or substance abuse in either parent represents risk for the disruption of family environments, researchers have, on a limited basis, begun to consider ways in which the clinical problems that affect men influence their ability to function as a parent. Given the epidemiology of behavioral health disorders among men in the general population, the existing literature is largely focused on ways that substance use, depression, and antisocial personality disorder affect men's parenting. However, it is important to note that although clear evidence indicates that children with a depressed, antisocial, or substance-abusing father are at risk for poor developmental outcomes, it is not clear to what extent the compromise of fathering contributes directly and indirectly to the risk children incur (McMahon and Rounsaville 2002). Moreover, there has been even less consideration of how men's socially responsible efforts to function as a parent—despite the presence of behavioral health problems—may mitigate the risk children incur, and there is little understanding of how treatment might enhance the functioning of fathers experiencing behavioral health problems (McMahon and Rounsaville 2002).

Substance Use

Acknowledging that substance use disorders are the most commonly occurring behavioral health problem for men (Kessler et al. 1994), researchers have begun to characterize the compromise of fathering when it is associated with substance abuse, particularly alcoholism. Within this literature, paternal alcoholism has been associated with 1) more conflictual, disorganized family environments; 2) poorer coparenting relationships; 3) more negative parenting behavior; 4) relatively poorer father–child relationships; and 5) poorer financial support of children. For example, Eiden and her colleagues (Eiden and Leonard 2000; Eiden et al. 1999, 2001, 2002) have shown that paternal alcoholism is associated with more negative attitudes toward infants, more negative and less positive affect during father–infant interaction, and more frequent disturbance in father–infant attachment. Similarly, Haugland (2005) recently found that while they are actively using, alcohol-dependent fathers are more likely to withdraw from family routines, less likely to set limits with their children, and more likely to be irritable during their interactions with their children. Dion et al. (1997) found that nonresident fathers abusing alcohol were less likely to contribute to the financial support of children, and Guterman and Lee (2005) recently outlined ways in which paternal alcohol abuse may contribute directly and indirectly to child abuse and neglect.

Although the data are even more limited, paternal drug abuse appears to be associated with similar, if not more serious, compromise of fathering. For example, McMahon and his colleagues (McMahon 2002; McMahon et al. 2001) recently found that when compared with men who have no history of alcohol or illicit drug abuse, drug-abusing fathers tend to have more limited personal definitions of the fathering role. They also have more children with more partners, report more conflict in coparenting relationships, are less able to provide financial support, and report less involvement in the lives of their children. As noted earlier, there are also open questions about how paternal drug abuse contributes directly and indirectly to child abuse and neglect (Guterman and Lee 2005).

Depression

After showing that depression represents a substantial risk for the compromise of mothering, researchers have also begun to consider how depression influences the quality of parenting that children receive from their fathers. However, the research is limited, and the findings are, to some extent, confounded by recent advances in understanding how depressive mood states may differ with gender. Although men typically present with the same primary symptoms as women, researchers have begun to identify gender-specific symptoms, like irritability, that may more completely characterize depressive disorders in men (for discussions see Cochran and Rabinowitz 2000 and Chapter 5 in this volume, "Depression"). Research examining the impact of depression on fathering has not yet acknowledged these broader conceptualizations of depressive symptoms in men.

Nevertheless, although Field et al. (1999) found that depressed fathers did not interact with their infant children much differently than fathers with no history of persistent depression, other researchers have found that depressed fathers consistently demonstrate less positive and more negative parenting behavior. For example, Lyons-Ruth et al. (2002) showed that depressed fathers are less likely than other fathers to play with their preschool children, read to them, hug them, cuddle with them, and participate in the maintenance of daily routines. Researchers (e.g., Conger et al. 1995; Jacob and Johnson 2001; Lyons-Ruth et al. 2002) have also shown that paternal depression tends to be associated with more hostile behavior toward children, more critical parenting, and more conflictual parent–child interaction. Researchers have also found that when men struggle with depression, father–child communication seems to become skewed, primarily through suppression of positive interaction, because fathers do not respond enthusiastically to positive interaction initiated by children (Jacob and Johnson 2001). Depression in men also influences fathering by affecting the quality of co-parenting relationships that seem to be so important to the maintenance of positive fathering. For example, Parke et al. (2004) recently showed that paternal depression contributed directly to an increase in marital conflict, which in turn increased the intensity of negative interactions with children.

Antisocial Personality Disorder

Antisocial personality disorder has been associated consistently with risk for early fatherhood, more difficulty during the transition to fatherhood, and negative parenting behavior. Researchers (e.g., see Capaldi et al. 1996; Fagot et al. 1998) repeatedly have shown that boys with antisocial orientations tend to become involved in sexual activity earlier and to become fathers earlier than their peers. Researchers (e.g., Florsheim et al. 1999; Jaffee et al. 2001) have also shown that as men with antisocial personality disorder become fathers, they are more likely to experience psychological and interpersonal problems during the transition to fatherhood and are less likely to be living with the child soon afterward. Patterson and Capaldi (1991) have shown that antisocial personality disorder in men is frequently associated with harsh, inconsistent discipline and poor supervision of children, and Dion et al. (1997) showed that men with antisocial personality disorder are less likely to contribute to the financial support of their children.

Beyond Deficit Perspectives on Fathering

Although research examining parenting issues within disenfranchised populations of men has begun to characterize the compromise of fathering, these findings sometimes also highlight men's efforts at socially responsible parenting. These findings are inconsistent with the popular stereotypes grounded in deficit perspectives on men's parenting. Similar findings are beginning to emerge in research being done with fathers with behavioral health problems. For example, although Eiden et al.

(2002) found that problematic attachment occurred more frequently in family systems affected by paternal alcoholism, approximately 50% of the infants examined still demonstrated secure attachment with an alcoholic father compared with approximately 65% of the infants in the control group. The finding suggests that despite their substance use, a substantial number of alcoholic men were still able to establish a positive affective connection with their child. Similarly, empirical study of drug-abusing fathers has begun to document socially responsible efforts to parent children in the context of ongoing drug use. For example, McMahon et al. (2000) found that within a small sample of fathers enrolled in methadone maintenance treatment, many of the men reported being present at the time their children were born, most had lived with their children at some point during their drug abuse career, most had made some attempt to provide financial support, and most had ongoing contact with at least some of their children.

Any compromise of fathering that occurs in the context of clinical problems may have a profound effect not only on the children but also on their fathers (McMahon and Rounsaville 2002). To the extent that men value fatherhood, failure to fulfill this important social role may contribute to affective distress that represents a risk for both the deterioration of these men's clinical status and the further compromise of their parenting (McMahon and Rounsaville 2002). For example, researchers (e.g., see Kearney et al. 1994) have written extensively about the guilt, shame, and depression that drug-abusing mothers experience when drug use compromises their ability to care for their children, and family scholars (e.g., see Lansky 1992; Rothe 2001) have repeatedly highlighted ways in which feelings of shame cause men to withdraw from their children in the context of divorce and other perceived failures. However, because of gendered assumptions about the nature of parenting (for a discussion see Phares 1996) and concerns about the degree of sociopathy among drug-abusing men (for a discussion see Parke and Brott 1999), the drug abuse treatment community does not acknowledge that drug-abusing fathers may also be distressed about their failure to function effectively as parents (McMahon and Rounsaville 2002). Like drug-abusing fathers, depressed men aware of their inability to function effectively as parents may also become mired in downward spirals involving guilt, irritable affect, and depressed mood that only aggravate both their depressive disorder and their problematic parenting (Jacob and Johnson 2001).

Finally, given that fatherhood is an important developmental milestone in the lives of many men, research done with special populations of fathers suggests that concern about parenting responsibilities does motivate some men to pursue help for psychosocial problems. Even when not actively involved with their children, estranged fathers are almost always interested in being more involved but often avoid making an effort to do so because of feelings, attitudes, stereotypes, and systemic issues that discourage greater involvement (Furstenberg 1995). Consistent with this finding, there is evidence that concern about their newfound status as fathers motivates some men to consider making changes in their lifestyle (Nelson et al. 2002; Palkovitz 2002). Men's concern about generative issues as they negotiate the developmental changes of middle age may also motivate some men to pursue positive change in their relationships with their children. Clearly, for men experiencing behavioral health problems, developmental transitions involving parenting issues may help some men mobilize themselves for behavior change.

PSYCHOSOCIAL ADJUSTMENT TO FAMILY TRANSITIONS AND FATHERING

Although considerable resources have been devoted to exploring the impact of family transitions on the psychosocial adjustment of mothers and children, the impact of family transitions on the well-being of men has received relatively little attention (Eggebeen 2002). At this time, an extensive literature describes the effect that pregnancy, delivery, and postnatal parenting have on women, but relatively little is known about how these parenting transitions affect the psychosocial adjustment of men. Furthermore, much of the existing knowledge base must be considered tentative because the findings have typically been based on data collected from small, poorly representative samples of parents, with the primary goal of comparing fathers with mothers. Although the results are not entirely consistent, much of this literature shows that men may be less vulnerable than women to emotional distress during parenting transitions. However, the lack of a comparison group composed of men not undergoing the same transition makes it difficult to characterize the extent to which these transitions still represent periods of vulnerability for men relative to other men. Furthermore, some researchers have argued that the existing literature tends to minimize the effects on men because men are not examined from a gender-sensitive perspective (Cook 1988). Therefore, although not intended to be exhaustive, or conclusive, the review that follows is presented simply to highlight ways in which parenting transitions may affect the mental health of men.

Pregnancy

Pregnancy is likely to provoke physical and psychological changes in men, although these changes are less overt than the changes that pregnant women experience. A common but poorly understood phenomenon is *couvade syndrome,* in which a man with a pregnant sexual partner begins to experience physiological symptoms involving complaints of appetite change, nausea, indigestion, weight gain, bowel changes, headache, insomnia, and backache (Klein 1991). These changes tend to begin during the first trimester and also often emerge late in the third trimester, and they usually resolve immediately after delivery (Klein 1991). Although these physiological changes have historically been attributed to psychological influences, there is at least limited evidence that they may be linked with hormonal changes men may experience during the pregnancy of a sexual partner (Storey et al. 2000).

During their partner's pregnancy, men are also likely to reconsider their own interest in being a parent, dramatically expand their personal definitions of fathering, and carefully consider their capacity to function as a parent (Marsiglio 2004). Although men may have considered these questions previously, the complexity and intensity of their thinking tend to increase dramatically during pregnancy as they become concerned about the meaning of the pregnancy for them (Pancer et al. 2000). As this occurs, many men develop visions of what their child will be like and what they will be like as fathers (Marsiglio 2004). Surprisingly, even when not wholly prepared to be a father, men seem to carefully and realistically evaluate their capacity to function as a parent (Nelson et al. 2002; Palkovitz 2002). It is also important to note that when considering what kind of father they would like to be, men often find themselves reconsidering early relationships with their parents, particularly their fathers. Although they may lack the social and psychological resources for change, some men decide to be a much different parent than their biological father or the other father figures in their lives (Furstenberg and Weiss 2000; Palkovitz 2002).

Loss of a Pregnancy

Although the potential impact of spontaneous abortion on the emotional and interpersonal world of women has been explored in detail, very little is known about the impact of spontaneous abortion on men. The limited data available suggest that, like women, many men mourn the loss of the unborn child, but they may not talk about the loss because of social restraints on the expression of grief by men and social expectations that men must support their partner (Puddifoot and Johnson 1997, 1999). Some men may also devote a great deal of mental energy trying to understand the reasons for a spontaneous abortion (Puddifoot and Johnson 1997). Having been present during an ultrasound scan of the fetus may aggravate risk for a grief reaction in men (Puddifoot and Johnson 1997, 1999), and after experiencing the loss of a pregnancy, men may be notably more anxious during a later pregnancy (Armstrong 2001).

Similarly, although a great deal is known about the emotional reaction to elective abortion in women, very little is known about the emotional reaction of men. Marsiglio and Diekow (1998) listed factors likely to influence the nature of the emotional reaction, and in one of the few explorations of the issue, Shostak et al. (1984) found that some men were affected deeply by the abortion process, with ongoing questions about the morality of elective abortion, persistent feelings of loss, and frequent thoughts about the fetus. Conversely, the researchers also found that some men were relieved that they would not have to assume the psychological, financial, and social obligations that come with the poorly timed birth of a child.

Childbirth

Although most men react positively to the arrival of a child, the postnatal period also represents a very stressful time for men and women. Both depressive and anxiety symptoms can occur in fathers during the postnatal period, with the prevalence of clinically significant depression ranging as high as 25% among new fathers (Ballard et al. 1993, 1994; Huang and Warner 2005; Matthey et al. 2000; Raskin et al. 1990; Soliday et al. 1999). Huang and Warner (2005) found that risk for clinically significant depression was lowest for married fathers and highest for fathers estranged from the mother of the child. Risk for depressive reactions in new fathers also seems to be aggravated by unplanned pregnancy, postpartum depression in a partner, substance abuse, unemployment, and depressive difficulty before the pregnancy (Areias et al. 1996; Atkinson and Rickel 1984; Huang and Warner 2005; Leathers and Kelley 2000; Soliday et al. 1999).

Clinically significant anxiety also seems to be fairly common among new fathers, with some indications that anxiety tends to occur concurrently with depression (Ballard et al. 1993). Anxiety about providing financial support seems to be a particularly salient concern for men (Nelson et al. 2002), and like women, men may experience anxiety about being separated from the newborn baby, particularly when living with a woman experiencing separation anxiety (Deater-Deckard et al. 1994;

Hock and Lutz 1998). Under circumstances in which men feel like they have had no voice in the decision to continue an unplanned pregnancy, the birth of the child may also leave men feeling angry that fatherhood has been forced upon them, and they may be particularly angry if they do not feel prepared to properly parent a biological child or if they have to provide financial support (Marsiglio and Diekow 1998).

Fathering

Once the child has been born, fatherhood continues to exert an influence on the psychosocial adjustment of men. Although the transition may be stressful, many scholars believe that fatherhood contributes to a consolidation of positive psychological changes as men become more and more involved in parenting, and accumulating evidence suggests that significant change does in fact occur (Palkovitz 2002; Snarey 1993). Most of the psychological changes involve an ongoing sense of commitment to fathering, a persistent sense of responsibility, and changes in internal representations of self as a father as children develop (Palkovitz 2002; Snarey 1993). Although the changes vary dramatically, there is agreement that fathering changes the nature of intimate relationships with sexual partners as men seek to balance the demands of being a father with the demands of being an intimate partner (Palkovitz 2002).

Psychological and dyadic changes associated with ongoing involvement in fathering also contribute to change in the social and vocational activity of men. For example, men who value the provider role may actually work more after the birth of a child, and time spent at work may actually increase with the birth of subsequent children (Kaufman and Uhlenberg 2000). Conversely, men who value direct involvement in child care may work less after the birth of a child, and time devoted to work may decrease further with the birth of subsequent children (Kaufman and Uhlenberg 2000). However, although some fathers may choose to work less, financial support of children remains an important responsibility for most fathers, and across ethnic groups, financial stress clearly contributes to depressed mood in men and deterioration of coparenting relationships (Conger et al. 2002; Parke et al. 2004). As might be expected, fathers living with children tend to organize their social activity around involvement with other parents and organizations that focus on the needs of children (Eggebeen and Knoester 2001; Snarey 1993).

Early Fatherhood

Teenage fathers typically demonstrate more psychosocial problems than both teens without children and men who become fathers later in the life cycle (Parke 2002). Moreover, not only do teenage fathers come to parenthood with more psychosocial problems, but early fatherhood also does not seem to improve psychosocial adjustment over the long term. Although fatherhood may motivate some teens to consider lifestyle changes, and teenage fathers may actually demonstrate some positive changes over the short term, psychosocial adjustment over the long term may actually worsen. For example, researchers (Brien and Willis 1997; Nock 1998) have found that men who become fathers early tend to earn more than their peers without children, but over time their vocational-educational adjustment tends to lag behind that of their peers as they complete less education, earn less money, and fail to maintain employment. Similarly, other researchers (e.g., Furstenberg 1995) have found that despite making an effort to be effective fathers early on, many teenage fathers become disillusioned and withdraw from parenting as they encounter social, economic, interpersonal, and psychological barriers to ongoing involvement in family life. Teenage fathers may also be at risk for subsequent problems with depression and illicit drug use (Christmon and Luckey 1994; Heath et al. 1995). Although researchers have not been able to establish direct links between early fatherhood and deterioration of psychosocial adjustment (e.g., see Heath et al. 1995), it is possible that failure to fulfill personal, familial, and social expectations of effective fatherhood may exacerbate the social and psychological problems of young fathers who were already at high risk for these difficulties. Moreover, it is important to note that although relatively poor psychosocial adjustment seems to be common in teenage males who become fathers, virtually nothing is known about the psychosocial changes that allow young men to successfully negotiate the challenges that come with early fatherhood.

Divorce

Review of the existing literature suggests that there is more information about the impact of divorce on the psychosocial adjustment of men than any other family transition. However, much of that literature focuses on patterns of father–child contact after divorce, with exploration of ways in which paternal involvement affects the well-being of children. As with most other family transitions, relatively little attention has been paid to how separation from children affects the well-being of fathers.

As might be expected, disruption of family relationships associated with divorce leaves fathers at risk for psychological, physical, and social difficulty. Feelings of anger, depression, and anxiety are common, and there is a risk for impulsive, antisocial behavior (Amato 2000; Hetherington and Stanley-Hagan 1997). As marriages deteriorate, men often experience confusion about family roles and feelings of powerlessness (Amato 2000; Hetherington and Stanley-Hagan 1997). During the divorce process, men are more vulnerable to depression than women (Kendler et al. 2001), and problematic use of alcohol is relatively common (Power et al. 1999). In high-conflict divorces, men are also at greater risk of physically or sexually assaulting their partners, particularly if a previous history of violence exists in the relationship and the men are abusing alcohol (DeKeseredy et al. 2004; Hardesty 2002).

Although marital separations are clearly stressful for men, their psychosocial adjustment typically improves over time. Ironically, ongoing contact with children seems to help men cope more effectively (Hetherington and Stanley-Hagan 1997). Historically, the frequency of contact with children declined after divorce, but there is accumulating evidence that men may be making more of an effort to maintain contact with children (Amato and Gilbreth 1999). The capacity to disentangle marital from parenting roles and the capacity to maintain a positive coparenting relationship seem, more than anything else, to help men maintain contact with their children. Social support, particularly from a new sexual partner, seems also to help promote positive psychosocial adjustment after divorce (Stone 2002).

Single Custodial Parenting

As the demographics of family life have changed in response to the changes in family law that made divorce more feasible, households headed by single custodial fathers have increased dramatically (Brown 2000). Although they still represent a small percentage of all households, single-parent households headed by fathers now make up approximately 20% of the single-parent households in this culture (Brown 2000). Moreover, just as men are more frequently assuming custody of children after divorce, more men are also assuming custody of children born outside of marriage (Brown 2000).

Given that single men–parented households represent a relatively new family structure, relatively little information exists about the impact of this parenting transition on men either from a comparative or longitudinal perspective. However, limited data suggest that single custodial fathers may experience less economic distress than single custodial mothers but more economic pressure than married fathers (Hetherington and Stanley-Hagan 1997). Likewise, although not as dramatic as the experience of single custodial mothers, single custodial fathers may also experience more psychological stress, more depression, and more conflict over the demands of work versus family life than married fathers (Hill and Hilton 1999) and may also frequently feel overwhelmed, socially isolated, and incompetent as they struggle with the demands of caring for children (Hetherington 1993; Simons 1996).

Children With Special Needs

Men who father children with special needs face unique challenges that can dramatically affect their psychosocial adjustment. Despite a degree of inconsistency in the empirical literature, Lamb and Laumann Billings (1997) noted that the initial diagnosis of a serious medical or developmental problem in a child may, as expected, be very stressful for fathers. Men may also have difficulty accepting the physical, cognitive, and behavioral limitations of a child with special needs (Keller and Honig 2004); men may have difficulty establishing a positive affective attachment to the child; and the quality of father–child interaction may suffer as men experience confusion about how to relate to the affected child (Bristol et al. 1988). Men may also experience a sense of loss as they realize that the child will not be able to meet their expectations, and they may have a loss of self-esteem, concern about social stigma, and feelings of guilt (Lamb and Laumann Billings 1997).

Over time, fathers—more so than mothers—seem to move from emotional distress to quiet acceptance, and they may become focused on financial and practical needs of the family (Hodapp 2002; Lamb and Laumann Billings 1997). Nevertheless, fathers of children with special needs may still experience more personal and family stress than other fathers. Satisfaction with family life may be diminished because of demands associated with the care of the affected child, but marital satisfaction and satisfaction with parenting may increase for fathers as the children grow older (Lamb and Laumann Billings 1997). However, fathers of children with special needs may be more at risk to leave the family (Lamb and Laumann Billings 1997).

When previously healthy children become seriously ill, fathers may also experience difficulty coping. As the family reorganizes to cope with the illness, fathers may feel frightened, powerless, angry, sad, and guilty (Chesler and Parry 2001). Delayed, unexpected, and overwhelming emotional reactions may be common (Chesler and Parry 2001), and a significant proportion of fathers may demonstrate symptoms of posttraumatic stress as the family struggles with the initial diagnosis and ongoing treatment of a potentially life-threatening medical illness in a child (Kazak et al. 2004; Landolt et al. 2003). Fathers may also feel like they need more medical information, they may struggle with the demands of work, they may feel alienated from the ill child, and they may quietly struggle with existential questions (Chesler and Parry 2001). As with other difficult family transitions, fathers may frequently feel as though they must cope alone and remain a stoic source of support for their partners and children (Chesler and Parry 2001).

Again, although fathering a child with special needs can be a source of social and psychological stress, psychosocial changes associated with the birth of a child with special needs or associated with serious threats to the well-being of a previously healthy child may not all be negative. In particular, some fathers may more clearly commit themselves to help with the care of the child, finding creative ways to relate to him or her (Brotherton and Dollahite 1997; Clarke 2005). Although they may have trouble explaining the nature of the change, some men may find they feel closer to their partners, closer to the affected child, closer to their other children, and better able to cope (Chesler and Parry 2001; Dollahite 2004). Fathers may also articulate other positive social, emotional, and spiritual changes that they relate directly to their experience of being the father of a child with special needs (Chesler and Parry 2001; Dollahite 2004). Dollahite (2004) noted that fathers of children with special needs often find special meaning in their personal situation. They often describe a special emotional tie to the affected child and find they can somehow make a unique contribution to the care of the child. They also frequently describe personal changes involving the development of empathy, patience, sensitivity, and humility. Fathers of children with special needs also frequently report that the experience caused them to reevaluate their priorities in life. This reevaluation often means deciding that religious beliefs are very important and that family is more important than work (Brotherton and Dollahite 1997; Dollahite 2004).

Death of a Child

Without question, the death of a child is the most distressing event in the life of a parent. Although women may be more likely to experience a major depressive episode in response to many other life events, men may be as likely as women to experience a major depressive episode in response to the death of a child (Maciejewski et al. 2001). Loss of a child because of accident, suicide, or homicide may also leave men vulnerable to posttraumatic stress reactions (Murphy et al. 2002), and as in many other situations, cultural norms that discourage men from expressing grief may complicate the loss for many men and leave them more likely to cope by withdrawing, being active, misusing alcohol, or being aggressive (for a discussion see Gray 2001). When men are involved in an intimate relationship with the mother of the child, the relationship may deteriorate as these men worry about the mental health of their partner, communicate less, become more irritable, and lose interest in sexual activity.

CONCLUSION

As the understanding of men's experience of fatherhood expands, professionals who work with men throughout the health care system need to begin using that knowledge in the assessment and treatment of men, women, and children. Within the mental health and substance abuse treatment systems, professionals need to acknowledge the extent to which parenting is an important treatment issue in the lives of men (McMahon and Rounsaville 2002). When doing so, clinicians need to find ways to better engage men in a dialogue about parenting issues, to build on whatever intrinsic motivation fathers may have for change, to support socially responsible efforts at fathering, and to address the parenting deficits men bring to treatment (McMahon and Rounsaville 2002). With accumulating evidence of the potential benefits of positive father–child relationships, clinical interventions designed to promote more effective parenting by men with behavioral health problems are clearly needed. These efforts would improve the psychosocial adjustment not only of fathers, but also of mothers and children too (McMahon and Rounsaville 2002).

Similarly, considering the extent to which family transitions affect the psychosocial adjustment of men, there is a clear need for health care professionals to be more sensitive to ways in which transitions involving the conception, birth, parenting, or death of a child affect the psychological and interpersonal worlds of men. Professionals must acknowledge that even when not the focus of service delivery, fathers are likely to be affected by whatever is happening and may be reluctant to share their thoughts and feelings even if provided an opportunity to do so. Sensitivity in health care settings must also be complemented by sensitivity in work, school, church, counseling, and other community settings. Clearly, there is a need for clinical intervention designed to support men struggling with parenting transitions. Professionals also must move beyond problem-oriented support for men experiencing difficulty to creative engagement of men in preventive interventions designed to minimize the psychosocial stress associated with parenting. Regardless of who the patient is in the health care system, professionals must think creatively about ways to help fathers, mothers, and children by being more responsive to the needs of men as parents.

KEY POINTS

- Fatherhood is an important developmental issue in the lives of all men.

- Fatherhood is best understood as a developmental process that unfolds in a social context.

- Although behavioral health problems undoubtedly contribute to compromise of fathering, men experiencing substance abuse, psychiatric, and personality problems may still be making an effort to parent children in a socially responsible manner, and concern about their status as fathers may motivate some men to pursue help.

- Family transitions involving the conception, birth, parenting, or death of a child may have a profound effect on the psychosocial adjustment of men.

PRACTICE GUIDELINES

1. Professionals working in mental health and substance abuse treatment systems should carefully evaluate parenting issues in the lives of men seeking help for behavioral health problems.

2. Professionals working in other health care settings should be sensitive to ways in which family transitions involving the conception, birth, parenting, or death of a child may affect the psychosocial adjustment of men.

3. Professionals working throughout the health care system should make an effort to help fathers, mothers, and children by being more responsive to the needs of men as parents.

REFERENCES

Amato PR: The consequences of divorce for adults and children. J Marriage Fam 62:1269–1287, 2000

Amato PR, Gilbreth JG: Nonresident fathers and children's well-being: a meta-analysis. J Marriage Fam 61:557–573, 1999

Areias ME, Kumar R, Barros H, et al: Correlates of postnatal depression in mothers and fathers. Br J Psychiatry 169:36–41, 1996

Armstrong D: Exploring fathers' experiences of pregnancy after a prior perinatal loss. MCN Am J Matern Child Nurs 26:147–153, 2001

Atkinson A, Rickel AU: Postpartum depression in primiparous parents. J Abnorm Psychol 93:115–119, 1984

Ballard CG, Davis R, Handy S, et al: Postpartum anxiety in mothers and fathers. The European Journal of Psychiatry 7:117–121, 1993

Ballard CG, Davis R, Cullen PC, et al: Prevalence of postnatal psychiatric morbidity in mothers and fathers. Br J Psychiatry 164:782–788, 1994

Bernard S, Knitzer J: Map and Track: State Initiatives to Encourage Responsible Fatherhood. New York, National Center for Children and Poverty, 1999

Brien MJ, Willis RJ: The partners of welfare mothers: earnings and child support potential. Future Child 7:65–73, 1997

Bristol MM, Gallagher JJ, Schopler E: Mothers and fathers of young developmentally disabled and nondisabled boys: adaptation and spousal support. Dev Psychol 24:441–451, 1988

Brotherton SE, Dollahite DC: Generative ingenuity in fatherwork with young children with special needs, in Generative Fathering: Beyond Deficit Perspectives. Edited by Hawkins AJ, Dollahite DC. Thousand Oaks, CA, Sage, 1997, pp 89–104

Brown BV: The single-father family: demographic, economic, and public transfer use characteristics. Marriage Fam Rev 29:203–220, 2000

Cabrera N, Peters HE: Public policies and father involvement. Marriage Fam Rev 29: 295–314, 2000

Capaldi DM, Crosby L, Stoolmiller M: Predicting the timing of first sexual intercourse for at-risk adolescent males. Child Dev 67:344–359, 1996

Chesler MA, Parry C: Gender roles and/or styles in crisis: an integrative analysis of the experience of fathers of children with cancer. Qual Health Res 11:363–384, 2001

Christmon K, Luckey I: Is early fatherhood associated with alcohol and other drug use? J Subst Abuse 6:337–343, 1994

Clarke J: Fathers' home health care work when a child has cancer: I'm her dad; I have to do it. Men and Masculinities 7:385–404, 2005

Cochran SV, Rabinowitz FE: Men and Depression: Clinical and Empirical Perspectives. San Diego, CA, Academic Press, 2000

Conger RD, Patterson GR, Ge X: It takes two to replicate: a mediational model for the impact of parents' stress on adolescent adjustment. Child Dev 66: 80–97, 1995

Conger RD, Wallace LE, Sun Y, et al: Economic pressure in African American families: a replication and extension of the family stress model. Dev Psychol 38:179–193, 2002

Cook JA: Dad's double binds: rethinking fathers' bereavement from a men's studies perspective. J Contemp Ethnogr 17:285–308, 1988

Deater-Deckard K, Scarr S, McCartney K, et al: Paternal separation anxiety: relationships with parenting stress, child-rearing attitudes, and maternal anxieties. Psychol Sci 5:341–346, 1994

DeKeseredy WS, Rogness M, Schwartz MD: Separation/divorce sexual assault: the current state of social scientific knowledge. Aggression and Violent Behavior 9:675–691, 2004

Dion MR, Braver SL, Wolchik S, et al: Alcohol abuse and psychopathic deviance in noncustodial parents as predictors of child-support payment and visitation. Am J Orthopsychiatry 67:70–79, 1997

Dollahite DC: A narrative approach to exploring responsible involvement of fathers with their special-needs children, in Conceptualizing and Measuring Father Involvement. Edited by Day RD, Lamb ME. Mahwah, NJ, Erlbaum, 2004, pp 109–127

Eggebeen DJ: The changing course of fatherhood: men's experiences with children in demographic perspective. J Fam Issues 23:486–506, 2002

Eggebeen DJ, Knoester CW: Does fatherhood matter for men? J Marriage Fam 63:381–393, 2001

Eiden RD, Leonard KE: Paternal alcoholism, parental psychopathology, and aggravation with infants. J Subst Abuse 11:17–29, 2000

Eiden RD, Chavez F, Leonard KE: Parent-infant interactions among families with alcoholic fathers. Dev Psychopathol 11:745–762, 1999

Eiden RD, Leonard KE, Morrisey S: Paternal alcoholism and toddler noncompliance. Alcohol Clin Exp Res 25:1621–1633, 2001

Eiden RD, Edwards EP, Leonard KE: Mother-infant and father-infant attachment among alcoholic families. Dev Psychopathol 14:253–278, 2002

Fagot BI, Pears KC, Capaldi DM, et al: Becoming an adolescent father: precursors and parenting. Dev Psychol 34:1209–1219, 1998

Field TM, Hossain Z, Malphurs J: "Depressed" fathers' interactions with their infants. Infant Ment Health J 20:322–332, 1999

Florsheim P, Moore D, Zollinger L, et al: The transition to parenthood among adolescent fathers and their partners: does antisocial behavior predict problems in parenting? Applied Developmental Science 3:178–191, 1999

Furstenberg FF: Fathering in the inner city, in Fatherhood: Contemporary Theory, Research, and Social Policy. Edited by Marsiglio W. Thousand Oaks, CA, Sage, 1995, pp 119–147

Furstenberg FF, Weiss CC: Intergenerational transmission of fathering roles in at risk families. Marriage Fam Rev 29:181–201, 2000

Gray K: Grieving reproductive loss: the bereaved male, in Men Coping With Grief. Edited by Lund DA. Amityville, NY, Baywood Publishing, 2001, pp 327–337

Guterman NB, Lee Y: The role of fathers in risk for physical child abuse and neglect: possible pathways and unanswered questions. Child Maltreat 10:136–149, 2005

Hardesty JL: Separation assault in the context of postdivorce parenting: an integrative review of the literature. Violence Against Women 8:597–625, 2002

Haugland BSM: Recurrent disruptions of rituals and routines in families with paternal alcohol abuse. Fam Relat 54:225–241, 2005

Hawkins AJ, Dollahite DC: Beyond the role inadequacy perspective on fathering, in Generative Fathering: Beyond Deficit Perspectives. Edited by Hawkins AJ, Dollahite DC. Thousand Oaks, CA, Sage, 1997, pp 3–16

Heath D, McKenry PC, Leigh GK: The consequences of adolescent parenthood on men's depression, parental satisfaction, and fertility in adulthood. J Soc Serv Res 20:127–148, 1995

Hetherington EM: An overview of the Virginia Longitudinal Study of Divorce and Remarriage with a focus on early adolescence. J Fam Psychol 7:39–56, 1993

Hetherington EM, Stanley-Hagan MM: The effects of divorce on fathers and their children, in The Role of the Father in Child Development, 3rd Edition. Edited by Lamb ME. New York, Wiley, 1997, pp 191–211

Hill LC, Hilton JM: Changes in roles following divorce: comparison of factors contributing to depression in custodial single mothers and custodial single fathers. J Divorce & Remarriage 31:91–114, 1999

Hock E, Lutz WJ: Psychological meaning of separation anxiety in mothers and fathers. J Fam Psychol 12:41–55, 1998

Hodapp RM: Parenting children with mental retardation, in Handbook of Parenting, Vol 1: Children and Parenting, 2nd Edition. Edited by Bornstein MH. Mahwah, NJ, Erlbaum, 2002, pp 355–381

Huang CC, Warner LA: Relationship characteristics and depression among fathers with newborns. Soc Serv Rev 79:95–118, 2005

Jacob T, Johnson SL: Sequential interactions in the parent-child communications of depressed fathers and depressed mothers. J Fam Psychol 15:38–52, 2001

Jaffee SR, Caspi A, Moffitt TE, et al: Predicting early fatherhood and whether young fathers live with their children: prospective findings and policy reconsiderations. J Child Psychol Psychiatry 42:803–815, 2001

Kaufman G, Uhlenberg P: The influence of parenthood on the work effort of married men and women. Soc Forces 78:931–947, 2000

Kazak AE, Alderfer M, Rourke MT, et al: Posttraumatic stress disorder (PTSD) and posttraumatic stress symptoms (PTSS) in families of adolescent childhood cancer survivors. J Pediatr Psychol 29:211–219, 2004

Kearney MH, Murphy S, Rosenbaum M: Mothering on crack: a grounded theory analysis. Soc Sci Med 38:351–361, 1994

Keller D, Honig AS: Maternal and paternal stress in families with school-aged children with disabilities. Am J Orthopsychiatry 74:337–348, 2004

Kendler KS, Thornton LM, Prescott CA: Gender differences in the rates of exposure to stressful life events and sensitivity to their depressogenic effects. Am J Psychiatry 158:587–593, 2001

Kessler RC, McGonagle KA, Zhao S, et al: Lifetime and 12-month prevalence of DSM-III-R psychiatric disorders in the United States: results from the National Comorbidity Survey. Arch Gen Psychiatry 51:8–19, 1994

Klein H: Couvade syndrome: male counterpart to pregnancy. Int J Psychiatry Med 21:57–69, 1991

Lamb ME, Laumann Billings LA: Fathers of children with special needs, in The Role of the Father in Child Development, 3rd Edition. Edited by Lamb ME. New York, Wiley, 1997, pp 179–190

Landolt MA, Vollrath M, Ribi K, et al: Incidence and associations of parental and child posttraumatic stress symptoms in pediatric patients. J Child Psychol Psychiatry 44:1199–1207, 2003

Lansky MR: Fathers Who Fail: Shame and Psychopathology in the Family System. Hillsdale, NJ, Analytic Press, 1992

Leathers SJ, Kelley MA: Unintended pregnancy and depressive symptoms among first-time mothers and fathers. Am J Orthopsychiatry 70:523–531, 2000

Lyons-Ruth K, Wolfe R, Lyubchik A, et al: Depressive symptoms in parents of children under age 3: sociodemographic predictors, current correlates, and associated parenting behaviors, in Child Rearing in America: Challenges Facing Parents With Young Children. Edited by Halfon NE, McLearn KT. New York, Cambridge University Press, 2002, pp 217–259

Maciejewski PK, Prigerson HG, Mazure CM: Sex differences in event-related risk for major depression. Psychol Med 31:593–604, 2001

Marsiglio W: Studying fathering trajectories: in-depth interviewing and sensitizing concepts, in Conceptualizing and Measuring Father Involvement. Edited by Day RD, Lamb ME. Mahwah, NJ, Erlbaum, 2004, pp 61–82

Marsiglio W, Diekow D: Men and abortion: the gender politics of pregnancy resolution, in The New Civil War: The Psychology, Culture, and Politics of Abortion. Edited by Beckman LJ, Harvey SM. Washington, DC, American Psychological Association, 1998, pp 269–287

Marsiglio W, Hutchinson S: Sex, Men, and Babies: Stories of Awareness and Responsibility. New York, New York University Press, 2002

Matthey S, Barnett B, Ungerer J, et al: Paternal and maternal depressed mood during the transition to parenthood. J Affect Disord 60:75–85, 2000

McMahon TJ: Drug dependence, psychological representations of fathering, and reproductive strategy. Paper presented at the annual meeting of the College on Problems of Drug Dependence, Quebec City, QC, Canada, June 2002

McMahon TJ, Rounsaville BJ: Substance abuse and fathering: adding poppa to the research agenda. Addiction 97:1106–1115, 2002

McMahon TJ, Luthar SS, Rounsaville BJ: Looking for poppa: a developmental-ecological perspective on fathers enrolled in methadone maintenance treatment (abstract), in Problems of Drug Dependence, 1999: Proceedings of the 61st Annual Scientific Meeting, the College on Problems of Drug Dependence, Inc. (NIDA Research Monograph 180, NIH Publ No 00-4737). Edited by Harris LS. Rockville, MD, National Institute on Drug Abuse, 2000, p 269

McMahon TJ, Luthar SS, Rounsaville BJ: Finding poppa: a comparative study of fathers enrolled in methadone maintenance treatment (abstract). Drug Alcohol Depend 63(suppl):S102–S103, 2001

Mincy RB, Pouncy HW: The responsible fatherhood field: evolution and goals, in Handbook of Father Involvement: Multidisciplinary Perspectives. Edited by Tamis-LeMonda CS, Cabrera N. Mahwah, NJ, Erlbaum, 2002, pp 555–597

Murphy SA, Johnson LC, Lohan J: The aftermath of the violent death of a child: an integration of the assessments of parents' mental distress and PTSD during the first 5 years of bereavement. Journal of Loss and Trauma 7:203–222, 2002

Nelson TJ, Clampet-Lundquist S, Edin K: Sustaining fragile fatherhood: father involvement among low-income, noncustodial African-American fathers in Philadelphia, in Handbook of Father Involvement: Multidisciplinary Perspectives. Edited by Tamis-LeMonda CS, Cabrera N. Mahwah, NJ, Erlbaum, 2002, pp 525–553

Nock SL: The consequences of premarital fatherhood. Am Sociol Rev 63:250–263, 1998

Palkovitz RJ: Involved Fathering and Men's Adult Development. Mahwah, NJ, Erlbaum, 2002

Pancer SM, Pratt M, Hunsberger B, et al: Thinking ahead: complexity of expectations and the transition to parenthood. J Pers 68:253–280, 2000

Parke RD: Fathers and families, in Handbook of Parenting, Vol 3: Being and Becoming a Parent, 2nd Edition. Edited by Bornstein MH. Mahwah, NJ, Erlbaum, 2002, pp 27–73

Parke RD, Brott AA: Throwaway Dads: The Myth and Barriers That Keep Men From Being the Fathers They Want to Be. Boston, MA, Houghton Mifflin, 1999

Parke RD, Coltrane S, Duffy S, et al: Economic stress, parenting, and child adjustment in Mexican American and European American families. Child Dev 75:1632–1656, 2004

Patterson GR, Capaldi DM: Antisocial parents: unskilled and vulnerable, in Family Transitions. Edited by Cowan PA, Hetherington EM. Hillsdale, NJ, Erlbaum, 1991, pp 195–218

Phares V: Fathers and Developmental Psychopathology. New York, Wiley, 1996

Pleck EH: Two dimensions of fatherhood: a history of the good dad–bad dad complex, in The Role of the Father in Child Development, 4th Edition. Edited by Lamb ME. New York, Wiley, 2003, pp 32–57

Pleck JH, Masciadrelli BP: Paternal involvement by U.S. residential fathers, in The Role of the Father in Child Development, 4th Edition. Edited by Lamb ME. New York, Wiley, 2003, pp 222–271

Power C, Rodgers B, Hope S: Heavy alcohol consumption and marital status: disentangling the relationship in a national study of young adults. Addiction 94:1477–1487, 1999

Puddifoot JE, Johnson MP: The legitimacy of grieving: the partner's experience at miscarriage. Soc Sci Med 45:837–845, 1997

Puddifoot JE, Johnson MP: Active grief, despair, and difficulty coping: some measured characteristics of male response following their partner's miscarriage. J Reprod Infant Psychol 17:89–93, 1999

Raskin VD, Richman JA, Gaines C: Patterns of depressive symptoms in expectant and new parents. Am J Psychiatry 147:658–660, 1990

Rothe EM: The challenge of maintaining the fathering role after divorce: overcoming shame, in Step-Parenting: Creating and Recreating Families in America Today. Edited by Cath SH, Shopper M. Hillsdale, NJ, Analytic Press, 2001, pp 94–101

Shostak AB, McLouth G, Seng L: Men and Abortion: Lessons, Losses, and Love. New York, Praeger, 1984

Simons RL: The effect of divorce on adult and child adjustment, in Understanding Differences Between Divorced and Intact Families: Stress, Interaction, and Child Outcome. Edited by Simons RL. Thousand Oaks, CA, Sage, 1996, pp 3–20

Snarey JR: How Fathers Care for the Next Generation: A Four-Decade Study. Cambridge, MA, Harvard University Press, 1993

Soliday E, McCluskey-Fawcett K, O'Brien M: Postpartum affect and depressive symptoms in mothers and fathers. Am J Orthopsychiatry 69:30–38, 1999

Stone G: Nonresidential father postdivorce well-being: the role of social supports. J Divorce & Remarriage 36:139–150, 2002

Storey AE, Walsh CJ, Quinton R, et al: Hormonal correlates of paternal responsiveness in new and expectant fathers. Evol Hum Behav 21:79–95, 2000

12

MEN, MARRIAGE, AND DIVORCE

SCOTT HALTZMAN, M.D.
NED HOLSTEIN, M.D., M.S.
SHERRY B. MOSS, M.A.

Case Vignette

Wesley was a 52-year-old engineer married for 29 years to his high school girlfriend. His wife, Ginger, first contacted the therapist with a chief complaint of marital stress and wished to schedule an appointment for Wesley. Early in their relationship, Wesley and Ginger had managed conflict related to in-laws and money, and in the decade before the couple's presentation, they celebrated a relatively conflict-free marriage. They raised two daughters (now in college) despite frequent moves around the country to accommodate his work designing factories for large corporations. In the months before the couple's presentation, the family had experienced increased stress related to financial concerns. The couple argued more frequently, with Ginger expressing sadness over Wesley's perceived lack of sensitivity to her concerns. Wesley was frustrated about the family problems but rather than discuss the situation with his wife, he attempted to resolve their financial duress by working more. As their marital stress increased, Ginger began to complain that Wesley was not home enough or "emotionally connected" to her. Rather than experiencing relief at his efforts to work more, she became unhappier and began to withdraw from him emotionally and sexually. She insisted that they find a therapist to "work through" their problems.

In 2004, 90% of Americans age 35 and over had married at least once (U.S. Census Bureau 2004). Marriage is a significant event in a person's life. It is a legal, social, and economic decision and, in Western culture, a romantic declaration. Although in comparison to the life span the marriage ceremony itself is quite brief, the act of marrying dramatically affects the course of a person's life.

There are myriad health and social benefits for married individuals and their children. Although both married men and women experience longer life expectancies, men appear to derive more life-extending benefits from marriage. Men who never marry are statistically more likely to have physical and mental health problems (Waite and Gallagher 2000). For men in particular, marriage increases the sense of community, improves financial security, and contributes to interpersonal growth and well-being (Nock 1998).

Becoming a husband marks a dramatic shift in sociological status. Marriage both empowers a man as a full-fledged adult and increases his sense of duty and responsibility. This responsibility frequently includes the expectation that he maintain a job and support his family. In 70% of American households, the man is the main breadwinner. Husbands' work commutes are on average 36% longer than those of their wives, and men who marry typically earn more money compared with men who never marry (Farrell 2005).

As men evolve into their new role as husbands, they generally find these changes ego-syntonic. In many cases, devoting themselves to work is not a significant change and merely solidifies a preconceived role. However, transitioning from bachelor to husband, despite keeping the same love object, frequently results in a dramatic change in a husband's mode of interaction with his wife. Most Western marriages are marked at onset by high levels of happiness and optimism. The couple find in each other a source of support and satisfaction. Yet as the marriage proceeds, warm and positive emotions that husbands and wives initially display typically decline (Lucas et al. 2003). And when a man fails to maintain a successful marital relationship, tremendous despair and psychological trauma frequently follow.

GENDER AND MARITAL CONFLICT

When two people share common living space and are contractually obligated to each other, interpersonal conflicts arise. When the nature of that bond is a heterosexual marriage, many typical conflicts involve or reflect gender differences. For instance, women are more likely to describe themselves as unhappy in the marriage (Waite et al. 2002) and lodge household complaints (Gottman and Silver 1999). Many wives' discontent stems from a perception that their husband is either inattentive to their efforts to communicate (e.g., "He never listens") or unable to meet their emotional needs (e.g., "I don't feel connected to him"). Although men are less likely to report marital discontent, they are sensitive to their wives' complaints. Men in couples counseling frequently state, "I don't know what to do make her happy."

Interpersonal communication and depth of emotional bond issues frequently emerge as predominant themes in marital relationships between men and women. Brain imaging scans and neuropsychological testing provide evidence that brain function, particularly visual-spatial and emotional processing, differs in men and women throughout the life span. For example, minutes after birth, girls are more likely to fix their gaze on a face, whereas boys are no more attracted to a face than they are to geometric shapes (Baron-Cohen 2003). The amount of testosterone a male fetus is exposed to by the time he is born is inversely proportional to the length of time he holds eye contact with his mother 1 year later (Baron-Cohen 2003), and fetal hormonal exposure influences gender-typical behavioral attributes of the child (Kimura 1999).

Gender-related behavioral differences persist into adulthood. Compared with women, men process emotional, visual, and verbal content differently. Men are less consistent and less rapid in their abilities to recognize and label facial expressions (Killgore and Yurgelun-Todd 2004). Whereas women demonstrated limbic activation in response to emotionally laden words, men activated left hemispheric verbal regions (Bremner et al. 2001). In contrast to women, men did not show increased hippocampal blood flow when negative emotions were triggered (Schneider et al. 2000), suggesting a diminished capacity to recall or process disturbing events.

Brain histopathological findings may explain some differences between men and women. The fibers of the corpus callosum connect the left hemisphere (thought to preferentially involve speech and logical mental processing) to the right hemisphere (thought to preferentially process emotion-related material). Although controversial, some findings suggest that fibers within the posterior splenium of the corpus callosum are thicker in women (Holloway et al. 1993; Hwang et al. 2004). It is hypothesized that increased capacity to transmit information from the "nonverbal" right brain to the "verbal" left brain may in part explain women's better ability to express feelings in words. This brain difference may also in part account for men having difficulty "hearing" emotionally charged words and having diminished arousal to these words. Although verbal skills typically appear stronger in females, visual-spatial cortical functioning is often superior in males (Gur et al. 2000).

Although no studies have directly examined the neural biology of marital discord, some aspects of marital stress likely involve gender differences in neurobiology and behavior. The relative lack of conflict during the early stages of courting may be due in part to the increased attentiveness of the man during courtship, at which time he typically demonstrates a heightened ability to attend to the emotional needs of his wife-to-be. Likewise, increased arousal levels on the woman's part allow her to enjoy more nonverbal time with her suitor and rely less on verbal communication. When conflict occurs early in dating or marriage it is usually quickly resolved because both parties want to perpetuate the good feelings that accompany the romantic phase of marriage. Early in relationships, partners tend to ignore their areas of difference.

After several months of marriage, spouses generally become more aware of their differences or the novelty of these differences diminishes. Women may have an increased desire for their men to feel emotionally connected through words, and men may be confused as to why their actions to support the marriage are less appreciated than they once were. Some men may not be able to express their feelings in a way that can be understood by their wives. As such, these men are labeled as "impaired" in their ability to contribute to the marriage. Men often desire mastery of a task, and being told by their wives they are not competent at relationship building often increases men's feelings of helplessness or anxiety. As demonstrated in the initial vignette, feelings of helplessness are often a central issue in marital relationships. Because women are more likely to express marital discontent, men who experience marital strife will frequently describe feeling unable to meet their wives' expectations. Husbands who learn to anticipate their wives' expectations and attend to them competently are more likely to achieve a successful marriage. Conflict management tools are essential to this task.

MANAGING CONFLICT

Conflict is an inevitable part of marriage—and how couples react to conflict is predictive of the success of their marriage. The most common areas of disagreement within a marriage are money, household chores, the first child, in-laws, and sex (Gottman and Silver 1999).

Arguably, the largest obstacle for couples to successfully negotiate marital conflict lies in differences in communication styles between men and women. Frequently, women emphasize verbal communication as a means of resolving problems, and many women expect that their mate will value this form of problem solving as well. A wife may assume that her husband can easily communicate his emotional experiences in response to her own. Some men report feeling frustrated because they feel overwhelmed by the quantity of their wives' verbalizations. Sociologists theorize that women communicate to develop networks and deepen their sense of cooperative alliance. Generally, men use fewer words than do women and tend to communicate to develop hierarchies of dominance (Tannen 1991). Thus a man may hear his wife's attempts to discuss problems as a challenge to him, and he may attempt to utilize problem-solving skills to construct solutions to "fix" the problems his wife enunciates. In order to avoid feelings of helplessness and decrease autonomic arousal, the husband may withdraw from the interaction. The man's withdrawal often inadvertently increases his spouse's anxiety and, in an effort to mend the riff, may lead her to seek further connection with him by talking more.

This approach-avoidance behavioral dyad is a multifactorial phenomenon emerging from neuropsychiatric traits (a relative impairment of men to recognize the emotional import of their wife's verbalizations or verbalize an emotion-based reaction), neurophysiological states (a wish to prevent autonomic arousal), and sociological influences (a lack of social training in handling domestic disputes). Many women are not aware of these gender-related differences in cognition, neuroendocrine function, or socialization and may expect their husbands to respond in an "appropriate fashion," where "appropriate" reflects a feminized view of social discourse. In order to avoid feeling impaired and prevent disappointing his wife, a husband may reflexively pull away.

All interactions provide a couple with opportunities either to improve or to disrupt their level of connectedness. Every communication is a complicated dialogue of "bids" to be recognized and heard (Gottman and DeClaire 2002). How a person responds to these bids informs an observer about the relationship. Husbands in stable relationships ignore 19% of their wives' bids for "connection." In couples headed for divorce, men ignore 82% of these bids. Women are less inclined to ignore their spouse's bids outright; rather, they focus on other household or their own interpersonal needs. In happy marriages, only 14% of the husband's bids are ignored. In troubled marriages, women ignore 50% of their husband's bids (Gottman and DeClaire 2002). Responding to a spouse's bid for connection is critical for making him or her feel cared for and important. Predictably, men who ignore these bids are more likely to have marital disruption or divorce.

Less than 25% of couples seek marital therapy before considering divorce (Doss et al. 2003). Clinicians may promote marital health in men in other psychiatric or medical settings. A substantial challenge for clinicians is finding ways to engage men in the process of developing good marital skills. Consistent with men less frequently seeking health care in general (see Chapter 17, "Overcoming Stigma and Barriers to Mental Health Treatment"), they are less likely than women to engage in therapy to improve their relationships. Men are typically less comfortable with feeling-based words and may respond more to action-based words, and providers who wish to generate change in men may inadvertently alienate them when they set objectives that do not resonate with male styles of mental processing. For instance, asking a man to foster a "deep emotional connection" with his wife may be met with confusion and avoidance. Likewise, suggesting that he should focus on "getting in touch with feelings" may fail to generate improvement and repel him from treatment. In order to connect with men, it is important to appeal to their style of communication. Clinicians should teach men how to improve their marriage by focusing on concrete and measurable conflict resolution approaches.

One operationalized example of action-based communication skills involves reflective listening. Reflective listening is a style of conflict resolution that can be readily applied to marriage. In PREP (Prevention and Relationship Enhancement Program), couples are taught to take turns: one partner talks about his or her areas of concerns while the other listens, and then the listening partner echoes back what he or she has heard. Only when the first partner has felt heard can the second partner "take the floor." Such systematized communications rely on certain ground rules. The first speaker must limit the scope of the discussion, and the second must be aware of certain "filters," such as inattention, bad moods, stylistic differences, or unrealistic beliefs or expectations.

When couples can learn to be aware of these filters, they better understand the intent of their partner's words, experience less subjective tension, and can better engage in cooperative discussions (Markman et al. 1993). Some features of PREP appear particularly appealing to men: it is structured, dialogue is goal oriented rather than free-floating, and the approach provides specific tasks (collecting data to reflect back to their partner). These features tend to help men maintain attention and not feel overwhelmed with emotional content. One drawback of this approach for many men is that it focuses on verbal communication and does not utilize positive effects of nonverbal communication.

Although intuitively attractive, approaches like PREP have been challenged with respect to their efficacies. Other, mathematical formulas have been used to predict the outcome of marriages based on the processes that occur during arguments in natural settings. A strong predictor of marital success is at least a 5:1 ratio of positive to negative interactions (Gottman and Silver 1999). Examples of positive interactions include expressing kind words, paying attention, providing a pleasant experience, making conciliatory gestures, and expressing compliments. Examples of negative behaviors include complaining, criticizing, mocking, insulting, whining, communicating contempt, and ignoring one's spouse. Therapists may teach couples to meet or exceed this 5:1 ratio to reduce their risk of divorce. As in PREP, men are likely to feel bolstered by a more measurable process, in this case a mathematical one. Other methods of managing or resolving conflict are described as follows:

- Teach the couple to focus on initiating arguments with a soft start-up. By toning down the initial phase of the discussion and using "I" statements (such as "I am upset when you leave the toilet seat up"), the couple are less likely to become distraught when discussing a conflictual topic.
- Once the couple engage in debate, certain behaviors (e.g., criticism, contempt, defensiveness, and stonewalling [a form of emotional avoidance and withdrawal]) are predictive of poor marital outcomes. By avoiding these behaviors, a couple greatly increases the chances that the marriage will thrive.
- The process of repair is essential after marital conflict. Couples who can successfully return to their spouse and display a desire to heal the wound of the argument have low rates (16%) of separation. Couples who fail to resolve issues have rates of divorce in excess of 90%. It is important to remind couples that autonomic arousal impedes conflict resolution and that a cooling-down period is often necessary.

SEXUAL ISSUES IN MARRIAGE

When people describe themselves as happily married, they report that their sexual relationship accounts for about 10%–20% of their happiness. When marital dissatisfaction is high, couples report that sexual problems account for up to 75% of their discontent (McCarthy 2004). Significantly more men describe themselves as having higher sex drives than their female partners (Baumeister et al. 2001). The presence of testosterone in men at levels 10–20 times greater than in women appears to underlie the differences in sex drives (Christiansen 2001). Other factors may include social pressure on men to be ever ready for sex; easy access to pornographic images; and a tendency for men to seek emotional connection through intercourse. Compared with women, men reach sexual peak early in life (usually before age 20) and thus may be more attuned to their sexual desires from an earlier age. Men's limbic systems may also be more adapted to promote sexual behaviors. In experiments involving sexually arousing visual stimuli, men demonstrated higher rates of blood flow to the amygdala (Hamann et al. 2004). It is hypothesized that this limbic activation results in increased arousal and engagement in sexual behavior.

When a man has a higher sex drive than his wife, therapeutic approaches have typically focused on the man's need to attend to his mate's perceived need for more "romance." By following this advice, the man is led to believe that frequent phone calls, gifts, or attention will increase his wife's level of sexual desire. To the extent that a woman wishes to feel cared for and loved as a prerequisite to arousal, increased courting behaviors on the part of a husband are appropriate. Intuitively, couples recognize that increasing romantic gestures may help the woman feel more relaxed, and (in both men and women) a decrease in anxiety correlates with improved sexual functioning. However, although this romantic approach has some validity, this course of action is not entirely helpful. (For example, studies show that men who engage in more housework—an activity not typically deemed romantic—report more frequent sex [Gottman and Silver 1999].)

Men who take the approach of increasing the intensity of romantic gestures and improving communication with their wives will frequently complain that they are trapped in a conundrum: their wives may not only feel courted but also feel an increased pressure for sex. The perceived demand for more sex may be met with the woman's resistance or anger and a decreased likelihood that the man's objective will be met. Moreover, an increase in romantic connectedness will not necessarily result in a dramatic heightening of sexual desire, nor will it automatically trigger a wish to engage in sexual intercourse as a means of positive feedback to the husband, especially if the romantic efforts are made when the woman is not in the high fertility part of her menstrual cycle. Therefore, men who employ the strategy of stepped-up courting may find that their sexual needs still are not met and feel even more frustrated than before they employed this technique.

Furthermore, when couples seek to increase their sexual connection by relying on closer bonds of friendship, their strategies may backfire. Intimacy and couple time are prime bridges to sexual desire, but too much intimacy may stifle erotic feelings and subvert desire (McCarthy 1999). Therefore, couples who have a "friendship" style of marriage may have a decrease, not an increase, in the frequency and intensity of sex (McCarthy 1999).

Therapeutic approaches to this issue of dissimilar sex drives are delicate. When men have higher sexual desires than their wives, therapists should communicate that these desires should not be scorned, deferred, or neglected. It is reasonable that women ask that men attend to their needs for romance, trust, respect, and safety (as well as sexual needs), but men should expect that women not dismiss their sexual needs as secondary or something that should only be addressed once all other aspects of the relationship are satisfactory. To help couples resolve sexual functioning, it is often important to use a multimodal approach that includes the following:

1. Help couples broaden the scope of sexual touch beyond the strict confines of sexual intercourse. If men can be taught to appreciate nongenital touch, massage, dance, and play as forms of sexual interaction, they may not be as focused on sexual intercourse as the only expected outcome of intimate interactions.
2. Eroticism should be encouraged and can take place as part of sexual intercourse or as an end in itself. Couples can be encouraged to explore erotic touch or engage in erotic fantasy play. Depending on the moral or religious beliefs of the couple, marital aids such as vibrators or pornographic movies may enhance the erotic connection between them.
3. The partner with the lower sex drive should be encouraged to regularly engage in sexual intercourse (or other forms of sexual interactions that lead to orgasm in the partner), even if he or she is not experiencing high levels of desire.
4. Partners who do experience higher sex drives and whose spouses are not willing or able to engage in sex as frequently as they would like should be encouraged to masturbate to reduce a sense of urgency and to minimize conflict with incongruent sexual desires.
5. Sex should not be avoided during times of relational conflict. Sexual connectedness should not be viewed as an end point of marital happiness; it ought to be considered as important to the relationship as verbal communication.

MALE-SPECIFIC ISSUES IN MARITAL THERAPY

Several environmental issues preferentially influence men and should be assessed when providing marital therapy. For example, although most American women work, men tend to work longer hours and are more likely to have full-time jobs. Many men therefore require appointments in the evening or on weekends (Farrell 2005).

Women often request psychiatric (or other medical) services for the couple because women typically perform household scheduling functions and are the ones to identify a need for marital therapy. The therapist should not draw conclusions that it is the wife who seeks contact; the wife's contacting does not necessarily reflect a passive-aggressive stance from the husband, nor does it mean that the wife is more motivated to change than is the husband.

The therapist may wish to provide "male friendly" decor in the consultation room. Male-oriented reading material in the waiting room and a general environment in which men will feel comfortable may help engage men in marital therapy.

The therapist should recognize that physical inactivity can reduce a man's creativity. The therapist might consider including action-oriented components in therapy: going outside for air (while addressing confidentiality concerns), bringing the couple to the basketball court, or making paper airplanes in the office and seeing who can throw them the farthest. If these activities cannot be done directly inside or outside of the office, prescribing time for physical activities to do at home is as important as prescribing time for talking.

Men's strong visual-spatial capacities promote a recognition of how processes work and their general trajectories. Because rules often appeal to men, it is important for them to understand the structure of the therapy and related aspects of time management. Men often find it helpful to know what to expect, from the timing of the sessions to the expected number of sessions.

The content of the session also benefits from structure imposed by the counselor. For example, a first session that proceeds without intervention by the therapist may give men the message that "there are no rules here." This message can cause a man to disengage and increase his anxiety. Imposing structure to placate the husband's anxieties may appear to minimize the wife's stylistic preferences and perpetuate a stereotype of the man needing to be in control. However, the clinician should remember that the husband who appears to have a strong degree of rigidity may not feel empowered at all: frequently such efforts to be "in charge" reflect his sense of loss and panic at the possibility of powerlessness. Imposing a structure on the couple from the first interview helps assure the man that one of his greatest worries, being out of control, will not happen in the therapist's office.

Marital therapists should be flexible in seeing husbands and wives separately. Having the wife present at each visit may create a dilemma for men, who might ask, "Đo I speak openly about my wife and thereby offend her and pay the price afterward, or do I keep my feelings to myself?" Men often do not have many models for discussing their feelings. However, clinicians should understand that men often discuss their feelings in settings in which they feel comfortable. Often when men do meet alone with a marital therapist, they report feeling less burdened.

Like women, men feel better when they are heard and validated. This feature holds even for men who are less comfortable with their verbal abilities. Using the therapeutic environment to allow the man to be heard provides a stronger therapeutic alliance and models the power of listening for him so that he can apply this skill to his own marriage.

A man is typically socialized to feel that if he talks badly about his wife, he betrays her and somehow lessens his own position in others' eyes. He often feels that his wife is a reflection of his status. When the therapist provides an encouraging, nonjudgmental setting, a man can learn how to verbalize without self-censoring some of the problems in the marriage.

When a husband meets alone with the counselor, he has an opportunity to learn about differences in how he and his wife perceive situations. Husbands can be instructed in how their wives may value verbal communication differently. They can also learn about gender differences in emotional reactivity and be given strategies for handling their own autonomic arousal that may accompany conflict.

When men experience heightened arousal, the therapist should consider cognitive-behavioral techniques in addition to psychodynamic strategies. These techniques might include self-soothing approaches, meditation, or prayer and regular exercise. Men can be encouraged to take time-outs if a discussion gets too heated and to return to the topic when they are feeling less emotionally charged. These techniques provide an action plan for men (e.g., "I will make my wife feel understood when she states what bothers her") and can help them develop a sense of mastery over these discussions.

In addition to hearing men alone, bringing wives into the office alone gives the therapist a chance to educate women so that they may benefit from the process of being heard in a supportive environment and learn gender-specific techniques for having successful relationships with their husbands.

During sessions when couples are seen together, the counselor should be cautious about allowing uninhibited self-revelation in the session. Although many women feel comfortable talking about their feelings vis-à-vis the marriage, most men do not easily express how they feel about relationships, and they may be tempted to use the therapist's office as a place to reveal their emotional state in front of their wives. Feelings of anger or hate may have fomented for long periods of time within the husband, and because he previously has not had such a forum for expressing these feelings, they may be magnified when he reveals them for the first time in therapy. The therapist should discourage a husband from ranting about emotions such as anger or frustration toward his wife until the wife demonstrates an ability to process these feelings without personalizing them. Equally, when a woman divulges her mounting frustrations without censure, her husband's increased autonomic arousal may prevent useful dialogue in the session.

The clinician may wish to avoid delving deeply into the husband's sense of vulnerability or insecurity early in treatment. Such revelations may provoke increased anxiety; the wife's reliance on her husband for safety and security exists on some level in nearly every marriage, even in those in which she is the main breadwinner. Early in treatment, a man's expression of fear may increase his wife's sense of instability.

Supportive psychotherapy is of minimal utility in couples therapy, particularly for men. Although many women describe therapeutic benefits that can evolve simply from being able to talk in a supportive environment (the therapist's office), many men prefer tangible tasks that allow them to feel a sense of accomplishment. Once objectives can be defined for the marriage (and these usually include communication issues), clear-cut and measurable assignments give each spouse a sense that he or she can generate beneficial change in the marriage. Teaching the couple listening skills and rules of engaging in conflict (as discussed earlier) gives the couple strategies to deal with stress and exercises that they can practice. The couple will progress to learning problem-solving techniques, including recognizing which problems may not be solved within the context of their relationship. The couple also may benefit from psychoeducation related to the health benefits of marriage and the positive influence of an intact family on the development and welfare of children. As therapy progresses, the therapist should be mindful that engaging a man's inherent wish to fix things may be the strongest asset for repairing the marriage.

If therapy is used prudently as a place to redefine commitment, learn about the nature of marriage (and the nature of conflict), and appreciate the unique qualities of each partner, it can give a couple the necessary tools to make their marriage better and stronger. If the marriage cannot be saved, the couple must deal with the often overwhelming consequences of divorce.

DIVORCE AND THE MENTAL HEALTH OF MEN

Divorce can be a profoundly disturbing process among couples with children and long-standing marriages. The psychological repercussions may last decades. The remainder of this chapter focuses on this type of divorce, rather than the approximate half of divorces in which the marriages were brief and childless.

Because of ubiquitous cultural myths that assign both blame and power to divorced men, many therapists have failed to grasp how dramatically the power balance in divorce has shifted against men since the late 1970s. Divorced men cannot be treated successfully without a realistic appreciation of the stressors they endure.

Common stressors of divorce for men include 1) loss of children, 2) loss of spouse, 3) loss of home, 4) loss of friends, 5) financial hardship, and 6) stressors of remarriage. Many divorced men experience additional stress because unfavorable societal stereotypes project an image of men thoughtlessly casting off women. As a consequence of these stressors, divorced men showed a ninefold increase in hospital admissions, difficulties at work, and depression (Bloom et al. 1978). In a large prospective study among men who experienced several work stressors, those who divorced had a 37% increase in total mortality compared with those who remained married (Matthews and Gump 2002).

Many divorced men employ defenses such as intellectualization, rationalization, or sublimation when describing their experience of the divorce. They may comment, "I don't see my children very often, but they are doing great with their mom and stepfather" or "Divorce isn't really such a big deal. That's all in the past." The therapist should not accept these kinds of assertions at face value, because they may represent a defensive cover for intense emotions.

Despite the many stressors of divorce, most men exhibit remarkable resiliency. Many divorced men assess their losses realistically and are able to move ahead. These men adapt more successfully. They are more likely to remain involved in their children's lives and to learn lessons that will help them in their next marriage. These men have the capacity to accept that life often falls short of their idealized image and that their own actions contributed to the marital dissolution.

Consequences of Divorce

The loss of frequent, predictable, and intimate relationships with their children is often particularly difficult for noncustodial parents. Family courts typically award sole physical custody of children to their mothers and award fathers parenting time consisting of every other weekend and a few hours for dinner on a weekday evening. Although it is increasingly apparent that this arrangement is less than optimal for most children (Amato and Gilbreth 1999; Bauserman 2002; Kelly and Lamb 2000; Lamb 2002; Thompson 1994), the deleterious effects on fathers have been explored much less (Dudley 1996).

Noncustodial parents quickly learn that they lose much of their ability to parent their children under these circumstances. They realize that no matter how adept they are in child care, it is difficult to be an effective parent with such limited contact. They often feel that they have little authority with their children. The noncustodial parent often feels a need to avoid parental conflict because they want the limited time with their children to be enjoyable. Thus they are frequently unable to discipline their children effectively.

Surveys of divorced mothers indicate that at least one-third have interfered with court-ordered parenting time of fathers (Pearson and Thoennes 1988). Within the first 4 years, between 25% (Ford 1997) and 61% (Braver et al. 2003) of custodial parents move significant distances away with the children. As children get into their preteen years, they increasingly desire time with their peers rather than with their parents. Thus even those fathers who maintain loving relationships with their children are likely to see them increasingly infrequently over time. Furstenberg et al. (1983) found that only 49% of children had seen their noncustodial parent within the past year and that only 16% of children had at least weekly contact.

The net result of these factors is, in many cases, ever-weakening ties with the children. Some therapists fail to understand that weekend visitations often become painful experiences rather than happy ones. Each visit may reopen old wounds in which both the noncustodial father and the child must confront the fact that they no longer have what they once had—an intimate relationship. Gradually, the father–child bond weakens and becomes superficial, until the highlight of their bond is reduced to a few hours at a restaurant.

A substantial minority of children of divorce go through varying periods of estrangement from their noncustodial parent, ranging from mild and temporary rejection to permanent estrangement (Marquardt 2005). A 4-year-old boy, for instance, regards his father as all-powerful. If he now sees his father only rarely and his father does not "magically" appear when he is mourning his absence, he feels abandoned by his father. This situation alone is enough in many cases to cause pain, anger, and rejection. If, in addition, his mother reinforces these feelings with negative verbalizations about his father, the likelihood of father–child estrangement becomes very strong.

The psychological effects of divorce depend in part on whether the person sought the divorce or was the discarded partner. The popular stereotype is that men initiate most divorces. However, women initiate most divorces (Ahrons 1994; Brinig and Allen 2000), and most men feel like the discarded partner, often remaining attached to their ex-wives (Berman 1985). Despite popular perception, male misbehavior, such as nonsupport, desertion, domestic violence, or alcoholism, is not the major cause of divorce. Women who initiated divorce cited the top three reasons as 1) "gradual growing apart, losing a sense of closeness"; 2) "serious differences in lifestyle and/or values"; and 3) "not feeling loved or appreciated by my husband" (Braver and O'Connell 1998).

In most cases, men actively oppose the dissolution of the marriage (Brinig and Allen 2000). Therapists should delve into this history, taking care to get past initial assertions that their patient desired the divorce, which are usually motivated by a man's reluctance to acknowledge a lack of control over his life. The man who has unwillingly lost his wife or who was ambivalent about the split usually experiences an intense sense of loss, often hidden behind a defensive mask. Once past the defenses, the therapist will often find that men who have left their spouses are likely to feel guilt and shame. Other men may express anger and blame toward the wife or self-righteousness as justification for the divorce. Many men with these feelings are taken by surprise by the other unanticipated losses they suffer in the divorce and may experience further distress as a result. Many experience disappointment or depression for which they may be unprepared, particularly if they left the marriage expecting improvements in their lives.

It is unusual for a divorced man to remain in the marital home, regardless of which party seeks the divorce. Few men can force their wives to leave, with or without the children, without a deep sense of guilt and betrayal of their masculine role as protector. Many men who leave from a sense of chivalry are thunderstruck when they realize that the courts, their friends, and, often most importantly, their children interpret their action as an abandonment of the family.

A particularly traumatic event is being evicted by a domestic restraining order when the man has not harmed or threatened the spouse. In such cases, police typically give the man approximately 10 minutes to gather a few belongings and then escort him from his home. He thereafter finds himself without financial records, checkbooks, car keys, household furnishings, or many of his personal effects.

Therapists should be particularly attentive to the emotions that result from this kind of eviction. Although a range of responses exists, many men consider their eviction to be one of the most traumatic events of their lives, even many years afterward. Occasionally, these men remain obsessed with the event and have accompanying feelings of rage, violation, betrayal, anger, anxiety, and humiliation that in some cases resemble posttraumatic stress disorder. Law-abiding men who were handcuffed and treated roughly by the police or who were incarcerated are especially prone to feelings of outrage, humiliation, betrayal, and violation, especially if any of these events occurred in front of their children.

Men typically become more isolated by divorce than do women. Many men in today's society actually have few close friends; for many, their "friends" are the husbands of their wife's friends, and these relationships typically do not survive divorce. Friends caught between conflicting loyalties are often compelled either to champion one party or lose contact altogether. Because it is usually the man who moves to a new residence, he may lose friendships among his neighbors, community associations, or place of worship. Because he usually does not gain custody of the children, he may find it difficult to maintain friendships with the parents of his children's friends.

The prevailing cultural belief is that compared with men, women experience a dramatic decrease in their standard of living after divorce. This widely held notion is no longer true. Since the 1980s, the economic circumstances of divorced women have changed dramatically because of the improved earning capacity of women, greatly increased and stringent enforcement of child support orders, and important changes in tax laws that favor single parents. The cumulative result of these changes is that most men who remain in the above-ground economy (i.e., those men whose income is taxed) are worse off after divorce than are their ex-wives. In a detailed analysis of seven representative states, Braver and Stockburger (2004) found that "under current child support guidelines, the majority of custodial parents have higher standards of living than their matched non-custodial parents" (p. 122). There is some evidence, however, that over time the economic status of both parties usually improves.

The economics of divorce have vast practical and emotional consequences. Men's parenting may be affected by the need to live some distance from their children in order to find affordable rent or by the need to work long hours that leave little time for the children. Sometimes the only housing divorced men can afford is too small to accommodate their children or is located in an undesirable neighborhood. They may be unable to date women of their former socioeconomic class because such women, either in the men's imagination or in reality, may devalue the men for their diminished status. The lack of control over these events is often extremely difficult for many men to process. Many of these men feel angry, depressed, hopeless, and emasculated, particularly those who must move in with their parents.

Remarriage may ameliorate some of the emotional turmoil of divorce, but it also introduces new difficulties. The divorced father often brings demands to his new wife as a result of the various stresses he continues to experience. He may depend excessively on his new wife for companionship, vent to her his anger, or behave miserably due to feelings of depression. Economic demands will sometimes require his new wife to work longer hours and postpone childbearing longer than she may have wished. When a new child does arrive, the husband often feels inadequate because after payment of child support, his earnings are often insufficient to support his new family.

As a father, a remarried man may feel he is lacking in authority in his new familial relations. Although he must learn to live amicably with stepchildren, he often feels he has little authority over them and that they are likely to resent his attempts to discipline them. He may feel like a visitor with little input into long-established routines and customs. Having little authority over his own children or his stepchildren, he feels a sense of loss about the nature of his domestic role.

Divorce may initiate an especially severe *downward spiral* among a few men, perhaps 1% or 2%, whose preceding psychological structure predisposes them to this pattern. The downward spiral may begin with intense fury and depression engendered by the various factors described earlier. This situation may lead to expensive and ill-fated legal battles. Some men become so emotionally depleted that their work suffers, and some lose their jobs. Without income, they may encounter child support arrearages. It is not unusual for these men to be incarcerated, because of either arrearages or heated exchanges with their ex-wives that are reported to the authorities as threats. Unemployed, financially depleted, depressed, and feeling pressure for child support payments they cannot make, they may lose their residence and contact with their children. As a result, they feel shame, guilt, or depression. Many with a prior history of substance abuse relapse, experience additional legal actions against them, feel more shame, and encounter more avoidance. Suicide becomes a significant risk among these men (Kposowa 2000).

Therapy for Divorced Men

Because cultural stereotypes about divorced men are prevalent, the therapist must be aware of his or her biases when attempting to create an empathic connection with the patient. This connection may be especially difficult to forge when the patient remains focused on that which was "done to him" while remaining blind to his own contributions to the problem.

The day of marital separation often marks the beginning of a period of acute crisis for many divorced men. Many feel overwhelmed by the multiple, simultaneous losses they incur as well as the new demands of finding a place to live, making ends meet, forging a new kind of relationship with their children, complying with the legal process, and other issues of general survival. Many previously well-functioning men become increasingly disorganized during the acute period, during which they may be in a near-constant state of limbic arousal. The intensity of their emotions may be unprecedented in their lives, and they may have strong, fluctuating emotions ranging from anger to helplessness.

In this stage, divorced men may be more receptive to supportive psychotherapy than ever before or after in their lives. Because family courts operate in a highly impersonal and peremptory manner, few individuals, male or female, feel that they have been heard in that venue. Even fewer feel validated there. Therapy offers an opportunity for validation, even if it involves simply attentive listening. Therapists should be open to seemingly far-fetched assertions, such as that a man was evicted from his home and incarcerated even though he had never threatened or assaulted his wife, that the court is indifferent to him having been prevented from seeing his children for months, or that the court is indifferent to his ex-wife selling his heirlooms. Some men may be unable to move past the need for supportive psychotherapy for an extended period of time. Frequently, these men are unable to see any prospect of improvement in their lives during the acute stage of therapy. They benefit from frequent reassurance that their lives will, in fact, improve.

During this acute crisis stage, emphasis should be placed on measures of crisis intervention. A psychopharmacological evaluation is usually indicated, with special attention to depression and anxiety. Because of the heightened state of arousal, cognitive-behavioral techniques such as self-soothing and meditation, prayer, and/or regular exercise may be of great benefit.

As soon as possible, therapy needs to move beyond simple crisis support to include structured, goal-oriented, and pragmatic tasks. Solution-focused therapy may be employed to help men understand the positive or negative effects of habitual coping skills. By asking men to define their goals in objective terms, a therapist can help them see that some of their activities may be counterproductive. For example, an obsession with obtaining justice through the court system may be particularly destructive in that it prolongs conflict, drains money and energy, and is rarely fruitful for men. Building positive bridges to the community, the children, and the ex-wife, in contrast, may help a man obtain his goal of more visitation with the children and a reduced internal state of anxiety.

Men who have recently separated also benefit from the identification of specific tasks for them to accomplish. For instance, men may be encouraged to get through the next visit with their child without creating a parental loyalty conflict for the child or without questioning the child about his or her mother. Other tasks might include refusing to be drawn into an argument with the ex-wife or refraining from attempts to seek cooperation from an ex-wife who appears intent on fighting.

Fathers should be helped to negotiate often radical changes in the nature of their relationships with their children. An empathic therapeutic alliance may help them to accept loss of authority while concurrently learning parenting skills they may not have needed in the past. For some men, it is extremely difficult, despite their best intentions, to appreciate the turmoil and pain their children are feeling. This situation is in part due to the brief parenting time they are usually allotted. Some fathers approach their children as though they are small adults who will understand the family's financial desperation, the perfidy of the child's mother, and the need for the child to take matters into his or her own hands. These men should be helped to abandon these unrealistic expectations of their children and to see their progeny as vulnerable and wounded and in need of security and love.

Among those ex-husbands who exhibit resiliency, the therapist should distinguish between those men who are achieving peace through defense mechanisms that may ultimately prove harmful and those men who are able to accept pain and loss realistically and move forward adaptively. The former are in danger of withdrawing from and perhaps abandoning their children, with delayed repercussions for the patient. These men are also in danger of terminating therapy without ever exploring underlying issues that may have contributed to the divorce and that may undermine their future relationships with women.

Divorced men who enter a downward spiral are at substantial risk for suicide, either immediately or after the passage of time. The clinician should remain alert to this very real danger in a small number of men.

Once a patient is able to apply cognitive and behavioral models to his emotional distress, he may be better prepared to work through many of the interpersonal and self-history issues that influenced the quality of his marriage. Most men who process the trauma of divorce eventually do well and become more available for psychodynamic therapy. At this stage, the therapist may fruitfully explore childhood experiences and other determinants of reactions to stress, dependency, narcissistic vulnerability, and other dynamics. Female therapists may be able to use the opportunity to explore issues of transference.

By employing a multimodal approach that attends to different stages of the emotional consequences of divorce, the clinician can assist men in coping with the ongoing demands of divorce and, if appropriate, in finding their way into a new and stronger marriage and dealing successfully with the inevitable conflicts of the new union. In doing so, the therapist may help the man not only have improved relationships in the future but also generate a better overall sense of self.

CONCLUSION

For men, marriage provides emotional and physical benefits. When marital conflict occurs, however, men appear to have different reactions, in part due to differences in communication styles and views of intimacy. When marriage ends in divorce, men face unique emotional, financial, and social challenges. Both marital therapy and therapy for men after divorce may be more beneficial if the issues unique to men are considered and addressed.

KEY POINTS

- Communication styles of men differ from those of women. Men's greater reliance on nonverbal communication and problem solving may be harnessed to foster the generation of a healthier marriage.

- Men and women experience intimacy differently. Men typically have stronger sex drives and women stronger desires for romance, and a healthy marital relationship involves strategies for maintaining intimacy despite these differences.

- Divorce is relatively common, and men who divorce experience particular challenges in the familial, social, financial, and occupational domains.

PRACTICE GUIDELINES

1. Successful marital therapy in men typically involves specific strategies for engaging men in treatment, providing an environment in which they feel comfortable, and validating their concerns.

2. Clinicians can help men process the trauma of divorce, examine contributions to the marital dissolution, and develop skills for maintaining father–child bonds and strengthening future intimate relationships.

REFERENCES

Ahrons C: The Good Divorce: Keeping Your Family Together When Your Marriage Comes Apart. New York, HarperCollins, 1994

Amato P, Gilbreth JG: Nonresident fathers and children's well-being: a meta-analysis. J Marriage Fam 61:557–573, 1999

Baron-Cohen S: The Essential Difference: The Truth About the Male and Female Brain. New York, Basic Books, 2003

Baumeister RF, Catanese KR, Vohs KD: Is there a gender difference in strength of sex drive? theoretical views, conceptual distinctions, and a review of relevant evidence. Pers Soc Psychol Rev 5:242–273, 2001

Bauserman R: Child adjustment in joint-custody versus sole-custody arrangements: a meta-analytic review. J Fam Psychol 16:91–102, 2002

Berman WH: Continued attachment after legal divorce. J Fam Issues 6:375–392, 1985

Bloom BL, Asher SJ, White SW: Marital disruption as a stressor: a review and analysis. Psychol Bull 85:867–893, 1978

Braver SL, O'Connell D: Divorced Dads: Shattering the Myths. New York, Tarcher Putnam, 1998

Braver SL, Stockburger D: Child support guidelines and equal living standards, in The Law and Economics of Child Support Payments. Edited by Comanor WS. Cheltenham, UK, Edward Elgar, 2004

Braver SL, Ellman IM, Fabricius WV: Relocation of children after divorce and children's best interests: new evidence and legal considerations. J Fam Psychol 17:206–219, 2003

Bremner JD, Soufer R, McCarthy G, et al: Gender differences in cognitive and neural correlates of remembrance of emotional words. Psychopharmacol Bull 35:55–78, 2001

Brinig MF, Allen DW: These boots are made for walking: why most divorce filers are women. American Law and Economics Review 2:126–169, 2000

Christiansen K: Behavioural effects of androgen in men and women. J Endocrinol 170:39–48, 2001

Doss BD, Atkins DC, Christensen A: Who's dragging their feet? husbands and wives seeking marital therapy. J Marital Fam Ther 29:165–177, 2003

Dudley JR: Noncustodial fathers speak about their parental role. Fam Concil Courts Rev 34:410–426, 1996

Farrell W: Why Men Earn More: The Startling Truth Behind the Pay Gap and What Women Can Do About It. New York, AMACOM, 2005

Ford C: Untying the relocation knot: recent developments and a model for change. Columbia J Gend Law 7:1–53, 1997

Furstenberg FF Jr, Nord CW, Peterson JL, et al: The life course of children of divorce: marital disruption and parental contact. Am Sociol Rev 48:656–668, 1983

Gottman JM, DeClaire J: The Relationship Cure. New York, Three Rivers Press, 2002

Gottman JM, Silver N: The Seven Principles for Making Marriage Work. New York, Crown Books, 1999

Gur RC, Alsop D, Glahn D, et al: An fMRI study of sex differences in regional activation to a verbal and a spatial task. Brain Lang 74:157–170, 2000

Hamann S, Herman RA, Nolan CL, et al: Men and women differ in amygdala response to visual sexual stimuli. Nat Neurosci 7:411–416, 2004

Holloway RL, Anderson PJ, Defendini R, et al: Sexual dimorphism of the human corpus callosum from three independent samples: relative size of the corpus callosum. Am J Phys Anthropol 92:481–498, 1993

Hwang SJ, Ji EK, Lee EK, et al: Gender differences in the corpus callosum of neonates. Neuroreport 15:1029–1032, 2004

Kelly JB, Lamb ME: Using child development research to make appropriate custody and access decisions for young children. Fam Concil Courts Rev 38:297–311, 2000

Killgore WD, Yurgelun-Todd DA: Sex-related developmental differences in the lateralized activation of the prefrontal cortex and amygdala during perception of facial affect. Percept Mot Skills 99:371–391, 2004

Kimura D: Sex and Cognition. Cambridge, MA, Bradford Book–MIT Press, 1999

Kposowa AJ: Marital status and suicide in the National Longitudinal Mortality Study. J Epidemiol Community Health 54:254–261, 2000

Lamb ME: Placing children's interests first: developmentally appropriate parenting plans. Va J Soc Policy Law 10:98–119, 2002

Lucas RE, Clark AE, Georgellis Y, et al: Reexamining adaptation and the set point model of happiness: reactions to changes in marital status. J Pers Soc Psychol 84:527–539, 2003

Markman HJ, Renick MJ, Floyd F, et al: Preventing marital distress through communication and conflict management training: a four and five year follow-up. J Consult Clin Psychol 62:1–8, 1993

Marquardt E: Between Two World: The Inner Lives of Children of Divorce. New York, Crown Books, 2005

Matthews KA, Gump BB: Chronic work stress and marital dissolution increase risk of posttrial mortality in men from the Multiple Risk Factor Intervention Trial. Arch Intern Med 162:309–315, 2002

McCarthy B: Marital style and its effects on sexual desire and functioning. J Fam Psychother 10:1–11, 1999

McCarthy B: Rekindling sexual desire. Paper presented at the Annual Conference of the Coalition for Marriage, Family and Couples Education, Dallas, TX, July 2004

Nock S: Marriage in Men's Lives. New York, Oxford University Press, 1998

Pearson J, Thoennes N: The denial of visitation rights: a preliminary look at its incidence, correlates, antecedents and consequences. J Law Policy 10:363–380, 1988

Schneider F, Habel U, Kessler C, et al: Gender differences in regional cerebral activity during sadness. Hum Brain Mapp 9:226–238, 2000

Tannen B: You Just Don't Understand. New York, Ballantine Books, 1991

Thompson RA: The role of the father after divorce. Future Child 4:210–235, 1994

U.S. Census Bureau: America's Families and Living Arrangements: 2004. Available at: http://www.census.gov/population/www/socdemo/hh-fam/cps2004.html. Accessed April 5, 2006.

Waite LJ, Gallagher M: The Case for Marriage: Why Married People Are Happier, Healthier, and Better Off Financially. New York, Doubleday, 2000

Waite LJ, Browning D, Doherty W, et al: Does Divorce Make People Happy? Findings From a Study of Unhappy Marriages. New York, Institute for American Values, 2002

13

BODY IMAGE AND MUSCULARITY

ROBERTO OLIVARDIA, PH.D.

I am a 14-year-old male. I used to have a "six-pack" when I was 11. Since then, I lost it. I still have muscle, but it seems buried under about a centimeter of fat. I can pinch about 1.2 inches under my belly button. Nobody has ever told me that I'm fat, but I need help to lose this!

I am 25 years old. Every night I sneak into my kitchen and eat tons of food, like bread, cakes, cookies, sticks of butter, and anything else I can get my hands on. I can't stop. Then I stick my finger down my throat and puke it up. I don't know if I'm the only guy who does it. I know lots of girls do it. Am I crazy?

I am 27 years old and hate the way I look. I am 5 feet 8 inches and feel too short. I would feel so much better about myself if I was 6 feet tall. Does anyone know of a drug or diet that I could do to get taller?

I'm 12 years old and I'm too skinny. I am always being picked on for being too skinny. I want to gain weight, so I have been eating lots of food. Anyone out there know where I can get steroids?

It has long been recognized that many girls and women experience body dissatisfaction and accompanying body image disorders (Striegel-Moore et al. 1989). Less attention has been given to similar issues in boys and men. The quotes at the beginning of this chapter are taken directly from various Internet Web sites and indicate that a substantial number of boys and men have body image concerns (Pope et al. 2000b). Males are not immune to the pressures of achieving an ideal body. Boys and men today long to be Adonis—the Greek half-man, half-god who represented the ideal of masculine beauty. Adonis had a full head of hair; perfect skin; rugged, masculine looks; and most importantly, a V-shaped, muscular body frame. The extreme pursuit of the perfect male body has been popularly dubbed the *Adonis complex* (Pope et al. 2000b), representing the various manifestations of how males struggle with their body image. Eating disorders, anabolic steroid use, and muscle dysmorphia are three extreme manifestations. Along the spectrum are boys and men who are dissatisfied with their appearance and judge their self-esteem and self-worth by their looks.

BODY IMAGE DISSATISFACTION

Although our body image begins in infancy, its importance increases significantly in adolescence (Alsaker 1992). Puberty results in voice changes, pubic hair growth, growth spurts, and increased muscle mass. How adolescents grapple with these biological changes differs among individuals. Research indicates that body image satisfaction and body image disturbance may rely more on pubertal development than previously thought. Alsaker (1992) conducted a study of pubertal timing and body satisfaction using a Norwegian sample of 1,256 boys and 1,109 girls ages 13–16. In this study, boys who matured early rated their bodies as more satisfactory than boys who entered puberty later. Among girls, those who matured early were more dissatisfied with their bodies than those who matured later. Other studies report similar findings (Blyth et al. 1981; Williams and Currie 2000).

Investigations of body satisfaction have found that boys report significant appearance discontent. Page and Allen (1995) asked male Mississippi high school students to rate their current weight as "much too thin," "a little too thin," "just right," "a little too fat," or "much too fat" and then asked them to rate their weight satisfaction on a five-point Likert scale. Boys who perceived themselves to be too thin were most dissatisfied, whereas the girls who perceived themselves as being too fat were most dissatisfied. In a large study conducted by Moore (1990), 895 males ages 12–22 were given questionnaires related to body dissatisfaction. In this sample, 42% of subjects were dissatisfied with their current weight, with 18% of subjects believing that they were underweight and 22% believing that they were too fat. Furthermore, 33% of the group were not content with their overall body shape. The study also found that 50% did not like the shape of their chests or waists, 40% did not like the way their chests looked, and 43% were dissatisfied with their arms. This finding is consistent with earlier studies showing that men consistently express greatest dissatisfaction with their chests, body fat, and waists (Berscheid et al. 1973).

Paxton et al. (1991) studied the body image of 221 Australian male high school students and found similar results: 66% of boys responded that being thin would have a negative impact on their lives. The authors found that 78% of boys had high scores on the Advantages of Being Fitter Scale, whereas only 9% of boys scored high on the Advantages of Being Thin Scale. Higher levels of exercise were related to body satisfaction in boys, suggesting that working out may be perceived to result in a socially sanctioned ideal male body. These findings reinforce the impression that being underweight for men is generally far from the ideal. One study reported that underweight men were comparable with or even worse off than overweight women in terms of negative self-view and low self-esteem. Men who were underweight were more dissatisfied with their build, perceived themselves to be less handsome, felt that they had less sex appeal, and were lonelier (Harmatz et al. 1985).

Many studies that assess body image use figure drawings that range from thin to fat (Stunkard et al. 1983). Participants are typically asked to select their perceived and ideal body size as well as the body they think others prefer. There does not seem to be a clear consensus with males when using this assessment. Some males idealize a heavier figure, whereas others prefer a thinner figure (Cohane and Pope 2001). One explanation for this lack of consistency may be that the figure drawings extend only on a thin-to-fat axis. Thus a boy who wants to be bigger and more muscular, but not bigger and fatter, has no suitable figure to choose. Unlike female body image, where being overweight equates to being overfat, males do not mind being overweight as long as their weight is in lean muscle mass. Bodybuilders, for example, are overweight but not overfat.

In an effort to rectify this problem, researchers developed the somatomorphic matrix, a computer instrument to measure body image (Gruber et al. 2000). The somatomorphic matrix offers the advantage of measuring body image along two separate axes, one for fatness and one for muscularity. One study using a small sample of 35 boys at a soccer camp found that boys chose a body that was 35 pounds more muscular than they actually were as their ideal body (Pope et al. 2000b). Olivardia et al. (2004) conducted a study of 154 male college students using the somatomorphic matrix. Men were asked to select the figure that corresponded to their perceived image, choose an image that represented their ideal body, and choose the image that they thought women desired. Height, weight, and body fat percentage of each student were measured. In addition, they were administered self-esteem, depression, and eating disorder inventories. Results demonstrated that men perceived themselves to be fatter than they actually were. They chose an ideal body with 25 pounds more muscle and 8 pounds less body fat than their own bodies. Subjects also thought that women desired a much more muscular build than women actually did.

Results also highlighted the importance of muscle in the body image of men. For example, depression positively correlated with feeling less muscular (what the authors referred to as "muscle belittlement") but did not correlate with perceiving oneself as fatter than one truly was ("fat exaggeration") (Olivardia et al. 2004). This finding varies from study results of women, in whom body fat plays a central role. The fatter a woman perceives herself, generally the more dissatisfaction she has with her body (Berscheid et al. 1973). Such does not seem to be the case with men. Instead, the less muscular a male feels, the more depressed he reports being. In men, scores on the Eating Disorder Inventory (such as drive for thinness; bulimia; ineffectiveness; and body dissatisfaction) were positively correlated with muscle belittlement but not fat exaggeration. How fat a man perceived himself did not elicit any significant correlations, whereas self-esteem significantly correlated negatively with muscle belittlement, body dissatisfaction, and feeling out of shape.

Although girls report greater body dissatisfaction than do boys (Cullari et al. 1998), the gender gap may be relatively narrow. It is thought that girls view their bodies along an aesthetic dimension and boys view their bodies along a functional one (Rodin and Larson 1992). However, the need for one's body to perform manual tasks has dramatically diminished since the early 1900s, a time when the strength and function of the male body were paramount. If this functionality were the source of historical gender differences in body image, then researchers might predict that an increasing number of boys will be evaluating their bodies in a manner similar to that of girls (Mishkind et al. 2000; Pope et al. 2000b). Many questionnaires and surveys created to evaluate body dissatisfaction were designed and validated using female samples and thus may be valid only for females. Some emerging research has attempted to correct this problem by implementing body image instruments that specifically assess body image concerns of boys and men (Gruber et al. 2000; McCreary and Sasse 2000). It is important to recognize and understand a patient's negative body image within a clinical setting before the negative image leads to development of a more serious problem, such as an eating disorder.

EATING DISORDERS

Eating disorders, including anorexia, bulimia, and binge eating disorder, are more prevalent among women than men. However, more men have these problems than ever before (Pope et al. 2000b). Although men account for approximately 5%–15% of individuals with eating disorders (Andersen 1990), epidemiological data on male eating disorders are scarce. Lucas et al. (1991) found a lifetime prevalence of anorexia nervosa of 22.5 per 100,000 men in Minnesota. Two studies of the prevalence of bulimia in the American population have yielded rates of nearly 0.2% in men, approximately 10 times the rate of anorexia nervosa found in the Minnesota study (Drewnowski et al. 1988; Striegel-Moore et al. 1989).

The phenomenological characteristics of eating disorders in men are generally similar to those in women (Margo 1987; Olivardia et al. 1995). In particular, men and women with eating disorders share an important core symptom of dissatisfaction with body shape and weight. Olivardia et al. (1995) found that groups of men with eating disorders and women with eating disorders resembled each other closely in terms of severe body dissatisfaction, but both groups differed sharply on all body satisfaction indices from comparison subjects of the same sex without eating disorders.

The prevalence of other mental disorders in men and women with eating disorders is also similar (Olivardia et al. 1995). Both men and women with eating disorders exhibit a high lifetime prevalence of major mood disorders—primarily major depressive disorder—that is significantly higher than that exhibited in matched comparison groups of the same sex who do not have eating disorders (Olivardia et al. 1995).

Differences between men and women with eating disorders have also been noted (Pope et al. 2000b). Men with eating disorders report greater weight fluctuations, a more frequent history of obesity, and a later age at onset. The later onset may coincide with the later onset of puberty. Men tend to abuse laxatives and diet pills less frequently than do women. However, compared with women, men binge more often and are more likely to use exercise as a purging method. Substance abuse and sexual conflicts are present more frequently in men versus women with eating disorders. Finally, men are less likely to seek treatment, a characteristic that contributes to the belief that men are immune to these problems (Olivardia et al. 1995).

Studies have also assessed subclinical features in boys, including dieting, binge-eating, and purging behavior. A study of adolescents in Connecticut found that adolescent males engaged in multiple eating-disordered behaviors, including dieting (12.4%), vomiting (1.7%), using laxatives or diuretics (1.6%), and taking diet pills (1.2%), to control their weight (Newmark-Sztainer et al. 1999). Arguably even more revealing, 21.2% of adolescent males reported eating more food or using food supplements to gain weight or muscle.

MUSCULARITY

Unlike the female ideal of thinness, muscularity is the male ideal (Mishkind et al. 2000). The ideal of muscularity influences men much in the way the ideal of thinness influences women. Men most often select the muscular mesomorphic shape as their ideal (Olivardia et al. 2004) and believe that women desire a much more muscular male body than women actually report preferring (Jacobi and Cash 1994). Similar studies with women demonstrate that women believe that men desire a thinner female body than men actually prefer (Jacobi and Cash 1994). The drive for muscularity has been associated with poorer self-esteem and depressive symptomatology (McCreary and Sadava 2001).

Males in the extreme pursuit of a muscular body often describe the importance of having a muscular body as a means of expressing their masculinity (Dutton 1995; Klein 1993; Mishkind et al. 2000). Interviews conducted with boys and men illustrate that the muscular body is a symbol of strength, sexual virility, attractiveness, confidence, admiration, control, and dominance (Dutton 1995; Klein 1993; Mishkind et al. 2000). Thus boys who feel that they lack these qualities may seek a muscular body as compensation. For example, an 18-year-old male with muscle dysmorphia states, "At least if I'm big, it would mean I was something. Without my muscles, I might as well be dead. No one would notice me." Another 25-year-old patient reported, "At least if I'm perfect on the outside, it would make up for the nothing I am on the inside. Muscles are a good illusion that you are brave. The fact is I feel so weak inside. I have no control over anything in my life, except my body build—and even that I don't feel I can totally control." This lack of internal control can lead many males to obsess about getting muscular and then act out those obsessions in the form of compulsive behaviors, a condition known as *muscle dysmorphia*.

MUSCLE DYSMORPHIA

Muscle dysmorphia is a newly recognized disorder characterized by the preoccupation that one's body is not muscular enough or is too small (Olivardia 2001). Men with muscle dysmorphia are often in top physical shape; however, they do not perceive themselves to be big enough. When they look in the mirror, they see someone who is too small. Muscle dysmorphia was first discussed in 1997 and conceptualized as a subtype of body dysmorphic disorder. The prevalence of the disorder in the United States is unknown at this time but is hypothesized to be at least 100,000 men, with tens of thousands more demonstrating subclinical aspects of it (Pope et al. 1997).

The preoccupation in muscle dysmorphia focuses on one's size. One study found that 50% of men with muscle dysmorphia spent more than 3 hours per day thinking about their muscularity (Olivardia et al. 2000). This obsession generates substantial anxiety that is somewhat managed by a compulsive need to maintain a rigorous workout or diet schedule. Men with the disorder may spend long hours lifting weights at the gym, often neglecting important events in their lives. They feel awful if they miss a workout, fearing that muscular shrinkage will result. They may continue training despite hernias, broken bones, torn joints and ligaments, or other injuries. Their strict adherence to a specific diet may preclude them from eating at restaurants because the caloric and nutritional content of the food is unknown.

These preoccupations cause significant anxiety, much like feeling fat can be devastating to someone struggling with anorexia nervosa (Pope et al. 2000b). The thoughts are very intrusive, consuming, and often detrimental to relationships. One man avoided sex with his wife for fear that he would waste energy that could better be used in workouts, and another abstained from kissing his girlfriend for fear that she might transmit calories through her saliva. Many men with muscle dysmorphia report sexual problems due to their negative body image, feeling they are too ugly and weak-looking for anyone to see their bodies.

Aside from working out, men with muscle dysmorphia engage in other compulsive behaviors (Olivardia 2001). They repetitively check mirrors and other reflective surfaces. They avoid situations in which their bodies may be exposed to others, or they endure such situations only with marked distress or intense anxiety. Unlike some muscular men who proudly remove their shirts to reveal their bodies, men with muscle dysmorphia tend to do the opposite. They do not remove their shirts at the beach and may wear multiple layers of clothing to look more muscular. One man refused to remove his shirt during a physical examination, requesting that the doctor place the stethoscope underneath his shirt. Some men remain housebound for days because they feel so out of shape.

Olivardia et al. (2000) found that 46% of men with muscle dysmorphia reported using steroids versus only 7% of weight lifters without the disorder, leading to the assumption that muscle dysmorphia may be a risk factor for steroid use.

ANABOLIC STEROID USE

Anabolic-androgenic steroids (commonly referred to as "steroids") are in a family of drugs that include the male hormone testosterone and are used to promote lean muscle growth (Pope and Brower 1999). Illegal in the United States, steroids are taken orally or intravenously. Once relegated to elite bodybuilders, steroids are now trickling down to high school students. Recent studies indicate that up to 6% of male high school students have already used anabolic steroids (Buckley et al. 1988; Durant et al. 1993). More than 66% of these youth report using them before age 16. It is estimated that 2 million to 3 million males have used steroids in the United States alone (Pope et al. 2000b). The short-term physical effects of these drugs include cystic acne, breast enlargement, testicular shrinkage, and impotence. Long-term effects can be fatal. Steroid use can lead to hardening of the arteries, which can lead to heart attacks, strokes, and other complications at an early age. Liver damage and risk of prostate cancer have also been implicated as adverse effects (Pope and Brower 1999).

Psychological effects can include depression, mania, psychosis, and increased aggression (commonly referred to as "roid rage") (Pope and Brower 1999). Some men with no prior history of violence, criminality, or psychiatric disorder will become uncharacteristically aggressive while on steroids—violently assaulting and injuring girlfriends and spouses and even committing murder (Choi and Pope 1994). Some scientists still question whether these phenomena represent a genuine biological effect of anabolic steroid use or may be due to expectational factors, premorbid personality factors, or sociocultural effects. However, in three placebo-controlled double-blind studies, supraphysiological doses of steroids produced clear instances of hypomanic symptoms in normal volunteers (Pope et al. 2000a). These findings strongly suggest that a frank biological effect, rather than a psychosocial effect, is responsible for the pathology observed.

Earlier studies cite performance enhancement in sports as the primary reason that males used steroids. Recent studies, however, report that the strongest predictor for steroid use is body dissatisfaction (Blouin and Goldfield 1995). Aside from steroids, many legal products or supplements available at health food stores claim to enhance muscle growth (Pope et al. 2000b). These products, including creatine, androstenedione, and dehydroepiandrosterone, are not regulated by the U.S. Food and Drug Administration and therefore are not subject to rigorous testing. In fact, there are questions regarding their ability to promote muscle growth. In addition, the long-term adverse effects are currently incompletely understood. However, some ingredients in these "all natural" supplements may be dangerous. One such ingredient is ephedrine, which causes many adverse effects, including death.

Steroid use has also increased among gay men, in which population a muscular build is a symbol not only for masculinity but also for health (Signorile 1997). Signorile (1997) observed that more gay men use steroids as a defense against the homophobic stereotype that being gay makes one less masculine. Another motivation is a reaction to the acquired immunodeficiency syndrome (AIDS) epidemic. The wasting syndrome associated with AIDS has made being very thin a possible cue of illness. Asserting a large, muscular frame signals that the person is healthy sexually, even though he may not be (Signorile 1997).

The diagnosis of steroid use is most effective through adequate drug testing (Pope and Brower 1999). However, attending to physical and psychological cues may alert clinicians as to whether their patient is using steroids. Cues include increased muscularity in a short period of time; increased aggressive, depressive, manic, or psychotic symptoms coupled with body dissatisfaction; low self-esteem; perfectionism; and an insecure sense of masculinity.

GAY MEN AND BODY IMAGE

Contrary to popular belief, both heterosexual and homosexual men are at risk for the Adonis complex (Pope et al. 2000b). Previous research reporting a high prevalence of gay men in samples of males with eating disorders suggested that gay men were at higher risk for experiencing the complex (Herzog et al. 1991; Silberstein et al. 1989). Recent data suggest that gay men are overrepresented in clinical settings, the environments in which many studies of men and eating disorders are conducted (Pope et al. 2000b). Community studies of men with eating disorders and other body image problems do not show a significantly higher percentage of gay men (Olivardia et al. 1995). Gay men, however, may be more willing to discuss these issues and seek treatment for them. The majority of men with these issues do not seek treatment for body image concerns, possibly out of fear that they will be labeled as gay, vain, or unmanly. Arguably, a greater dialogue is available in gay communities for men to discuss body image concerns (Signorile 1997).

ETIOLOGY

Muscle dysmorphia has been conceptualized as part of the obsessive-compulsive spectrum, which posits that disorders such as obsessive-compulsive disorder, body dysmorphic disorder, and muscle dysmorphia share an underlying biological or genetic predisposition (Phillips 1996). These disorders share common phenomenological features and may run in families. Eating disorders have been theorized as being part of an affective spectrum that groups eating disorders in a similar physiological category with mood disorders (Hudson et al. 1983). Research assessing the presence of these disorders within families is being conducted. Although someone can be born with a genetic tendency for a disorder, environmental circumstances often contribute to its expression.

Relatively little is known about the psychological factors that influence men to develop eating disorders and muscle dysmorphia. Common personality traits include perfectionism, low self-esteem, and obsessive-compulsive personality features (Andersen 1990; Phillips 1996). Some men with eating disorders report having been underweight or overweight as children and adolescents; they were often harassed or teased by peers and felt socially uncomfortable about their weight (Pope et al. 2000b). Family data have shown that men with eating disorders report a distant relationship with their fathers (Herzog et al. 1991). Steroid users, as well as men with eating disorders and muscle dysmorphia, typically have concerns about their sense of masculinity (Pope et al. 2000b). Males striving to be an "Adonis" may be struggling with a sense of inferior masculinity. If they feel less masculine than their peers, for example, they may seek to develop a large, fit body as a means of compensating for their lack of internal masculinity. It is not clear whether feeling inadequate as a man leads the person to pursue a specific body as a means of expressing maleness in a purely physical and aesthetic dimension, or whether having these problems affects the person's experience as a man. More research is needed to elucidate these findings.

Images from television, movies, and video games often highlight the V-shaped muscular body considered ideal by society. The popularity of World Wrestling Entertainment and its well-muscled superstars is in large part a result of the adolescent male demographic who admire not only the sport but also the impressive physiques of the wrestlers. Various advertisements and the covers of health and fitness magazines feature muscular men—often well-built models—who are considered indicative of physical perfection. Pope et al. (2001) found that men's bodies are used increasingly in advertisements for products unrelated to the body. The authors found that the proportion of undressed women in popular women's magazines (such as *Cosmopolitan* and *Glamour*) has remained fairly steady over the last three or four decades, whereas the proportion of undressed men in such magazines has skyrocketed from as low as 3% in the 1950s to 35% in 1 year in the 1990s. Just as *Playboy* centerfolds have been documented as getting thinner over the decades (Garner et al. 1980), *Playgirl* models were found to be increasingly muscular between 1973 and 1997 and to have less fat (Leit et al. 2000). In fact, the study revealed that in the 25 years since the mid-1970s, the average *Playgirl* centerfold man shed about 12 pounds of body fat while putting on approximately 27 pounds of muscle. Increasing attention to the muscular physique has even been documented in department store mannequins, who are now sporting larger genital bulges and more chiseled, muscular builds (Rodin and Larson 1992).

Action figures also send boys messages about their appearance (Pope et al. 1999). If a 1998 G.I. Joe action figure were a real-life human male, his waist and biceps would both measure 26 inches and his chest would be 55 inches. These measurements are a sharp contrast to his 1982 counterpart, which would sport more ordinary dimensions. Researchers have reported the conscious attempt on the part of toy companies to "beef up" certain figures (Pope et al. 1999). When the popular movie *Star Wars* was originally released in 1977, an accompanying action figure line was released of the main characters, including Luke Skywalker and Han Solo. When *Star Wars* was rereleased in movie theaters in the mid-1990s in digitally remastered form, an action figure line of the same characters was sold to capture a new generation of fans. However, Luke's and Han's dimensions changed dramatically. Luke's figure, once characterized as boyish looking, with average physique, a closed robe, and soft facial features, changed into a man with a chiseled, more masculine face; defined, muscular legs; and an open robe showing sport-defined, muscular pectorals and a much smaller waist. Toy companies may have felt a need to change the figure to correspond with the current societal view of the ideal physical form. More research needs to be conducted as to the specific effects that media have on body image and body satisfaction. Some studies have demonstrated that exposure to muscular male images may quickly influence a man's body image. Leit et al. (2002) found that men who were exposed to advertisements featuring muscular men demonstrated higher body dissatisfaction versus men exposed to neutral advertisements, as reflected in an increased difference between the level of muscularity that they perceived themselves to have and their ideal level of muscularity.

Although the media may greatly influence how men and boys view their bodies, it would be inaccurate to consider media as the sole etiological factor. Overly focusing on the media also does a disservice to patients, because clinicians may neglect or de-emphasize other important social, psychological, or psychiatric factors.

INTERVENTIONS

Men with poor body image rarely present for treatment (Pope et al. 2000b). If they do, it may be for depression or substance abuse (although they rarely seek treatment for steroid abuse). The small number of men who seek treatment for body image disorders appears to reflect the intense shame and embarrassment that men who have this condition feel about their bodies. They often feel emasculated, vain, and effeminate, feelings that may prevent them from disclosing the problem to anyone. In addition, men with muscle dysmorphia may fear treatment because treatment would include decreasing time at the gym and ceasing steroid use, both of which could result in some decrease of muscle mass—often their biggest fear. Men with anorexia fear that treatment will make them fat.

When men do engage in treatment, the clinician should establish a strong rapport with the patient, validate his experience, recognize his courage in seeking help, and acknowledge his reservations about treatment. Through this process, the clinician gains credibility and strengthens the therapeutic alliance.

Important elements for treatment include assessment of the patient's body image, perception, and ideals; nutritional habits; steroid usage; and view of media influences (Pope et al. 2000b). Psychotherapy can explore the patient's peer experiences or important events that may have contributed to or resulted from appearance concerns. For some men, a discussion of gender and sexual identity may be relevant. Cognitive-behavioral strategies appear effective for men with eating disorders and muscle dysmorphia (Phillips 1996). Serotonin reuptake inhibitors may be effective for the obsessions and compulsions characteristic of the disorders (Phillips 1996).

Little has been written about treatment of steroid use, largely because steroid users rarely seek treatment (Pope et al. 2000b). Classical models of drug abuse rarely apply to "body image" drugs such as steroids; unlike other drugs of abuse, which reward the user with an immediate high, steroids produce a delayed reward in the form of a more muscular body that will presumably impress others. As modern society places an increasing value on an idealized male body, steroid users are unlikely to perceive their drug use as a pathological behavior that requires remediation. A substance abuse model may be appropriate for steroid use, although no published studies describe specific, empirically validated intervention strategies for this population (Pope et al. 2000b).

In the rare instances in which a steroid user seeks treatment, perhaps the best advice is for the clinician to consider the possibility of a treatable underlying body image disorder. Although ceasing steroid use is the ultimate goal in treatment, this process must be monitored carefully and requires medical supervision (Pope and Brower 1999). Men who cease steroid use may develop a major depressive episode as a withdrawal syndrome, sometimes progressing to the point of suicidal ideation and/or suicide (Thiblin et al. 1999).

Parents and educators can engage in preventive dialogues with the young men in their lives. Before this interaction, adults must educate themselves on the social context of male body image and recognize that boys and men are affected by how they feel about their bodies. Parents and educators can listen and talk to young men about the images they are faced with and explain to young men how body dissatisfaction is spurred by a multimillion-dollar industry. Many companies engage in advertising that heightens the insecurities of those individuals who feel that their bodies are not ideal.

Other conversations can include topics of masculinity, the need to fit in, and the various ways to embrace gender identity without resorting to obsessive or unhealthy behaviors. Gender identity appears particularly salient to males, because females struggling with eating and body dysmorphic disorders typically do not feel less feminine. Most importantly, parents and educators can help boys increase their self-esteem by giving praise that does not exacerbate concerns about their physical appearance. Last, if issues about body image have already adversely affected a boy, parents and educators can validate his experience by explaining that many of his peers feel similarly but likely do not openly discuss their feelings because of societal taboos about men discussing their emotions. Adults can reassure the boy that he is not vain, self-centered, or a "sissy" for having these feelings. In fact, it would be abnormal in today's culture not to feel insecure or self-conscious about appearance given the excessive attention it is paid in the media. Working with a professional who specializes in body image is preferable, especially those who have experience working with males.

HEALTH VERSUS HARM: WHERE'S THE LINE?

Although exercise, grooming, and other body image–related activities can be taken to extremes, every man has a valid "normal" level of preoccupation with his body. There is certainly nothing wrong with wanting to look one's best. Eating healthy, exercising regularly, and buying grooming products are not pathological behaviors for men. The difference between health and harm can be categorized by four criteria (Olivardia 2001):

1. Healthy self-esteem is generated from many different life factors, including relationships, occupational achievements, and personality strengths. Although these components do not diminish the role of body satisfaction in a person's self-esteem, men with the Adonis complex virtually rest their entire self-esteem on their appearance. This focus is particularly problematic because there is no permanence to appearance. To these men, aging, injuries, or lack of gym access can be completely devastating, crushing any sense of self-worth.
2. The presence of body image distortions can differentiate healthy versus unhealthy behavior. If the patient does not accurately perceive himself, he is more likely to turn to unhealthy behaviors to remedy a perceived defect.
3. The patient's pursuit of the perfect body interferes with normal life functioning. This focus contrasts to a healthier perspective of working out as part of a balanced day complete with other activities.
4. The patient engages in unhealthy behaviors (steroid use, purging) to achieve a desired body. A balanced pursuit of a healthy and fit body is generally positive, whereas the extreme pursuit is not. Even with proper nutrition and regular exercise, many males will still not be able to reach the ideals set forth in media images. Self-acceptance and the recognition of the large role that genetics plays in the way bodies are shaped and built are paramount.

CONCLUSION

Men are becoming increasingly preoccupied and dissatisfied with their body image. This preoccupation has manifested in various ways, including eating disorders, muscle dysmorphia, and steroid use. Boys are learning at a young age of the societal standards of being muscular as a means of expressing masculinity. This message carries a price with many consequences.

Because the issue of men's body image and muscularity is an area of research that is still relatively new, much undiscovered empirical terrain remains. Further research can examine accurate prevalence rates of muscle dysmorphia and steroid use as well as etiological influences. This research will serve as the important foundation for strengthening treatment interventions.

In the meantime, men will continue to wrestle with questions similar to the one posed by a steroid-using patient with muscle dysmorphia: "Why be Clark Kent when I can be Superman?" The resounding answer is that as long as the person is healthy, it should be perfectly acceptable to look like Clark Kent.

KEY POINTS

- Males are not immune to body image problems such as eating disorders. Contrary to popular belief, self-esteem and body image are related in boys and men.

- Muscle dysmorphia is a pathological preoccupation with muscularity. This preoccupation results in various compulsive behaviors and obsessive thoughts about one's body that often interfere with normal life functioning.

- Anabolic steroids have become an increasing problem among boys and men. Body image dissatisfaction is the main reason males resort to these dangerous drugs, which carry a host of physical and psychological consequences.

PRACTICE GUIDELINES

1. Clinicians must acknowledge and educate themselves about body image issues in males. They are often the first, and sometimes only, person a boy or man will disclose their problem to.

2. An understanding of popular culture and media images is important for clinicians, because these will undoubtedly be discussed in the course of therapy with males struggling with body image.

3. When working with a steroid user, it is very important that the process of discontinuing steroids be monitored medically, because withdrawal symptoms can include depression and suicidality.

REFERENCES

Alsaker FD: Pubertal timing, overweight, and psychological adjustment. J Early Adolesc 12:396–419, 1992

Andersen AE (ed): Males With Eating Disorders. New York, Brunner/Mazel, 1990

Berscheid E, Walster E, Bohrnstedt G: The happy American body: a survey report. Psychol Today 7:119–131, 1973

Blouin AG, Goldfield GS: Body image and steroid use in male bodybuilders. Int J Eat Disord 18:159–165, 1995

Blyth DA, Simmons RG, Bulcroft R, et al: The effects of physical development on self-image and satisfaction with body image for early adolescent males. Res Community Ment Health 2:43–73, 1981

Buckley WA, Yesalis CE, Friedl KE, et al: Estimated prevalence of anabolic steroid use among male high school seniors. JAMA 260:3441–3445, 1988

Choi PYL, Pope HG Jr: Violence towards women and illicit androgenic-anabolic steroid use. Ann Clin Psychiatry 6:21–25, 1994

Cohane G, Pope HG Jr: Body image in boys: a review of the literature. Int J Eat Disord 29:373–379, 2001

Cullari S, Rohrer JM, Bahm C: Body image perception across sex and age groups. Percep Mot Skills 87:839–847, 1998

Drewnowski A, Hopkins SA, Kessler RC: The prevalence of bulimia nervosa in the U.S. college student population. Am J Public Health 78:1322–1325, 1988

Durant RH, Rickert VI, Ashworth CS, et al: Use of multiple drugs among adolescents who use anabolic steroids. N Engl J Med 328:922–926, 1993

Dutton KR: The Perfectible Body: The Western Ideal of Male Physical Development. New York, Continuum, 1995

Garner DM, Garfinkel PE, Schwartz D, et al: Cultural expectations of thinness in women. Psychol Rep 47:483–491, 1980

Gruber AJ, Pope HG Jr, Borowiecki JJ, et al: The development of the somatomorphic matrix: a bi-axial instrument for measuring body image in men and women, in Kinanthropometry VI. Edited by Olds TS, Dollman J, Norton KI. Sydney, Australia, International Society for the Advancement of Kinanthropometry, 2000, pp 217–231

Harmatz MG, Gronendyke J, Thomas T: The underweight male: the unrecognized problem group of body image research. Journal of Obesity and Weight Regulation 4:258–267, 1985

Herzog DB, Newman KL, Warshaw M: Body image dissatisfaction in homosexual and heterosexual males. J Nerv Ment Dis 170:356–359, 1991

Hudson JI, Pope HG Jr, Jonas JM, et al: Phenomenologic relationship of eating disorders to major affective disorder. Psychiatry Res 9:345–354, 1983

Jacobi L, Cash T: In pursuit of the perfect appearance: discrepancies among self-ideal percepts of multiple physical attributes. J Appl Soc Psychol 24:379–396, 1994

Klein AM: Little Big Men: Bodybuilding, Subculture and Gender Construction. New York, State University of New York Press, 1993

Leit RA, Pope HG Jr, Gray JJ: Cultural expectations of muscularity in men: the evolution of Playgirl centerfolds. Int J Eat Disord 29:90–93, 2000

Leit RA, Gray JJ, Pope HG Jr: The media's representation of the ideal male body: a cause for muscle dysmorphia? Int J Eat Disord 31:334–338, 2002

Lucas AR, Beard CM, O'Fallon WM, et al: 50-year trends in the incidence of anorexia nervosa in Rochester, Minn: a population-based study. Am J Psychiatry 148:917–922, 1991

Margo JL: Anorexia nervosa in males: a comparison with female patients. Br J Psychiatry 151:80–83, 1987

McCreary DR, Sadava SW: Gender differences in relationships among per-ceived attractiveness, life satisfaction, and health in adults as a function of body mass index and perceived weight. Psychology of Men and Masculin-ity 2:108–116, 2001

McCreary DR, Sasse DK: An exploration of the drive for muscularity in adoles-cent boys and girls. J Am Coll Health 48:297–304, 2000

Mishkind ME, Rodin J, Silberstein LR, et al: The embodiment of masculinity: cultural, psychological and behavioral dimensions. Am Behav Sci 29:545–562, 2000

Moore DC: Body image and eating behavior in adolescent boys. Am J Dis Child 144:475–479, 1990

Newmark-Sztainer D, Story M, Falkner NH, et al: Sociodemographic and per-sonal characteristics of adolescents engaged in weight loss and weight/muscle gain behaviors: who is doing what? Prev Med 28:40–50, 1999

Olivardia R: Mirror, mirror on the wall, who's the largest of them all? Harv Rev Psychiatry 9:254–259, 2001

Olivardia R, Pope HG Jr, Mangweth B, et al: Eating disorders in college men. Am J Psychiatry 152:1279–1285, 1995

Olivardia R, Pope HG Jr, Hudson JI: Muscle dysmorphia in male weightlifters: a case-control study. Am J Psychiatry 157:1291–1296, 2000

Olivardia R, Pope HG Jr, Borowiecki JJ, et al: Biceps and body image: the rela-tionship between muscularity and self-esteem, depression, and eating dis-order symptoms. Psychology of Men and Masculinity 5:112–120, 2004

Page RM, Allen O: Adolescent perceptions of body weight and weight satisfac-tion. Percep Mot Skills 81:81–82, 1995

Paxton SJ, Wertheim EH, Gibbons K, et al: Body image satisfaction, dieting be-liefs and weight loss behaviors in adolescent girls and boys. J Youth Ado-lesc 20:361–379, 1991

Phillips KA: The Broken Mirror: Recognizing and Treating Body Dysmorphic Disorder. New York, Oxford University Press, 1996

Pope HG Jr, Brower KJ: Anabolic-androgenic steroid abuse, in Comprehensive Textbook of Psychiatry, VII. Edited by Sadock BJ, Sadock VA. Baltimore, MD, Williams & Wilkins, 1999, pp 1085–1096

Pope HG Jr, Gruber AJ, Choi P, et al: Muscle dysmorphia: an underrecognized form of body dysmorphic disorder. Psychosomatics 38:548–557, 1997

Pope HG Jr, Olivardia R, Gruber AJ, et al: Evolving ideals of male body image as seen through action toys. Int J Eat Disord 26:65–72, 1999

Pope HG Jr, Kouri EM, Hudson JI: The effects of supraphysiologic doses of tes-tosterone on mood and aggression in normal men: a randomized con-trolled trial. Arch Gen Psychiatry 57:133–140, 2000a

Pope HG Jr, Phillips KA, Olivardia R: The Adonis Complex: The Secret Crisis of Male Body Obsession. New York, Free Press, 2000b

Pope HG Jr, Olivardia R, Borowiecki J, et al: The growing commercial value of the male body: a longitudinal survey of advertising in women's magazines. Psychother Psychosom 70:189–192, 2001

Rodin J, Larson L: Social factors and the ideal body shape, in Eating, Body Weight and Performance in Athletes: Disorders of Modern Society. Edited by Brownell KD, Rodin J, Whitmore JH. Philadelphia, PA, Lea & Febiger, 1992, pp 146–158

Signorile M: Life Outside: The Signorile Report on Gay Men—Sex, Drugs, Muscles and the Passages of Life. New York, HarperCollins, 1997

Silberstein LR, Mishkind ME, Striegel-Moore RH, et al: Men and their bodies: a comparison of homosexual and heterosexual men. Psychosom Med 51: 337–346, 1989

Striegel-Moore RH, Silberstein LR, Frensch P, et al: A prospective study of disordered eating among college students. Int J Eat Disord 8:499–509, 1989

Stunkard A, Sorenson T, Schulsinger F: Use of the Danish Adoption Register for the study of obesity and thinness, in The Genetics of Neurological and Psychiatric Disorders. Edited by Kety S, Rowland LP, Sidman RL, et al. New York, Raven, 1983, pp 115–120

Thiblin I, Runeson B, Rajs J: Anabolic androgenic steroids and suicide. Ann Clin Psychiatry 11:4:223–231, 1999

Williams JM, Currie C: Self-esteem and physical development in early adolescence: pubertal timing and body image. J Early Adolesc 20:129–149, 2000

14

AGGRESSION, VIOLENCE, AND DOMESTIC ABUSE

CAROLINE J. EASTON, PH.D.

TARA M. NEAVINS, PH.D.

DOLORES L. MANDEL, L.C.S.W.

Case Vignette

James was referred by family relations for court-mandated substance abuse evaluation and treatment after he was charged with disorderly conduct and assault in the third degree. James reported drinking and arguing with his wife. He said that they began arguing about money. He recalled trying to leave the apartment, but his wife wanted to discuss how they would pay the bills. He stated that he was extremely angry and started yelling, swearing, and pushing her out of his way. A neighbor heard the yelling and called the police. James went to court and was seen by a family relations official, and his pending court case required a substance abuse evaluation and treatment for substance use and anger management.

Some emotionally distressed men use violence and antisocial behaviors to express their emotions. This chapter reviews biological factors that underlie violent behaviors, describes issues that are associated with violence in men, and provides an overview of psychosocial and pharmacological interventions for violence in men. Evidenced-based therapies that focus on men who are physically violent are highlighted and promising emerging therapies are explored. Significant attention is given to men with co-occurring substance abuse and intimate partner violence (IPV) because of the prevalence of this group in substance abuse and mental health treatment settings and the criminal justice system.

The term *violence* is frequently used within the legal, forensic, mental health, and criminal justice systems, whereas the term *aggression* tends to be used within the clinical and animal research literatures. Both terms are used interchangeably throughout this chapter. The terms *domestic violence, domestic abuse,* and *intimate partner violence* are also used interchangeably to describe male-to-female violence in intimate relationships. Violence includes verbal, emotional, psychological, sexual, and physical behaviors that invoke fear or cause injury (Alpert et al. 1987).

Most violence described within this chapter involves behaviors causing physical harm or injury that are perpetrated by a man and directed toward a woman. Physical violence is the behavior that has been targeted and treated in most randomized clinical trials performed to date. Examples of physical violence include kicking, biting, scratching, pushing, slapping, choking, grabbing, hair pulling, punching, and causing a bruise. Assessing the severity and frequency of physical violence at treatment entry serves as a method of monitoring treatment outcome (i.e., abstinence from violence, including amount and type of physical violence committed).

EPIDEMIOLOGY AND CLINICAL CHARACTERISTICS

Violence Committed by Men in the United States: Epidemiological Data

Much violence reported in the literature involves IPV committed by men toward women (Bureau of Justice Statistics 1998b). Partner physical aggression is a pervasive problem in a significant proportion of U.S. families. According to the Department of Justice, roughly 1,500 instances of homicide and manslaughter between intimate partners occur annually, with more than 1,200 of these involving women as victims (Bureau of Justice Statistics 1998b). The findings of the National Crime Victimization Survey (Bureau of Justice Statistics 2006), which is a survey of the victimization experiences of a nationally representative sample of the U.S. population, indicate that there are nearly 1 million female victims of IPV each year. Surveys of representative samples of couples include less severe instances of aggression (e.g., single episodes of pushing or slapping one's partner) and suggest that 8.7 million couples experience an incident of physical violence from within the dyad each year (Straus and Gelles 1990). A recent survey of U.S. couples indicated that more than 1 in 5 had experienced at least one episode of violence during the previous year (Schafer et al. 1998).

Female-to-Male Perpetration of Violence

Although incidents of female-to-male physical aggression are more rare than incidents involving male aggression toward women (Bureau of Justice Statistics 1998a, 1998b), it is important to understand the dynamics and clinical implications of IPV perpetrated by women against men. Women who are violent toward men in their intimate relationships often have problems with alcohol or drugs (Stuart et al. 2003). Similarly, these women's partners are often hazardous drinkers (Stuart et al. 2003). Investigators have found that a hazardous drinking status among women is associated with more drug problems, relationship aggression, general violence, and marital dissatisfaction and is predictive of women's perpetrating physical assault toward their partners (Stuart et al. 2003, 2004). Integrated substance abuse and anger management treatment for women arrested for domestic violence is important (Stuart et al. 2004). Little research has evaluated men who are victims of domestic violence, and more research is needed to provide clinical recommendations as to how best to help these men.

Typologies of Men Who Are Physically Violent and the Role of Antisocial Personality Disorder

Holtzworth-Munroe and colleagues (Holtzworth-Munroe and Meehan 2004; Holzworth-Munroe and Stuart 1994) described three groups or typologies of men who batter. The three descriptive dimensions of men with IPV include 1) family-only batterers, 2) borderline-dysphoric batterers, and 3) generally violent–antisocial batterers. *Family-only batterers* engage in the least severe form of marital violence, violence outside the home, and criminal behavior. These men evidence little or no psychopathology. *Borderline-dysphoric batterers* engage in moderate to severe abuse. Their violence is primarily confined to the wife or partner, although some extrafamilial violence might be evident. These batterers are often psychologically distressed, demonstrate borderline personality characteristics, and abuse substances. *Generally violent–antisocial batterers* engage in moderate to severe abuse and have the highest levels of extrafamilial aggression and criminal behavior. They are the most likely to have antisocial characteristics and problems with substance abuse.

Holtzworth-Munroe and colleagues suggested that typologies 1 and 2 respond to treatment, whereas typology 3 shows a limited response.

Although some researchers support the typologies of batterers just described, others posit a *threshold approach* as underlying the link between substance use, antisocial personality disorder, and IPV (Fals-Stewart and Stappenbeck 2003; Fals-Stewart et al. 2005). Fals-Stewart et al. (2003) described a multiple threshold model that integrates the main and interactive effects of alcohol use and antisocial personality characteristics to predict the occurrence of IPV among male partners with a history of male-to-female physical aggression. First, this model posits that aggression occurs when the strength of the provocation exceeds the strength of aggressive inhibitions. Second, aggressive inhibitions are believed to be higher for severe violence than for nonsevere violence. Third, aggressive inhibitions are thought to be lower for men with antisocial personality disorder than for those without antisocial personality disorder. Finally, alcohol intoxication, largely through its deleterious impact on cognitive processes, is viewed as leading to a reduction in aggressive inhibitions.

Fals-Stewart et al. 2005) examined the moderating effects of antisocial personality disorder and the day-to-day relationship between male partner alcohol consumption and male-to-female physical aggression for married or cohabiting men entering a domestic violence treatment program ($n = 170$) and those entering an alcoholism treatment program ($n = 169$). Alcohol use was related to increased nonsevere forms of male partner violence among men without a diagnosis of antisocial personality but not in men with the disorder. In men with antisocial personality disorder, alcohol use was more strongly associated with a likelihood of *severe* male partner violence, compared with men without antisocial personality disorder who also consumed alcohol.

Intimate Partner Violence and Substance Abuse

General Issues

IPV is common and constitutes a significant public health concern. Substance use is involved in 40%–60% of incidents of IPV (Easton et al. 2000a, 2000b; Fals-Stewart 2005; Murphy and O'Farrell 1996). Several lines of evidence suggest that substance use plays a facilitative role in IPV by precipitating or exacerbating violence (Fals-Stewart 2003b). Furthermore, several studies suggest the promise of interventions that target substance use in men who have histories of IPV (Fals-Stewart 2003b, 2005).

A large percentage of IPV episodes involve alcohol or drug consumption. Kaufman-Kantor and Straus (1990) found that more than 20% of males were drinking before their most recent and severe act of violence. Fals-Stewart (2003b) found that on days of heavy drug use, physical violence was 11 times more likely to occur. Victims of IPV frequently report that the offender was drinking (Bureau of Justice Statistics 1998a) or using illicit drugs (Miller 1990). Miller (1990) reported that IPV offenders typically use alcohol and have a dual problem with drugs. A strong relationship between substance use and perpetration of IPV has been found in primary health care settings (McCauley et al. 1995), family practice clinics (Oriel and Flemming 1998), prenatal clinics (Muhajarine and D'Arcy 1999), and rural health clinics (Van Hightower and Groton 1998).

Conceptual Models and Evidence for a Proximal Effects Model

Three conceptual models have been posited to explain the observed relationship between substance use and spousal violence: 1) the spurious model, 2) the indirect effects model, and 3) the proximal effects model (K.E. Leonard and Quigley 1999). These models are discussed below:

1. The *spurious model* suggests that substance use and IPV co-occur due to other factors that influence both drinking and violence. For example, as compared with other groups, young men tend to be violent and use drugs; thus drug use and violence may appear directly related when they are not. Several studies suggest that alcohol and other drug use is associated with partner violence after controlling for factors thought to be associated with both behaviors, such as age, education, socioeconomic or occupational status, and race or ethnicity (e.g., C. Leonard et al. 1988; Pan et al. 1994). The relationship between substance use and violence remains strong after controlling for levels of general hostility (e.g., K.E. Leonard and Senchak 1993) and normative views of aggression (Kaufman-Kantor and Straus 1990).

2. In the *indirect effects model,* substance use is viewed as corrosive to relationship quality. Thus long-term substance use creates an environment that sets the stage for partner conflict and, ultimately, partner violence. When marital satisfaction, relationship discord, or other similar variables are controlled for, the relationship between substance use and violence remains strong (e.g., McKenry et al. 1995).

3. According to the *proximal effects model* (Fals-Stewart 2003b), individuals who consume psychoactive substances are more likely to engage in partner violence because intoxication facilitates violence, which

may be mediated through the psychopharmacological effects of drugs on cognitive processing (Chermack and Taylor 1995) or the expectancies associated with intoxication (Critchlow 1983). It follows from this theory that 1) substance use should precede the episodes of IPV and 2) the episode of violence should occur closely in time to the consumption of the drug. Several longitudinal studies support temporal ordering consistent with the proximal effects model. For example, Fals-Stewart (2003b) collected daily diaries from partners with histories of IPV entering either an alcoholism or domestic violence treatment program over a 15-month period. These data allowed for a detailed examination of the daily temporal relationship between male-to-female aggression and drinking. The findings suggested that alcohol and male-to-female aggression were linked only on days when the drinking occurred before the IPV episode. The odds of severe male-to-female physical aggression were more than 11 times higher on days of men's drinking than on days of no drinking. Moreover, more than 60% of all episodes occurred within 2 hours of drinking by the male partner. These findings were recently replicated with another sample of men entering treatment for drug abuse (Fals-Stewart et al. 2003).

In sum, three conceptual models have been put forth to explain the relationship between alcohol use and violence. Although each may have some merit and may, in fact, serve to explain some part of the relationship between substance use and violence, the greatest empirical support rests with the proximal effects model (Fals-Stewart 2003b). Hence, interventions that target substance use among men with histories of IPV and substance use may lead to reductions in partner violence.

TREATMENT OF SUBSTANCE-USING PATIENTS WHO ENGAGE IN INTIMATE PARTNER VIOLENCE

Referral to Domestic Violence Treatment

Currently, men convicted of IPV are referred to batterer or IPV programs. The Duluth Domestic Abuse Intervention Project was established by an activist group associated with a women's shelter in Duluth, Minnesota. The core of a perpetrator program is to change the behavior of men convicted or accused of domestic assault. The program uses a psychoeducational structure in which actual behaviors are identified and challenged by facilitators who model alternative behaviors and alternative solutions to conflict.

The methodology is based on a two-part map of violent and nonviolent behaviors, displayed in a wheel format (the Duluth Wheel). One wheel divides violence and abuse into eight categories: 1) coercion and threats, 2) intimidation, 3) economic abuse, 4) emotional abuse, 5) gender-privilege, 6) isolation, 7) using children, and 8) minimizing, denying, and blaming. On the other wheel, the respective target behaviors shown for each category include 1) negotiation and fairness, 2) nonthreatening behavior, 3) economic partnership, 4) respect, 5) shared responsibility, 6) trust and support, 7) responsible parenting, and 8) honesty and accountability. However, it should be noted that there is very little empirical support regarding the effectiveness of the Duluth model in reducing violence or substance use, which suggests that many offenders are likely to repeat the cycle of violence (Babcock and La Taillade 2000). Meta-analytic reviews of outcomes for these approaches have consistently found them to be of very limited effectiveness, with effect sizes near zero (Babcock and La Taillade 2000). Moreover, many batterer programs do not address substance use, are highly confrontational in nature, and reach far fewer individuals than substance abuse treatment programs. Hence, it is likely that focusing on IPV with men who batter within the context of a substance abuse treatment facility may reach a comparatively larger number of individuals with IPV.

Standard Substance Abuse Treatment

Several studies suggest that treatment-associated reductions in substance use are related to reductions in violence. O'Farrell et al. (2003) examined partner violence in the year before and the year after individually based, outpatient alcoholism treatment for male alcoholic patients compared with a demographically matched nonalcoholic comparison group. In the year before treatment, 56% of the alcoholic patients had been violent toward their female partner, four times the rate of the comparison sample (14%). In the year after treatment, violence decreased significantly to 25% of the alcoholic sample but remained higher than in the comparison group. In a parallel study, Fals-Stewart et al. (2003) examined partner violence among a sample of married or cohabiting men entering outpatient treatment for drug abuse. During the year before treatment, the prevalence of IPV was roughly 60%, but it dropped to 35% during the 1-year posttreatment follow-up period. In both studies, the treatments were standard 12-step facilitation interventions that did not address partner violence (e.g., Schumacher et al. 2003). Nonetheless, participation in the programs resulted in significant reductions in interpersonal violence, consistent with what would be expected from the proximal effects model.

Nevertheless, the levels of IPV during the posttreatment period for participants in both groups remained comparatively high. Because substance use is only one of several factors likely to influence the occurrence of IPV (e.g., negative mood states such as anger and hostility are other factors), interventions designed to address the other issues may further reduce IPV.

Evidence-Based Psychotherapies

Behavioral Couples Therapy

Several studies suggest that interventions targeting substance use and skill deficits have particular promise in men with co-occurring substance abuse and IPV. Behavioral couples therapy has demonstrated effectiveness in several populations (Fals-Stewart et al. 2002; O'Farrell and Fals-Stewart 2000). Although not designed specifically as an intervention for IPV, behavioral couples therapy has demonstrated efficacy in reducing alcohol and drug use and improving dyadic functioning (for a review, see O'Farrell and Fals-Stewart 2000). Participation in behavioral couples therapy led to significantly reduced levels of frequency and incidence of IPV during a 1-year posttreatment follow-up period compared with standard treatment (Fals-Stewart et al. 2002). The effects of behavioral couples therapy on the frequency of maladaptive methods of conflict resolution used by male partners were examined during the 12-week treatment. Compared with men who received standard treatment, men who received behavioral couples therapy reported more rapid reductions in the frequency of maladaptive methods of conflict resolution and, by the end of treatment, reported a lower frequency of these methods. Changes in drinking and in the frequency of maladaptive methods of conflict resolution were both significant mediators of posttreatment frequency of IPV.

Couples learn and practice several techniques in behavioral couples therapy, both within and outside treatment. One example is a sobriety contract in which the substance-using partner verbally commits not to consume any alcohol or to take any illicit drugs that day (O'Farrell and Fals-Stewart 2000). In return, the nonusing partner expresses verbal support for the substance-using partner. The nonusing partner records all information on a calendar.

A second technique of behavioral couples therapy is the development of more effective communication skills. Active listening skills are taught to the couple, and each partner takes turns in session practicing the newfound skills and making reflective statements (O'Farrell and Fals-Stewart 2000).

A third and related topic of behavioral couples therapy is helping the couple to engage in shared positive activities while minimizing their negative interactions. One assignment, for instance, is entitled "Catch Your Partner Doing Something Nice," in which each partner points out each day one specific thing that he or she appreciated that the other partner did; couples are taught to focus on compliments rather than criticisms (O'Farrell and Fals-Stewart 2000). Couples also are encouraged to contemplate leisure activities they both enjoy and to schedule time each week to do these activities together. Focusing on specific activities is most useful because many substance abusers are no longer involved in many healthy activities.

The final section of behavioral couples therapy focuses on relapse prevention. Each partner develops a continuing recovery plan to specify abstinence-based activities. Possible difficult or challenging situations are considered so that individuals are less likely to relapse if they encounter these situations in the future.

Although there is ample evidence that behavioral couples therapy is effective with couples willing and motivated to participate in this treatment, behavioral couples therapy may not be applicable to all male participants with co-occurring substance abuse and IPV. In some cases, behavioral couples therapy may be contraindicated (e.g., the relationship is over). Hence, there is a need for other evidence-based approaches that do not rely on couples-focused interventions.

Cognitive-Behavioral Therapy

Cognitive-behavioral therapy (CBT) has been effective at treating a range of substance abuse disorders (Carroll 1996; DuRubeis and Crits-Christoph 1998; Irvin et al. 1999; National Institute on Drug Abuse 2000). Based on social learning theories of substance use disorders, CBT focuses on the implementation of effective coping skills for recognizing, avoiding, and coping with situations that increase the risk of drug use. CBT is one of comparatively few empirically supported therapies that have been demonstrated to be effective across a range of substance use disorders, including alcohol- (Morgenstern and Longabaugh 2000; Project MATCH Research Group 1997), marijuana- (Marijuana Research Treatment Group 2004), and cocaine- (Carroll 1998, Carroll et al. 1994, 1998; Maude-Griffin et al. 1998; McKay et al. 1997; Monti et al. 1997) related disorders. CBT is well accepted by the clinical community and can be implemented effectively by "real world" clinicians (Morgenstern et al. 2001.

An Emerging Psychotherapy Showing Promise and Efficacy: An Integrated Substance Abuse–Domestic Violence Intervention

A substance abuse–domestic violence behavior therapy approach (SADV) was developed out of a community need for an integrated intervention. Men with co-occurring substance use and domestic violence problems are rarely motivated for one treatment program, let alone referral to separate programs located across town (Easton et al. 2000b). Evidence suggests that cross-referrals to separate agencies do not work (Easton et al. 2000a). SADV is grounded in evidence-based treatments (e.g., CBT for substance users), with additional sessions that pertain to the target population (awareness of anger, anger management, communication skills training, coping with criticisms) from the Project MATCH Elective Session Modules (Project MATCH Manual Series 1995).

SADV is an integrated treatment designed to target both substance use and aggression in each session at one location. Cognitive-behavioral skills training in SADV is used to target substance use, interpersonal violence and conflict, and the relationship between the two. SADV interventions include understanding patterns of substance use, coping with craving, problem-solving skills, drug refusal skills, and managing cognitions. First, participants are asked to monitor their substance use as well as any difficulty they may be having controlling violent behavior and angry feelings. This step highlights relationships between substance use and violent behavior and helps patients understand behavior patterns (e.g., how substance use may trigger anger or violent behavior and how anger or violence may lead to relapse). Second, skills are taught that are directly relevant to the reduction of IPV, including communication and management of anger.

SADV differs from standard CBT for substance use because of SADV's dual focus on substance use and interpersonal violence, as well as the relationship between these two behaviors. SADV differs from behavioral couples therapy in inclusion of specific skills for anger, and it differs from drug counseling (Mercer and Woody 1999) because the focus is on interpersonal violence, skills training, and extra session practice exercises.

The key ingredients that distinguish SADV from other therapies—and that must be delivered to ensure adequate exposure to SADV—include the following: 1) dual focus on treatment strategies for substance use and IPV (e.g., identify triggers for substance use and for violence); 2) individualized training that emphasizes that complete abstinence from substances is likely to lead to abstinence from IPV; 3) development of unique anger management skills for each client in preparation for a high-risk situation (this essential ingredient emphasizes that a substance use slip or relapse does not need to result in violence); 4) in each session, increased emphasis on role plays and practice exercises that pertain to anger management, communication, and conflict resolution skills training; and 5) no requirement for the female partner to be involved in the intervention but flexibility to allow for couples modules when feasible and therapeutically indicated.

To date, SADV has shown promising results in a recently completed randomized, controlled study (C.J. Easton, unpublished manuscript). Alcohol-dependent men with a domestic violence arrest within the past 6 months were recruited and evaluated. Male participants were randomly assigned to either 12 weeks of the integrated SADV group treatment or 12 weeks of the group 12-step facilitation. Of the 78 individuals who were eligible, 77 were randomized and 75 started treatment. Out of the 75 starters, 62 completed the full 12 weeks of treatment. Across treatments, participants completed an average of 9 of the 12 offered sessions. There were no significant differences between the SADV group and the 12-step group in number of sessions attended. Follow-up interviews were conducted 6 months after randomization; the follow-up rate was 80% across conditions. SADV participants showed significantly more days abstinent from alcohol use as compared with participants in the 12-step group. SADV participants also showed a significant decline in aggressive behavior from pre- to posttreatment as compared with the 12-step group. To date, SADV is one of the first integrated group treatments found to be efficacious. However, this study needs to be replicated with a larger sample of substance-dependent men with co-occurring physical violence in both individual and group treatment modalities.

Pharmacological Treatments

To date, few large-scale randomized trials have assessed the safety and efficacy of pharmacological agents in treating domestic violence offenders with and without substance-related problems. Some medications that have been used to treat various forms of aggressive behavior are briefly mentioned in the following discussion.

Drugs that enhance serotonin neurotransmission or decrease dopamine neurotransmission are indicated in specific cases of aggression (acute vs. chronic). For example, serotonin reuptake inhibitors such as fluoxetine have been used among patients with anger, hostility, and mood lability problems (New et al. 2004). Dopamine antagonists such as clozapine are useful in treating forms of acute aggression and violence, whereas other medications are indicated for the treatment of chronic aggression and organic brain syndromes (De Leon 1994). Mood stabilizers such as carbamazepine and valproic acid have yielded promising results in placebo-controlled studies (Coccaro and Siever 2002).

Few randomized clinical trials have assessed effective pharmacotherapies among substance-using men with IPV. Regarding medication compliance, Timothy O'Farrell and William Fals-Stewart have used behavioral couples therapy in patient populations receiving methadone maintenance treatment, naltrexone, and medications for human immunodeficiency virus (HIV). These researchers assessed whether behavioral couples therapy would increase medication compliance, decrease substance use, and increase relationship adjustment. Fals-Stewart et al. (2001) found that men in a methadone maintenance program who were assigned to behavioral couples therapy had fewer urine screenings positive for drugs, better relationship adjustment, and greater reductions in drug use severity. Men assigned to behavioral couples therapy had greater reductions in both family and social problems than did men who were assigned to an individual behavior therapy modality. In another study, Fals-Stewart (2003a) found that among male patients receiving naltrexone, men who were assigned to behavioral couples therapy complied with more doses of naltrexone, attended more sessions, remained abstinent longer, and had more days abstinent from drug use than men who were assigned to the individual behavior therapy group. O'Farrell and Fals-Stewart (2001) found that HIV-positive drug users reported significantly more days in which they took all their HIV medications as compared with men who were not in the behavioral couples therapy condition.

CONCLUSION

Although behavioral couples therapy has been shown to be the most effective therapy to date, it may have limited application to IPV in substance abuse treatment facilities. An alternative approach is needed for the following reasons: 1) involving all female partners in couples treatment is not clinically feasible (e.g., the female partner has left the relationship and has no involvement with the offender); 2) a male offender may refuse to have his partner participate in his treatment; 3) a female partner may refuse to participate in the offender's treatment; 4) there may be imposed restraining or protective orders that limit contact between the offender and the victim; and 5) offenders and victims may separate and have no further contact. Thus even if behavioral couples therapy may be an effective approach to dually address substance use and IPV, there is a clear need for an integrated IPV–substance abuse treatment that is *not* solely couples based. Research lags in the development of both behavior therapies and pharmacological treatments for substance-using males who commit domestic violence. Alternative approaches such as SADV show promise, and future investigations would include more randomized studies with larger samples of patients. Other directions include assessing SADV with and without various pharmacotherapies, because adjunctive medication may further improve treatment outcomes with this population and lead to prolonged abstinence from substances and violence.

KEY POINTS

- Male-to-female aggression is a pervasive problem.

- Substance use has been shown to facilitate or exacerbate physical aggression and commonly occurs among men who are physically violent toward their partners.

- Although substance abuse treatment alone has been shown to decrease physical aggression among men who have co-occurring substance use and domestic violence problems, integrated approaches (behavioral couples therapy, SADV) appear particularly promising in targeting a broader range of problematic behaviors.

PRACTICE GUIDELINES

1. Screen for substance-related disorders in men presenting for domestic violence and vice versa, and assess multiple domains of social and functional impairment in men with co-occurring substance abuse and domestic violence.

2. Provide a thorough evaluation of the type and frequency of IPV (e.g., physical, psychological, verbal, sexual violence), utilizing such instruments as the Conflict Tactics Scale or Timeline Followback Spousal Violence Interview.

3. Consider both pharmacological and behavioral treatment interventions.

REFERENCES

Alpert DB, Niaura RS: Social learning theory, in Psychological Theories of Drinking and Alcoholism. Edited by Blane HT, Leonard KE. New York, Guilford, 1987, pp 131–178

Babcock JC, La Taillade JJ: Evaluating interventions for men who batter, in Domestic Violence: Guidelines for Research-Informed Practice. Edited by Vincent J, Jourilles E. Philadelphia, PA, Jessica Kingsley, 2000, pp 37–77

Bureau of Justice Statistics: Alcohol and Crime: An Analysis of National Data on the Prevalence of Alcohol Involvement in Crime. Washington, DC, U.S. Department of Justice, 1998a

Bureau of Justice Statistics: Violence by Intimates (NCJ Publ No 167237). Washington, DC, U.S. Department of Justice, 1998b

Bureau of Justice Statistics: National Crime Victimization Survey. Washington, DC, U.S. Department of Justice. Available at: http://www.ojp.usdoj.gov/bjs/cvict.htm#ncvs. Accessed May 23, 2006.

Carroll KM: Relapse prevention as a psychosocial treatment approach: a review of controlled clinical trials. Exp Clin Psychopharmacol 4:46–54, 1996

Carroll KM (ed): A Cognitive-Behavioral Approach: Treating Cocaine Addiction (NIH Publ 98–4308). Rockville, MD, National Institute on Drug Abuse, 1998

Carroll KM, Kadden RM, Donovan DM, et al: Implementing treatment and protecting the validity of the independent variable in treatment matching studies. Special issue: alcoholism treatment matching research: methodological and clinical approaches. J Stud Alcohol Suppl 12:149–155, 1994

Carroll KM, Nich C, Ball SA, et al: Treatment of cocaine and alcohol dependence with psychotherapy and disulfiram. Addiction 93:713–728, 1998

Chermack ST, Taylor SP: Alcohol and human physical aggression: pharmacological versus expectancy effects. J Stud Alcohol 56:449–456, 1995

Coccaro EF, Siever LJ: Pathophysiology and treatment of aggression, in Neuropsychopharmacology: The Fifth Generation of Progress. Edited by Davis K, Charney D, Coyle J. Philadelphia, PA, Lippincott Williams & Wilkins, 2002, pp 1709–1723

Critchlow B: Blaming the booze: the attribution of responsibility for drunken behavior. Pers Soc Psychol Bull 9:451–473, 1983

De Leon OA: The neurobiological bases of aggression: the pharmacotherapeutic implications (in Spanish). Rev Med Panama 19:106–116, 1994

DeRubeis RJ, Crits-Christoph P: Empirically supported individual and group psychological treatments for adult mental disorders. J Consult Clin Psychol 66:37–52, 1998

Easton C, Swan S, Sinha R: Motivation to change substance use among offenders of domestic violence. J Subst Abuse 19:1–5, 2000a

Easton C, Swan S, Sinha R: Prevalence of family violence in clients entering substance abuse treatment. J Subst Abuse Treat 18:23–28, 2000b

Fals-Stewart W: Behavioral family counseling and naltrexone for male opioid dependent patients. J Consult Clin Psychol 71:432–442, 2003a

Fals-Stewart W: The occurrence of partner physical aggression on days of alcohol consumption: a longitudinal diary study. J Consult Clin Psychol 71:41–52, 2003b

Fals-Stewart W, Stappenbeck CA: Intimate partner violence and alcohol use: the role of drinking in partner violence and implications for intervention. Family Law Psychology Briefs 4(4), 2003

Fals-Stewart W, O'Farrell TJ, Birchler GR: Behavioral couples therapy for male methadone maintenance patients: effects on drug-using behavior and relationship adjustment. Behav Ther 32:391–411, 2001

Fals-Stewart W, Kashdan TB, O'Farrell TJ, et al: Behavioral couples therapy for drug-abusing patients: effects on partner violence. J Subst Abuse Treat 22:87–96, 2002

Fals-Stewart W, Golden J, Schumacher J: Intimate partner violence and substance use: a longitudinal day-to-day examination. Addict Behav 28:1555–1574, 2003

Fals-Stewart W, Leonard KE, Birchler GR: The occurrence of male-to-female intimate partner violence on days of men's drinking: the moderating effects of antisocial personality disorder. J Consult Clin Psychol 73:239–248, 2005

Holtzworth-Munroe A, Meehan JC: Typologies of men who are maritally violent: scientific and clinical implications. J Interpers Violence 19:1369–1389, 2004

Holtzworth-Munroe A, Stuart G: Typologies of male batterers: three subtypes and the differences among them. Psychol Bull 116:476–497, 1994

Irvin JE, Bowers CA, Dunn ME, et al: Efficacy of relapse prevention: a meta-analytic review. J Consult Clin Psychol 67:563–570, 1999

Kaufman-Kantor G, Straus M: The "drunken bum" theory of wife beating, in Physical Violence in American Families: Risk Factors and Adaptations to Violence in 8,145 Families. Edited by Straus MA, Gelles RJ. New Brunswick, NJ, Transaction Publishers, 1990, pp 203–224

Leonard C, Puranik C, Kuldau J, et al: Normal variation in the frequency and location of human auditory cortex landmarks. Heschl's gyrus: where is it? Cereb Cortex 8:397–406, 1998

Leonard KE, Quigley BM: Drinking and marital aggression in newlyweds: an event-based analysis of drinking and the occurrence of husband marital aggression. J Stud Alcohol 60:537–545, 1999

Leonard KE, Senchak M: Alcohol and premarital aggression among newlywed couples. J Stud Alcohol 11(suppl):96–108, 1993

Marijuana Research Treatment Group: Brief treatments for cannabis dependence: findings from a randomized multisite trial. J Consult Clin Psychol 72:455–466, 2004

Maude-Griffin PM, Hohenstein JM, Humfleet GL, et al: Superior efficacy of cognitive-behavioral therapy for crack cocaine abusers: main and matching effects. J Consult Clin Psychol 66:832–837, 1998

McCauley J, Kern DE, Kolodner K, et al: The "battering syndrome": prevalence and clinical characteristics of domestic violence in primary care internal medicine practices. Ann Intern Med 123:737–746, 1995

McKay JR, Alterman AI, Cacciola JS, et al: Group counseling versus individualized relapse prevention aftercare following intensive outpatient treatment for cocaine dependence. J Consult Clin Psychol 65:778–788, 1997

McKenry PC, Julian TW, Gavazzi SM: Toward a biopsychosocial model of domestic violence. J Marriage Fam 57:307–320, 1995

Mercer DE, Woody GE: Individual Drug Counseling. Treating Cocaine Addiction Therapy Manual 3 (NIH Publ No 99-4380). Rockville, MD, National Institute on Drug Abuse, 1999

Miller B: The interrelationships between alcohol and drugs and family violence, in Drugs and Violence: Causes, Correlates, and Consequences (NIDA Research Monograph 103). Edited by De La Rosa M, Gropper B. Rockville, MD, National Institute on Drug Abuse, 1990, pp 177–207

Monti PM, Rohsenow DJ, Michalec E, et al: Brief coping skills treatment for cocaine abuse: substance use outcomes at three months Addiction 92:1717–1728, 1997

Morgenstern J, Longabaugh R: Cognitive-behavioral treatment for alcohol dependence: a review of the evidence for its hypothesized mechanisms of action. Addiction 95:1475–1490, 2000

Morgenstern J, Morgan TJ, McCrady BS, et al: Manual-guided cognitive behavioral therapy training: a promising method for disseminating empirically supported substance abuse treatments to the practice community. Psychol Addict Behav 15:83–88, 2001

Muhajarine N, D'Arcy C: Physical abuse during pregnancy: prevalence and risk factors. CMAJ 160:1007–1011, 1999

Murphy CM, O'Farrell TJ: Marital violence among alcoholics. Current Directions in Psychological Science 5:183–186, 1996

New AS, Buchsbaum MS, Hazlett EA, et al: Fluoxetine increases relative metabolic rate in prefrontal cortex in impulsive aggression. Psychopharmacology (Berl) 176:451–458, 2004

National Institute on Drug Abuse: Principles of Drug Abuse Treatment: A Research Based Guide. Bethesda, MD, National Institute on Drug Abuse, 2000

O'Farrell TJ, Fals-Stewart W: Behavioral couples therapy for alcoholism and drug abuse. J Subst Abuse Treat 18:51–54, 2000

O'Farrell TJ, Fals-Stewart W: Family-involved alcoholism treatment: an update. Recent Dev Alcohol 15:329–356, 2001

O'Farrell TJ, Fals-Stewart W, Murphy M, et al: Partner violence before and after individually based alcoholism treatment for male alcoholic patients. J Consult Clin Psychol 71:92–102, 2003

Oriel KA, Flemming MF: Screening men for partner violence in a primary care setting: a new strategy for detecting domestic violence. J Fam Pract 46:493–498, 1998

Pan HD, Neidig PH, O'Leary KK: Predicting mild and severe husband-to-wife physical aggression. J Appl Behav Sci 36:108–122, 1994

Project MATCH Manual Series: Cognitive Behavioral Coping Skills Therapy Manual: A Clinical Research Guide for Therapists Treating Individuals With Alcohol Abuse and Dependence, Vol 3. Bethesda, MD, National Institute on Alcohol Abuse and Alcoholism, 1995

Project MATCH Research Group: Matching alcoholism treatments to client heterogeneity: Project MATCH posttreatment drinking outcomes. J Stud Alcohol 58:7–29, 1997

Schafer J, Caetano R, Clark C: Rates of intimate partner violence in the United States. Am J Public Health 88:1702–1704, 1998

Schumacher JA, Fals-Stewart W, Leonard KE: Domestic violence treatment referrals for men seeking alcohol treatment. J Subst Abuse Treat 24:279–283, 2003

Straus MA, Gelles R: How violent are American families? estimates from the National Family Violence Survey and other studies, in Physical Violence in American Families. Edited by Straus MA, Gelles R. New Brunswick, NJ, Transaction Publishing, 1990, pp 95–112

Stuart GL, Moore TM, Ramsey SE, et al: Relationship aggression and substance use among women court-referred to domestic violence intervention programs. Addict Behav 28:1603–1610, 2003

Stuart GL, Moore TM, Ramsey SE, et al: Hazardous drinking and relationship violence perpetration and victimization in women arrested for domestic violence. J Stud Alcohol 65:46–53, 2004

Van Hightower NR, Groton J: Domestic violence among patients at two rural health care clinics: prevalence and social correlates. Public Health Nurs 15:355–362, 1998

15

CULTURE, ETHNICITY, RACE, AND MEN'S MENTAL HEALTH

DECLAN T. BARRY, PH.D.

Case Vignette

Emilio was a 28-year-old, single American male of Puerto Rican descent who presented at a northwest Ohio university-based psychology clinic because of "difficulty studying." At intake, Emilio reported that his parents had immigrated to Ohio from Puerto Rico when he was 5 years old and that a part of him would prefer to live there. Upon initial assessment, Emilio was administered intellectual and achievement tests that indicated an IQ of 122 ("superior range") and absence of a learning disorder. Emilio was informed that his testing scores did not explain his difficulty studying. His clinician suggested that further psychological assessment focusing on Emilio's feelings and his characteristic way of interacting with people might illuminate the reason(s) for his difficulty studying. After the clinician reviewed how people's psychological functioning may influence their ease or difficulty in studying, Emilio agreed to further testing.

Emilio was next administered semistructured clinical interviews for diagnosing Axis I and Axis II DSM-IV (American Psychiatric Association 1994) psychiatric disorders and was subsequently diagnosed with dysthymic disorder and borderline personality disorder. Emilio was informed of the diagnosis, and his clinician suggested that his mood and characteristic style of interacting with people might, in part, explain his difficulty studying. The clinician recommended that Emilio begin psychotherapy so that he could learn additional skills to regulate his mood, which would improve his ability to study. Emilio agreed to participate in five sessions and then reconsider if he wished to proceed.

Emilio completed a trial of 50 weekly sessions of individual psychotherapy, which largely comprised cognitive-behavioral and experiential therapy interventions. In early sessions, Emilio exhibited a "separation" mode of acculturation (i.e., he socialized and communicated primarily with individuals of Latino descent and largely eschewed communication or socialization with those of non-Latino descent), an interdependent self-construal (i.e., self-concept viewed as flexible, variable, and guided by external factors, such as roles, status, and relationships), and a strong Puerto Rican ethnic identity. During treatment, Emilio began making friends with non-Latino university peers and began dating an African American female student from one of his classes. The focus in the sessions was on identifying cognitions that appeared to influence Emilio's mood and style of interaction with others, including his initial strong traditional sex-role identification (e.g., "A woman needs to cook for her man") and reduced empathy for others (e.g., "Black women prefer white and black men; they don't like men like me"). Sessions also involved examining the relative advantages and disadvantages of his assumptions and prescribing "homework" to test his cognitions and assumptions.

Treatment ended with the mutual agreement of the patient and clinician. Emilio reported better grades, decreased difficulty studying, improved mood, and increased enjoyment interacting with Latino and non-Latino individuals. By the end of treatment, Emilio exhibited an integrated mode of acculturation (i.e., he socialized and communicated with ethnic and nonethnic peers with comparable ease); salient independent (i.e., self is viewed as a separate, stable, autonomous, and bounded entity) and interdependent self-construals; salient (but weaker in comparison with treatment initiation) Puerto Rican ethnic identity; and a weaker traditional sex-role ideology.

In recent years, mental health professionals have increasingly recognized the role of cultural factors in psychiatric diagnosis and treatment (Lewis-Fernandez and Kleinman 1995). DSM-IV-TR (American Psychiatric Association 2000) now includes sections related to capturing patients' cultural contexts, including a general introductory cultural statement, information concerning cultural considerations for the use of diagnostic categories and criteria, a listing of culture-bound syndromes and idioms of distress, and a suggested outline for a cultural formulation. In 2001, the U.S. Department of Health and Human Services issued a supplement to the Surgeon General's report on mental health. The supplement highlighted the role of ethnicity and race in accounting for several disparities in mental health care in the United States, including limited access to effective mental health services for Americans of ethnic/racial minority descent compared with Americans of European descent. In addition, researchers have highlighted the importance of attending to gender differences nested within cultural variables (Barry and Grilo 2002; Johnson and Glassman 1998) and to patients' gender when attempting to individualize treatment for ethnic/racial minority individuals (U.S. Department of Health and Human Services 2001). This chapter discusses issues related to culture, ethnicity, and men's mental health and offers practice recommendations for clinicians who work with male patients of ethnic/racial minority descent.

DEFINITIONS OF CULTURE, ETHNICITY, AND RACE

Considerable debate exists concerning culture and its nature and influence on human behavior (Brislin 1993; Greenfield et al. 2003; Segall et al. 1998). *Culture* has been defined as "the man-made part of the environment" comprising accepted behaviors, beliefs, and institutions that exhibit great variability but that make sense to members of the cultural group (Herskovits 1948). Individuals use culture as a lens to filter information and to make sense of the world, other people, and themselves (Barry and Bullock 2001). Culture may also act as a buffer to minimize human awareness of vulnerability (Solomon et al. 1991) and may satiate our basic human need to belong (Baumeister and Leary 1995). Although many authors have emphasized the importance of culture, its usefulness as an explanatory concept in examining psychological phenomena resides in the investigator's ability to "unpackage" or deconstruct it (Poortinga et al. 1989; Whiting 1976). Mental health researchers have traditionally deconstructed culture by using two categorical variables: ethnicity and race.

Ethnicity is a designation commonly used by mental health professionals to classify group membership. Betancourt and Lopez (1993) noted that ethnicity is typically used to assign group membership based on cultural, nationality, or linguistic factors. *Race* was initially viewed as a biological category based on shared, fixed, immutable inborn traits (e.g., skin color) that could classify individuals into mutually exclusive groups. It is important to consider the history and origin of the construct of race when discussing possible racial differences in mental health outcomes (Smedley and Smedley 2005). Many scientists in the 1800s and 1900s employed an essentialist approach to argue that traits, such as morality and intelligence, could be hierarchically arranged by racial group membership, with whites composing the apex (e.g., Porteus 1926). This position was used to justify government-sanctioned discrimination against racial minority group members (Davenport 1923). Increased public criticism of race-based research, especially in the civil rights era, coupled with researchers' inability to identify putative biological markers of race resulted in its decreased use (Owens and King 1999); instead of race differences, researchers increasingly examined constructs such as socioeconomic status (Takeuchi and Gage 2003). However, human genome investigation has revitalized interest in the genetic foundations of race (Collins 2004; Henig 2004). Decisions about the inclusion and exclusion criteria of ethnicity and race occur within a sociopolitical context and are as much based on domestic and foreign policy concerns of the day as they are on scientific or anthropological data (Takeuchi and Gage 2003; Yanow 2003).

In the 1970s, the U.S. federal government issued a directive to standardize census data collection efforts that were, in part, required by the Voting Rights Act and affirmative action (U.S. Office of Management and Budget 1978). Revisions by the U.S. Office of Management and Budget in 1997 resulted in the inclusion of six racial categories in Census 2000: American Indian or Alaska Native, Asian, Native Hawaiian and Other Pacific Islander, Black or African American, White, and "Some Other Race." Census 2000 also employed two categories for ethnicity: Hispanic or Latino and Not Hispanic or Latino, with the stipulation that Hispanics or Latinos may be of any race. The existence of such ethnic/racial group categories facilitates intergroup comparison on different indicators, including mental health and mental illness, and has been instrumental in documenting mental health disparities (see Mays et al. 2003).

MENTAL HEALTH DISPARITIES

Beginning in the 1970s, Sue et al. (1974, 1978) began documenting that extant mental health systems in the United States were not adequately serving the needs of ethnic/racial minority groups. The landmark *Report of the Secretary's Task Force on Black and Minority Health* (U.S. Department of Health and Human Services 1985) documented a disparity in a variety of health indicators (e.g., hospital admissions, physician visits) among ethnic/racial minority groups. Epidemiological findings concerning significant differences in morbidity and mortality between ethnic/racial groups focused attention on health disparities (Hummer et al. 2004), and this area has become a major priority for federal health research funding (National Institutes of Health 2002). Differences in access to effective mental health services across ethnic/racial groups (i.e., mental health disparities) have also garnered increased research attention. In particular, two issues have shaped the debate surrounding mental health disparities among men from different ethnic/racial minority groups: comparative prevalence rates of psychiatric disorders and comparative rates of mental health service utilization.

In the 2000 U.S. census, 4.1 million Americans (1.5%) identified themselves as American Indian or Alaska Native solely or in combination with one or more ethnic/racial categories (U.S. Census Bureau 2002). Similar to African American men, American Indian or Alaska Native men are disproportionately represented in at-risk populations, including populations with low socioeconomic status and populations with low educational level (U.S. Department of Health and Human Services 2001). Although large epidemiological and randomized, controlled trials have advanced the field of mental health, information regarding American Indian or Alaska Native status has traditionally not been measured or has been measured in such small numbers as to obviate relevant statistical analyses (Manson 2003). To address such gaps in the literature, the American Indian Service Utilization, Psychiatric Epidemiology, Risk and Protective Factors Project was conducted in two American Indian reservation populations (Southwest and Northern Plains tribes). Among these men, the lifetime prevalence of having any DSM-IV psychiatric disorder was approximately 50% for both tribes; for the Southwest and Northern Plains tribes, respective lifetime prevalence rates were high for alcohol abuse (21.7%, 20.5%), alcohol dependence (17.0%, 20.5%), any depressive and/or anxiety disorder (19.2%, 14.7%), posttraumatic stress disorder (PTSD; 11.7%, 8.9%), drug abuse (8.1%, 10.7%), and drug dependence (5.9%, 4.8%) (Beals et al. 2005). In comparison with other population-based psychiatric epidemiology studies, alcohol use disorders and PTSD were more common in the two American Indian populations. Furthermore, lifetime exposure to at least one trauma (62.4%–67.2% among men) was common. In comparison with results of the National Comorbidity Survey, men from both tribes were more likely to report that they had witnessed trauma, including trauma to loved ones, and were often victims of physical attacks (Manson et al. 2005). In addition to alcohol use disorders and PTSD, American Indian men appear to have elevated rates of suicide and suicide attempts (May et al. 2005).

In the 2000 U.S. census, 10.2 million (3.6%) people in the American population identified themselves as Asian and approximately 400,000 (0.1%) identified themselves as Native Hawaiian and Other Pacific Islander (U.S. Census Bureau 2002). Although Census 2000 distinguished between Asian and Native Hawaiian and Other Pacific Islander, most of the relevant mental health research on these populations has used the term "Asian American and Pacific Islander." In contrast to other ethnic/racial minority groups, this category has traditionally been characterized as a "model minority," who rarely use mental health services because of purported low rates of psychopathology (Hu et al. 1991)—although more recently, the myth of the model minority has been disputed (Association of Asian Pacific Community Health Organizations 1995). One of the few Epidemiologic Catchment Area studies to examine prevalence rates of psychiatric disorders among Asian Americans and Pacific Islanders found that lifetime prevalence rates for major depression (6.9%) and dysthymia (5.2%) among Chinese Americans in Los Angeles, CA, were much lower than those rates reported for whites in the National Comorbidity Survey (Kessler et al. 1994; Takeuchi et al. 1998). Studies to date indicate that Asian Americans and Pacific Islanders are less likely than whites to use mental health services (Matsuoka et al. 1997; Zhang et al. 1998). A study of Chinese, Japanese, and Korean immigrants in the United States found that men were significantly less willing than women to use psychological services or to recommend such services to distressed friends (Barry and Grilo 2002). Assessment of psychiatric problems in Asian American and Pacific Islander men is further complicated because DSM-IV diagnostic categories and indigenous group labels of subjective distress may not correspond well. Unlike Western medicine, some Asian cultures have not traditionally dichotomized body and mind; this characteristic, coupled with reticence regarding emotional expression, may result in exclusive reporting of somatic symptoms (Lin and Cheung 1999). However, the finding that Asian Americans may have difficulty identifying psychological symptoms is not unequivocal (Chun et al. 1996). Conclusions about prevalence rates of psychiatric disorders and mental health utilization rates in Asian American and Pacific Islander men are difficult to make given the relative dearth of relevant large-scale epidemiological studies.

In the 2000 U.S. census, 34.7 million Americans (12.3%) identified themselves as black or African American (U.S. Census Bureau 2002). Although the prevalence rates of psychiatric disorders for African Americans who live in the community parallel those of European Americans, many more African American men belong to at-risk groups (e.g., homeless, incarcerated) that typically have higher rates of psychopathology (U.S. Department of Health and Human Services 2001). In comparison with men from other ethnic/racial groups, African American men are more likely to report having been shot or shot at (Turner and Lloyd 2004). In a study of 920 rural youth, Angold et al. (2002) found no difference in the prevalence rates of DSM-IV psychiatric disorders among African American and white participants; however, African Americans, especially boys, were less likely to use specialty mental health services. One area of clinical concern is the escalating suicide rate among young African American males (ages 15–19), which according to one estimate increased 70% between 1979 and 1997 (Joe and Kaplan 2001).

According to the U.S. Census Bureau (2003), the Hispanic population rose from approximately 22 million (9.1%) in 1990 to 39 million (13.4%) in 2003 and now outnumbers the African American population. Mexican Americans, many of whom are immigrants, compose the largest Hispanic subgroup in the United States. Two large-scale epidemiological studies have examined the mental health status of Mexican Americans: the Los Angeles, CA, site of the Epidemiologic Catchment Area (Burnam et al. 1987) and the Mexican American Prevalence and Services Survey (Vega et al. 1998). Both studies found higher rates of anxiety, mood, and substance use disorders among U.S.-born versus foreign-born Mexican Americans. More recently, Grant et al. (2004), using data from the National Epidemiologic Survey on Alcohol and Related Conditions (Grant et al. 2003), found that Mexican Americans were at significantly lower risk than U.S.-born non-Hispanic whites of psychiatric comorbidity; foreign-born Mexican Americans and foreign-born non-Hispanic whites were at significantly lower risk of DSM-IV mood, anxiety, and substance use disorders than their U.S.-born counterparts.

Two national surveys—the National Ambulatory Medical Care Survey (NAMCS) and the National Hospital Ambulatory Medical Care Survey (NHAMCS)—have played a pivotal role in documenting health care disparities in the United States. Both surveys were designed to collect information about the provision and use of ambulatory medical care services, the former in primary care settings and the latter in hospital emergency and outpatient departments. Snowden and Pingitore (2002), using data from the 1997 NAMCS, found that African Americans were more likely to seek mental health care from primary care physicians than psychiatrists and were less likely to receive psychotropic medications from primary care providers. In a separate analysis of NAMCS and NHAMCS databases regarding prescription of atypical antipsychotic medications from 1992 through 2000, Daumit et al. (2003) found that whereas African Americans and Hispanics were significantly less likely than whites to receive an atypical antipsychotic medication in the early 1990s, by the end of the decade there was no disparity between Hispanics and whites across psychiatric diagnoses; however, the adjusted odds of African Americans receiving these medications in visits specified for psychotic disorders was still 25% lower than whites. Atypical antipsychotic medications (e.g., olanzapine, risperidone) appear to be more effective than traditional antipsychotic medications for negative symptoms of psychosis and carry fewer serious adverse side effects (Kapur and Remington 2000). Richardson et al. (2003) examined racial differences in psychosocial and pharmacotherapy interventions from the 1997 NHAMCS and found that after controlling for diagnosis and other factors, African Americans were more likely to receive pharmacotherapy and less likely to receive psychotherapy than were whites.

CRITIQUE OF THE USE OF ETHNICITY AND RACE IN MENTAL HEALTH RESEARCH

Whereas ethnicity and race-based categories have been useful in drawing attention to mental health care disparities in the overall American population (Mays et al. 2003), the degree to which these categories are useful to mental health practitioners is debatable. Not only is there controversy over whether ethnicity and race may be social constructs that do not accurately capture the differences among Americans (Williams 1994, 1997), the common practice of attributing putative cultural, biological, or social etiologies to reported ethnicity- and race-based differences on psychosocial functioning measures is flawed; rather than inferring such causation, it is incumbent on mental health researchers to measure putative causal variables directly (Barry and Garner 2001). To illustrate this point, consider the categorization of Asian American and Pacific Islander—a term used by many mental health professionals—whose members comprise 43 ethnic groups and speak more than 100 languages. The extent of shared heritage, values, rituals, and traditions between individuals of Filipino and Pakistani descent, for example, is debatable, as is any assumption that differences in psychosocial functioning found between men from these two groups can (without testing) be attributed to cultural, biological, or social causation (see Foster and Sharp 2002; Lee et al. 2001; Shields et al. 2005). Problems with solely relying on categorical measures of culture, such as ethnicity and race, have prompted researchers to recommend that (similar to the notion of culture itself) the constructs of ethnicity and race be deconstructed. Phinney (1996) outlined three dimensions of ethnicity and race: cultural values and norms; salience and meaning of ethnic or racial identity; and experiences associated with ethnic/racial minority status. Barry and colleagues (Barry and Beitel, in press; Barry and Garner 2001; Barry et al. 2000) have outlined a three-factor model to better assist mental health clinicians and researchers in deconstructing the concept of culture. The three factors—acculturation, self-construal, and ethnic identity—are cultural variables that have been shown to be related to human psychosocial functioning among individuals of ethnic/racial minority status (Berry 1980; Markus and Kitayama 1991; Phinney 1996; Singelis et al. 1999).

THREE-FACTOR APPROACH

Barry's three factors—*acculturation, self-construal,* and *ethnic identity*—provide mental health professionals who work with men from diverse ethnic/racial backgrounds a dimensional approach to examining culture. This approach acknowledges that culture is not static but rather dynamic and complex, and this approach may provide a more differentiated measure of culture than such categorical variables as race and ethnicity (Barry and Garner 2001; Barry and Grilo 2002). The three factors allow researchers and clinicians to directly measure issues related to culture rather than inferring them in a post hoc fashion based on findings related to ethnicity and race differences (Barry and Garner 2001; Barry and Grilo 2003). A brief overview of the three components follows.

Acculturation is defined as social interaction and communication styles that individuals adopt when interacting with individuals and groups from another culture (Barry and Garner 2001). It comprises competence and ease or comfort in communicating with both ethnic/racial group peers and out-group members. Communication difficulty resulting from cultural differences between ethnic/racial minority patients and their providers has been associated with minority patients' underutilization of and unwillingness to use health care services (Barry and Grilo 2002; Ma 1999). The process and outcome of acculturation may also influence how symptoms are expressed and, in turn, subsequent entry into or use of the mental health system (Aponte and Barnes 1995). Berry's (1980) schema may be used to classify socialization and communication patterns: *assimilation* for socialization and communication primarily with individuals from the majority culture, *separation* for socialization and communication primarily with ethnic/racial peers, *integration* for socialization and communication with members of both minority and majority cultural groups, and *marginalization* for absence of socialization and communication with ethnic/racial minority peers or majority culture members.

Self-construal refers to two types of self-concept, independent and interdependent, that appear to be linked to the degree to which one's culture makes a distinction between the individual and the group (Markus and Kitayama 1991). Variations in self-construal may influence recognition and reporting of psychiatric symptoms, communication styles, and use of mental health services (Lin and Cheung 1999; Oetzel 1998; Yeh 1999). *Independent self-construal* refers to a self that is viewed as a separate, stable, autonomous, and bounded entity, whereas *interdependent self-construal* is described as a self that is flexible, variable, and guided by external factors such as roles, status, and relationships. Americans of ethnic/racial minority status may differ from those of European descent in terms of the salience of their self-construals. For example, Asian Americans, unlike Americans of European descent, tend to have more salient interdependent rather than independent self-construals (Chung 1992).

The third factor—*ethnic identity*—may be a more useful psychological construct than ethnicity (Phinney 1996). *Ethnic identity* may be viewed as the ethnic component of social identity, defined by Tajfel (1981) as "that part of an individual's self-concept which derives from his knowledge of his membership of a social group (or groups) together with the value and emotional significance attached to that membership" (p. 255). Ethnic identity has been identified as an important cultural variable in examining psychosocial functioning and health care utilization among ethnic/racial minority men (Pierre and Mahalik 2005; Pillay 2005).

CULTURAL SENSITIVITY AND CULTURAL COMPETENCE

Because it is now common for mental health providers to encounter male patients from diverse cultural backgrounds, mental health specialists are now called to have increased cultural sensitivity and cultural competence. Some researchers have suggested that ethnicity- and race-based mental health care disparities are, in part, a function of clinicians' disregard of patients' cultural backgrounds (Sue and Zane 2005). However, the constituent elements of cultural sensitivity and cultural competence are ambiguous, and the steps involved in conducting culturally sensitive and culturally competent clinical interventions are unclear (see O'Donohue 2005). For the purposes of this chapter, *cultural sensitivity* is defined as being aware of and having knowledge about "otherness" (i.e., people who are different from oneself) with the view of fostering or maintaining empathy for individuals who hail from different cultural backgrounds. *Cultural competence* is viewed as developing and effectively incorporating cultural expertise into clinical practice.

Currently, the standard methods of teaching cultural sensitivity to mental heath professionals comprise 1) documenting similarities and differences between indigenous and mainstream cultural values, beliefs, and behaviors; 2) examining different ethnic/racial minority groups' history of immigration, including the perceived prejudice and discrimination against them, relative socioeconomic standing, and sociopolitical factors associated with group membership; and 3) performing experiential exercises in which participants share their personal histories of being members of their respective ethnic/racial groups.

Many researchers use the terms *cultural sensitivity* and *cultural competence* interchangeably. Rather than providing specific guidelines about how to provide culturally sensitive or culturally competent mental health services, many researchers simply list a plethora of potentially defining cultural values and historical markers targeting different ethnic/racial minority groups. This practice may paradoxically engender overgeneralizing and stereotyping on the part of clinicians and has been termed the "cookbook" approach to cultural sensitivity and cultural competence (Barry et al. 2000). Simply put, good intentions and knowledge about cultural differences do not confer cultural competence (see Barry and Bullock 2001; Dumas et al. 1999).

RECOMMENDATIONS FOR DEVELOPING CULTURAL COMPETENCE WITH ETHNIC/RACIAL MINORITY MEN

Given that research on evidence-based practices with ethnic/racial minority populations is scant (Chambless et al. 1996), the following recommendations for mental health professionals are tentatively suggested and are based on my understanding of the relevant research and my experiences working with men from diverse ethnic/racial backgrounds.

1. Clinicians should consider expanding their knowledge about different cultures through informal (e.g., travel, social interaction) and formal (e.g., reading multicultural psychology/psychiatry research, attending relevant lectures) activities.

2. Clinicians should consider using their current knowledge and clinical impressions to generate hypotheses that are then tested when conducting psychotherapy or other clinical interventions with men from different cultures. A primary task for clinicians who wish to conduct culturally competent interventions is to become aware of their own cultural assumptions and to use a hypothesis-driven scientific approach to test them (Barry 2005; Betancourt and Lopez 1993; Sue 1998). A cardinal feature of this approach is that preconceived notions about individuals from one's own or other ethnic/racial groups are

natural. Cognitive science researchers have long understood that given the potentially overwhelming array of information that humans face, we tend to filter information using cognitive sets or schemata (Bartlett 1932; Stein 1992). Thus, cultural competence does not automatically emerge from exposure to or memorization of lists of values or facts related to culture; rather, cultural competence emerges from systematically becoming aware of one's culture-related assumptions and testing them empirically in a clinically meaningful manner. This approach leads the clinician to be scientifically minded (Sue 1998) and to become a "culture broker" (Abudabbeh 1998; Barry et al. 2000). Consequently, rather than being a pejorative stance toward clinician assumptions and impressions, this cultural competence approach frees clinicians from second-guessing their culture-related hunches and knowledge and instead emphasizes scientifically testing clinical and cultural assumptions. This approach often involves creativity and is likely to be experienced by clinicians as positive rather than overwhelming (Barry and Bullock 2001). The previously described three-factor approach may be useful in guiding hypothesis testing related to cultural factors.

3. Clinicians should consider providing male patients with a rationale for clinical interventions. Some mental health professionals may not provide patients with an explicit context or rationale for such interventions—an approach that may, in part, reflect the clinician's assumption that his or her patients are socialized to clinical encounters or to find the clinician and clinical interventions to be credible. However, clinicians who work with men—and especially men of ethnic/racial minority descent—should consider that men have been found, in comparison with women, to have more doubts or suspicions about the efficacy or rationale for psychotherapy, appear less willing to reveal information about themselves (a key prerequisite of counseling), and seem less willing to seek mental health services (Barry and Grilo 2002; Dindia and Allen 1992; Kahn and Hessling 2001; Kessler et al. 1981; Rabinowitz and Cochran 2001). Thus when clinicians provide a concrete, credible rationale for clinical interventions, it may allay the initial doubts and misconceptions of ethnic/racial minority men and consequently increase the likelihood of treatment engagement (see case of Emilio described earlier).

4. Clinicians should consider framing their clinical interventions (at least until a solid working alliance has been established) in terms of enhancing patients' preexisting skills or strengths. Traditional psychosocial interventions may inadvertently challenge normative mas-

culinity messages by stressing the patients' problems and ignoring preexisting strengths (see Addis and Mahalik 2003; Cervantes 2006).

5. In addition to deconstructing the construct of culture, clinicians should consider deconstructing male gender. For example, clinicians may informally or formally assess dimensions of "maleness," such as sex-role ideology (see case vignette) and masculinity, because these factors may assist clinicians in conceptualizing multiple areas of patient change over the course of treatment (see Addis and Mahalik 2003).

CONCLUSION

Ethnic/racial minority men make up an important clinical group whose psychological functioning and mental health needs are poorly understood. Findings from recent epidemiological studies suggest that men from ethnic/racial minority groups have higher rates of specific psychiatric disorders than do their female and/or white male counterparts. Evidence-based treatments for ethnic/racial minority men are not well understood given the relative dearth of relevant controlled trials of psychosocial and pharmacological interventions. Future research on psychologically meaningful dimensions of culture and gender may inform the development of culturally competent services for this population.

KEY POINTS

- Ethnic/racial minority men, particularly those born in the United States, appear at high risk for specific psychiatric disorders.

- It is often difficult for ethnic/racial minority men to self-disclose personal information and utilize mental health services.

- Although ethnicity and race are commonly used constructs, knowledge regarding clinically relevant facets of culture is still limited. However, true knowledge and sensitivity to ethnicity and race is clinically relevant to treatment.

- Developing and effectively incorporating cultural expertise into clinical practice with ethnic/racial minority men involves an understanding that cultural values and data are dynamic and complex.

PRACTICE GUIDELINES

1. Empirically test culture-related assumptions in a clinically meaningful manner.
2. Assess multiple psychologically meaningful dimensions of culture and gender.
3. Frame clinical interventions to emphasize strengths and/or building skills and avoid focusing on weaknesses. Provide a concrete, convincing rationale for culturally informed clinical interventions.

REFERENCES

Abudabbeh N: Counseling Arab-American families, in The Family and Family Therapy in International Perspective. Edited by Gielen PU, Comunian L. Trieste, Italy, Edizioni Lint Trieste, 1998, pp 115–126

Addis ME, Mahalik JR: Men, masculinity, and the contexts of help seeking. Am Psychol 58:5–14, 2003

American Psychiatric Association: Diagnostic and Statistical Manual of Mental Disorders, 4th Edition. Washington, DC, American Psychiatric Association, 1994

American Psychiatric Association: Diagnostic and Statistical Manual of Mental Disorders, 4th Edition, Text Revision. Washington, DC, American Psychiatric Association, 2000

Angold A, Erkanli A, Farmer EMZ, et al: Psychiatric disorder, impairment, and service use in rural African American and white youth. Arch Gen Psychiatry 59:893–901, 2002

Aponte JF, Barnes JM: Impact of acculturation and moderator variables on the intervention and treatment of ethnic groups, in Psychological Interventions and Cultural Diversity. Edited by Aponte JF, Rivers RY, Wohl J. Boston, MA, Allyn & Bacon, 1995, pp 19–39

Association of Asian Pacific Community Health Organizations: Taking Action: Improving Access to Health Care for Asians and Pacific Islanders. Oakland, CA, Association of Asian Pacific Community Health Organizations, 1995

Barry DT: Measuring acculturation among male Arab immigrants in the United States: an exploratory study. J Immigr Health 7:179–184, 2005

Barry DT, Beitel M: Sex role ideology among East Asian immigrants in the United States. Am J Orthopsychiatry, in press

Barry DT, Bullock WA: Culturally creative psychotherapy with a Latino couple by an Anglo therapist. J Fam Psychother 12:15–30, 2001

Barry DT, Garner DM: Eating concerns in East Asian immigrants. Eat Weight Disord 6:90–98, 2001

Barry DT, Grilo CM: Cultural, psychological, and demographic correlates of willingness to use psychological services among East Asian immigrants. J Nerv Ment Dis 190:32–39, 2002

Barry DT, Grilo CM: Cultural, self-esteem, and demographic correlates of perception of personal and group discrimination among East Asian immigrants. Am J Orthopsychiatry 73:223–229, 2003

Barry DT, Elliot R, Evans EM: Foreigners in a strange land: ethnic identity and self-construal in male Arab immigrants. J Immigr Health 2:133–144, 2000

Bartlett FC: Remembering. Cambridge, England, Cambridge University Press, 1932

Baumeister RG, Leary MR: The need to belong: desire for interpersonal attachments as a fundamental human motivation. Psychol Bull 117:479–529, 1995

Beals J, Manson SM, Whitesell NR, et al: Prevalence of DSM-IV disorders and attendant help-seeking in 2 American Indian reservation populations. Arch Gen Psychiatry 62:99–108, 2005

Berry JW: Acculturation as varieties of adaptation, in Acculturation: Theory, Models and Some New Findings. Edited by Padilla A. Boulder, CO, Westview, 1980, pp 9–25

Betancourt H, Lopez SR: The study of culture, ethnicity, and race in American psychology. Am Psychol 48:629–637, 1993

Brislin RW: Understanding Culture's Influence on Behavior. Orlando, FL, Harcourt College Publishing, 1993

Burnam MA, Hough RL, Karno M, et al: Acculturation and lifetime prevalence of psychiatric disorders among Mexican Americans in Los Angeles. J Health Soc Behav 28:89–102, 1987

Cervantes JM: A new understanding of the macho male image: explorations of the Mexican-American man, in In the Room With Men: A Casebook of Therapeutic Change. Edited by Englar-Carlson M, Stevens MA. Washington, DC, American Psychological Association, 2006, pp 197–224

Chambless DL, Sanderson WC, Shoham V, et al: An update on empirically validated therapies. Clin Psychol 49:5–18, 1996

Chun CA, Enomoto K, Sue S: Health care issues among Asian Americans: implications of somatization, in Handbook of Diversity in Health Psychology. Edited by Kato PM, Mann T. New York, Plenum, 1996, pp 439–467

Chung D: Asian cultural commonalities: a comparison with mainstream American culture, in Social Work Practice With Asian Americans. Edited by Furuto S, Biswas R, Chung D, et al. Newbury Park, CA, Sage, 1992, pp 27–44

Collins FS: What we do and don't know about race, ethnicity, genetics, and health at the dawn of the genome era. Nat Genet 36(suppl):1–3, 2004

Daumit GL, Crum RM, Guallar E, et al: Outpatient prescriptions for atypical antipsychotics for African Americans, Hispanics, and whites in the United States. Arch Gen Psychiatry 60:121–128, 2003

Davenport CB: Eugenics in Race and State, Vol 2. Scientific Papers of the Second International Conference of Eugenics. Baltimore, MD, Williams & Wilkins, 1923

Dindia K, Allen M: Sex differences in self-disclosure: a meta-analysis. Psychol Bull 112:106–124, 1992

Dumas JE, Rollock D, Prinz RJ, et al: Cultural sensitivity: problems and solutions in applied and preventive intervention. Appl Prev Psychol 8:175–196, 1999

Foster MW, Sharp RR: Race, ethnicity, and genomics: social classifications as proxies of biological heterogeneity. Genome Res 12:844–850, 2002

Grant BF, Moore TC, Shepard J, et al: Source and Accuracy Statement: Wave 1 National Epidemiologic Survey on Alcohol and Related Conditions (NESARC). Bethesda, MD, National Institute on Alcohol Abuse and Alcoholism, 2003

Grant BF, Stinson FS, Hasin DS, et al: Immigration and lifetime prevalence of DSM-IV psychiatric disorders among Mexican Americans and non-Hispanic whites in the United States: results from the National Epidemiological Survey on Alcohol and Related Conditions. Arch Gen Psychiatry 61:1226–1233, 2004

Greenfield PM, Keller H, Fuligni A, et al: Cultural pathways through universal development. Annu Rev Psychol 54:461–490, 2003

Henig RM: The genome in black and white (and gray), in The New York Times Magazine, October 10, 2004, pp 47–51

Herskovits MJ: Man and His Works. New York, Knopf, 1948

Hu T, Snowden LR, Jerrell JM, et al: Ethnic populations in public mental health services: choices and level of use. Am J Public Health 81:1429–1434, 1991

Hummer RA, Benjamins MR, Rogers RG: Racial and ethnic disparities in health and mortality among the U.S. elderly population, in Critical Perspectives on Racial and Ethnic Differences in Health in Late Life. Edited by Anderson N, Bulatao R, Cohen B. Washington, DC, National Academies Press, 2004, pp 53–94

Joe S, Kaplan MS: Suicide among African American men. Suicide Life Threat Behav 31(suppl):106–121, 2001

Johnson PB, Glassman M: The relationship between ethnicity, gender and alcohol consumption: a strategy for testing competing models. Addiction 93: 583–588, 1998

Kahn JH, Hessling RM: Measuring the tendency to conceal versus disclose psychological distress. J Soc Clin Psychol 20:41–65, 2001

Kapur S, Remington G: Atypical antipsychotics. BMJ 321:1360–1361, 2000

Kessler RC, Brown RL, Broman CL: Sex differences in psychiatric help-seeking: evidence from four large-scale surveys. J Health Soc Behav 22:49–64, 1981

Kessler RC, McGonagle KA, Zhao S, et al: Lifetime and 12-month prevalence of DSM-III-R psychiatric disorders in the United States: results from the National Comorbidity Survey. Arch Gen Psychiatry 51:8–19, 1994

Lee S, Mountain J, Koenig BA: The meanings of "race" in the new genomics: implications for health disparities research. Yale J Health Policy Law Ethics 1:33–75, 2001

Lewis-Fernandez R, Kleinman A: Cultural psychiatry: theoretical, clinical, and research issues. Psychiatr Clin North Am 18:433–448, 1995

Lin K-M, Cheung F: Mental health issues for Asian Americans. Psychiatr Serv 50:774–780, 1999

Ma GX: Access to health care by Asian Americans, in Ethnicity and Health Care: A Sociocultural Approach. Edited by Ma GX, Henderson G. Springfield, IL, Charles C Thomas, 1999, pp 99–121

Manson SM: Extending the boundaries, bridging the gaps: crafting Mental Health: Culture, Race, and Ethnicity, a Supplement to the Surgeon General's Report on Mental Health. Cult Med Psychiatry 27:395–408, 2003

Manson SM, Beals J, Klein SA, et al: Social epidemiology of trauma among 2 American Indian reservation populations. Am J Public Health 95:851–859, 2005

Markus HR, Kitayama S: Culture and the self: implications for cognition, emotion, and motivation. Psychol Rev 98:224–253, 1991

Matsuoka JK, Breaux C, Ryujin DJ: National utilization of mental health services by Asian Americans/Pacific Islanders. J Community Psychol 25:141–145, 1997

May PA, Serna P, Hurt L, et al: Outcome evaluation of a public health approach to suicide prevention in an American Indian Tribal Nation. Am J Public Health 95:1238–1244, 2005

Mays VM, Ponce NA, Washington DL, et al: Classification of race and ethnicity: implications for public health. Annu Rev Public Health 24:83–110, 2003

National Institutes of Health: Strategic Research Plan and Budget to Reduce and Ultimately Eliminate Health Disparities, Vol 1. Washington, DC, U.S. Department of Health and Human Services, 2002

O'Donohue WT: Cultural sensitivity: a critical examination, in Destructive Trends in Mental Health: The Well-Intentioned Path to Harm. Edited by Wright RH, Cummings NA. New York, Routledge, 2005, pp 29–44

Oetzel JG: The effects of self-construals and ethnicity on self-reported conflict styles. Communication Reports 11:133–144, 1998

Owens K, King MC: Genomic views of human history. Science 286:451–453, 1999

Phinney JS: When we talk about American ethnic groups, what do we mean? Am Psychol 51:918–927, 1996

Pierre MR, Mahalik JR: Examining African self-consciousness and Black racial identity as predictors of Black men's psychological well-being. Cultur Divers Ethnic Minor Psychol 11:28–40, 2005

Pillay Y: Racial identity as a predictor of the psychological health of African American students at a predominantly White university. J Black Psychol 31:46–66, 2005

Poortinga Y, van de Vijver F, Joe R, et al: Peeling the onion called culture: a synopsis, in Growth and Progress in Cross-Cultural Psychology. Edited by Kagitcibasi C. Berwyn, PA, Swets North America, 1989, pp 22–34

Porteus SD: Temperament and Race. Boston, MA, Richard G Badger, 1926

Rabinowitz FE, Cochran SV: Deepening Psychotherapy With Men. Washington, DC, American Psychological Association, 2001

Richardson J, Anderson T, Flaherty J, et al: The quality of mental health care for African Americans. Cult Med Psychiatry 27:487–498, 2003

Segall MH, Lonner WJ, Berry JW: Cross-cultural psychology as a scholarly discipline: on the flowering of culture in behavioral research. Am Psychol 53:1101–1110, 1998

Shields AE, Fortun M, Hammonds EM, et al: The use of race variables in genetic studies of complex traits and the goal of reducing health disparities: a transdisciplinary perspective. Am Psychol 60:77–103, 2005

Singelis TM, Bond MH, Sharkey WF, et al: Unpackaging culture's influence on self-esteem and embarrassability. J Cross Cult Psychol 30:315–341, 1999

Smedley A, Smedley BD: Race as biology is fiction, racism as a social problem is real: anthropological and historical perspectives on the social construction of race. Am Psychol 60:16–26, 2005

Snowden LR, Pingitore D: Frequency and scope of mental health service delivery to African Americans in primary care. Ment Health Serv Res 4:123–130, 2002

Solomon S, Greenberg J, Pyszczynski T: A terror management theory of social behavior: the psychological functions of self-esteem and cultural worldviews. Advances in Experimental Social Psychology 24:93–159, 1991

Stein DJ: Schemas in the cognitive and clinical sciences: an integrative construct. Journal of Psychotherapy Integration 2:45–63, 1992

Sue S: In search of cultural competence in psychotherapy and counseling. Am Psychol 53:440–448, 1998

Sue S, Zane N: How well do both evidence-based practices and treatment as usual satisfactorily address the various dimensions of diversity? in Evidence Based Practices in Mental Health: Debate and Dialogue on the Fundamental Questions. Edited by Norcross JC, Beutler LE, Levant RF. Washington, DC, American Psychological Association, 2005, pp 329–337

Sue S, McKinney H, Allen D, et al: Delivery of community mental health services to black and white clients. J Consult Clin Psychol 42:794–801, 1974

Sue S, Allen DB, Conaway L: The responsiveness and equality of mental health care to Chicanos and Native Americans. Am J Community Psychol 6:137–146, 1978

Tajfel H: Human Groups and Social Categories. Cambridge, England, Cambridge University Press, 1981

Takeuchi DT, Gage S-JL: What to do with race? changing notions of race in the social sciences. Cult Med Psychiatry 27:435–445, 2003

Takeuchi DT, Chung RC-Y, Lin K-M, et al: Lifetime and twelve-month prevalence rates of major depressive episodes and dysthymia among Chinese Americans in Los Angeles. Am J Psychiatry 155:1407–1414, 1998

Turner RJ, Lloyd DA: Stress burden and the lifetime incidence of psychiatric disorders in young adults: racial and ethnic contrasts. Arch Gen Psychiatry 61:481–488, 2004

U.S. Census Bureau: The American Indian and Alaska Native Population: 2000. Hyattsville, MD, U.S. Census Bureau, 2002. Available at: http://www.cdc.gov/omh/Populations/AIAN/AIAN.htm. Accessed June 20, 2006.

U.S. Census Bureau: Annual Resident Population Estimates of the United States by Age, Race, and Hispanic or Latino Origin: April 1, 2000 to July 1, 2003. Hyattsville, MD, U.S. Census Bureau, 2003

U.S. Department of Health and Human Services: Report of the Secretary's Task Force on Black and Minority Health. Washington, DC, U.S. Department of Health and Human Services, 1985

U.S. Department of Health and Human Services: Mental Health: Culture, Race, and Ethnicity. A Supplement to Mental Health: A Report of the Surgeon General. Rockville, MD, U.S. Department of Health and Human Services, 2001

U.S. Office of Management and Budget: Directive No. 15: Race and Ethnic Standards for Federal Statistics and Administrative Reporting. Washington, DC, U.S. Office of Management and Budget, 1978

Vega WA, Kolody B, Anguilar-Gaxiola S, et al: Lifetime prevalence of DSM-III-R psychiatric disorders among urban and rural Mexican Americans in California. Arch Gen Psychiatry 55:771–778, 1998

Whiting BB: The problem of the packaged variable, in The Developing Individual in a Changing World. Edited by Riegel KF, Meecham JA. New York, Hawthorne, 1976, pp 303–309

Williams DR: The concept of race in Health Services Research: 1966 to 1990. Health Serv Res 29:261–274, 1994

Williams DR: Race and health: basic questions, emerging directions. Ann Epidemiol 7:322–333, 1997

Yanow D: Constructing "Race" and "Ethnicity" in America: Category-Making in Public Policy and Administration. Armonk, NY, ME Sharpe, 2003

Yeh CJ: Invisibility and self-construal in African American men: implications for training and practice. Couns Psychol 27:810–819, 1999

Zhang AY, Snowden L, Sue S: Differences between Asian and white Americans' help seeking and utilization patterns in the Los Angeles area. J Community Psychol 26:317–326, 1998

16

MENTAL HEALTH OF GAY MEN

MICHAEL KING, M.D., PH.D., F.R.C.P., F.R.C.G.P., F.R.C.PSYCH.

Case Vignette

Gary was 28 when he first consulted his general practitioner with depression and sexual difficulties. For more than 1 year he had experienced low mood, tearfulness, and thoughts of self-harm. He lacked motivation or interest in life, could not work or sleep, and had lost his appetite. He was adamant that his feelings were due to his loss of sexual desire for his wife. When referred to a sexual medicine specialist, he asserted that his loss of sex drive was difficult to understand but that he was anxious to ensure that it was restored.

In therapy Gary gradually revealed that he had always been primarily sexually attracted to men, but despite the fact that his brother was gay and accepted by the family, Gary had been unable to come to terms with his own sexuality. He was terrified of how his wife and their respective parents would react and feared for his marriage if his sexuality were to be revealed. Individual and couples therapy helped Gary and his wife realize the situation fully and agree to a separation that would allow Gary unrestricted visitation with his daughter.

Although his wife was very supportive of the adjustments he had to make, she in her turn was extremely distressed at the change in their relationship and took a considerable time to adjust. On follow-up, Gary was living with a male partner in a neighborhood close to his wife and daughter and had joined a gay football team. His depression had completely resolved, and his sex drive and function were normal. Gary's story illustrates the great difficulty many gay men have in accepting their sexuality, how they dread the opinion of the outside world, and how this dilemma has major mental health consequences not only for the men involved but also for the people close to them.

HISTORY

Gay men's mental health and their approach to help seeking can only be understood in the context of homosexuality's particular history. Religious and moral objections to sexual attraction between men have existed since at least the Middle Ages (Davenport-Hines 1990). Men who desired sex with other men were regarded as sinful or depraved, if not ill or abnormal (Weeks 1989), and same-sex contacts were not distinguished from lewd behaviors. The idea of homosexuality as illness, even if not widely held among early physicians, has a long history. Homosexuality was listed as an affliction of the mind or soul by the Greek physician Soranus of Ephesus, who practiced medicine in Rome between 98 and 138 A.D. Although Soranus only regarded "passive" male homosexuality (and lesbianism) as disease, he believed it could not be cured and might be hereditary (Bullough 1976). Interestingly, neither Hippocrates nor Plato mentions homosexuality as madness or pathology (Mendelson 2003).

Legal objection to sodomy was first endorsed in Britain in the 1533 Act of Henry VIII, which classified sodomy as an illegal act between man and woman, man and man, or man and beast (Weeks 1990). This law, which was reenacted in 1563, was the basis for all male homosexual convictions until 1885, when an amendment to the new Criminal Assessment Act extended the legal sanction to *any* form of sexual contact between men (Weeks 1990). This amendment greatly expanded the circumstances under which men could be arrested and tried for same-sex contacts. The prosecution of Oscar Wilde was the first and most famous instance of this law in action. For multiple cultural and historical reasons, lesbian sexual behavior was never subject to legal sanction.

Science and Same-Sex Desire

The scientific study of same-sex desire that began in the nineteenth century evolved through three distinct phases in the Western world and continues up through the present time (Cochran and Mays 2000). These phases are described below.

Sexology

In the first phase of study, the discipline of *sexology* emerged in the late nineteenth century; sexology drew on scientific discourse to provide a medical explanation for the development of same-sex desire. Thus, the work of sexologists in Europe such as Ulrichs, Krafft-Ebing, and Ellis, coupled with the legal discourses of the time, had a profound effect by defining someone who was homosexual as a distinctive kind of person. Karl Ulrichs, a German civil servant who was dismissed from his post for homosexual activity, published 12 pieces on his scientific theory of homosexuality between 1864 and 1879. In this work, he propounded the "natural," biological basis for what he regarded as a human characteristic (Kennedy 1997). The notion of the *homosexual* had materialized, an identity expressed in both physical appearance and personality. Making same-sex desire into a condition was optimistically used to justify appeals for greater tolerance toward homosexual persons and campaigns for legal reform. If homosexuality was determined before birth or by biological anomaly, then individuals should not be denigrated and shunned for what was simply a physiological variation (Felski 1995; Kennedy 1997). Of greater impact, however, was the negative view of homosexuality as medical aberration.

A new kind of opposition to homosexuality arose in the late nineteenth century based on scientific-medical opinion that sexual contact between men was both pathological and criminal (Weeks 1989). Official sanction of homosexuality as illness hindered the development of a gay and lesbian identity and led to oppression, shame, guilt, and fear for many men and women and their families. Between the 1950s and early 1980s in Britain and the United States, unknown numbers of gay men underwent psychoanalytic and psychiatric "treatments" to become heterosexual. Men were sometimes encouraged to accept treatment to avoid a term of imprisonment. These interventions, particularly those using behavioral methods, had a negative impact on homosexual men's sense of identity, self-esteem, mental health, and well-being (King and Bartlett 1999; King et al. 2004; Smith et al. 2004).

Reconsidering the Diagnosis

In 1951, Lemert suggested that both the prejudice and the social discrimination against homosexual men were likely to have a negative impact on their mental health. This theory began the second identifiable phase in scientific understanding of homosexuality, when the validity of homosexuality as a diagnosis of mental illness was examined in psychological research and found to be lacking (Bayer 1981). Of particular influence was the pioneering work of Evelyn Hooker, a young psychologist in the United States who first questioned the inclusion of homosexuality as a "sexual deviation" in DSM. She was among the first to describe the fallacy in drawing inferences based on psychoanalytic theory from samples of men seeking to change their homosexual behavior. Data collected using better sampling and statistical methods led to the publication of her influential paper in which she discarded the notion that homosexuality was pathological (Hooker 1957; Kirby 2003). Interest in the study of homosexuality accelerated in the psychiatric and psychological professions, and parallels were drawn between these professions' views of homosexuality and the misuse of psychiatry to punish political dissidents in countries such as the former Soviet Union. Medicalization of homosexuality was increasingly seen as punishment of a sexual minority that did not conform to the religious and moral view of the majority (Kirby 2003).

These studies, together with social changes whereby gay, lesbian, and bisexual people became increasingly visible in Western society, eventually led the American Psychiatric Association to remove homosexuality as a mental disorder from DSM-III (American Psychiatric Association 1980). (The Association also decided in 1973 that subsequent printings of DSM-II [American Psychiatric Association 1968] would no longer contain homosexuality as a disorder.) However, it was not until the early 1990s that homosexuality was removed from the International Classification of Diseases (ICD; World Health Organization 1992). Even now, reference to sexual orientation is still included as "F66.1 Egodystonic sexual orientation" to indicate when a person's "gender identity or sexual preference…is not in doubt but the individual wishes it were different because of psychological and behavioral disorders, and may seek treatment in order to change it" (World Health Organization 1994, pp. 254–255). This muddle conflates gender identity with sexual orientation and suggests that sexual orientation may be "treated." The silent assumption behind the classification is that gay and lesbian people will want to change. Heterosexuals seeking treatment to become homosexual is presumed to be illogical.

Environment and Mental Health

Later research that concentrated on the psychological and social status of lesbian, gay, and bisexual people constituted the third phase of scientific understanding of homosexuality. Data arising from opportunity samples of lesbian, gay, and bisexual people, together with the judgments of mental health professionals, suggested that mental health problems as a consequence of social stigma might be common in the lesbian, gay, and bisexual populations (Faulkner and Cranston 1998; Garofalo et al. 1998; King et al. 2003; Pillard 1998; Skegg et al. 2003). However, the inadequacy of available samples made it difficult to know whether such elevated risks could be generalized to all gay men (Cochran and Mays 2000).

EPIDEMIOLOGY OF MENTAL DISORDERS

Defining Sexual Orientation

Research into the prevalence of mental disorders in any minority group is controversial and complex. One difficulty involves determining the prevalence of same-sex attraction. Estimates of the prevalence of male homosexuality have generated considerable debate. A common assumption is that there are homosexual and nonhomosexual men. However, scientists have long been aware that sexual responsiveness to others of the same sex, like most human traits, is continuously distributed in the population (Kinsey et al. 1948; McConaghy and Blaszczynski 1991). A second difficulty involves the presumption that such traits are stable within each man over time (Michaels 1996). A third problem is encountered in conflating same-sex sexual experiences with a categorization of the man as homosexual. Defining sexuality solely on the basis of sexual experience (Kinsey et al. 1948) excludes people who fantasize about sex with others of the same sex but never have sexual contact (Gilman et al. 2001). Most modern conceptions of sexual orientation consider personal identification, sexual behavior, and sexual fantasy (McWhirter et al. 1990). One widely established definition of a *homosexual* is a person "with an orientation towards people of the same gender in sexual behavior, affection, or attraction, and/or self-identity as gay/lesbian or bisexual"_ (Dean et al. 2000, p. 102). Given these qualifications, there is evidence that at least 5% of men in Western countries are gay or bisexual (Johnson et al. 2001; Michaels 1996; Sell et al. 1995).

Sampling

Once a definition of what constitutes being gay has been agreed on, the subsequent obstacle of recruiting a large, broad-based sample of gay men is encountered. Random population research requires very large surveys in order to find adequate numbers of gay men (Gilman et al. 2001). Furthermore, many gay men may not be open about their sexuality, and even when open about sexuality, many people do not always tell the truth about sex (Sharp 2002). An alternative method of recruitment is snowball sampling, which involves recruiting an initial convenience sample and asking each recruit to approach, on behalf of the researchers, as many others as possible who might be interested in participating. The sample "snowballs" recruit people who may not be contacted otherwise. This method is useful when there is no adequate sampling frame and the population is relatively dispersed (Gilbert 1993). Although snowball sampling does not constitute an epidemiological framework, it reaches men who might not respond to newspaper and magazine advertisements. However, snowball sampling is likely to miss those men who are not open about their sexuality to at least one or two friends or family members.

Many studies of gay men have not included comparison groups, making it difficult to place the findings in the context of the wider population (Pillard 1998). The observation that half of gay men have at some time considered harming themselves, for example, is of concern, but this observation has greater impact if researchers know how it compares with heterosexual men. This comparison helps determine whether gay men are different than or similar to the larger male population with regard to ideas of self-harm. Studies have been criticized for employing convenience samples unlikely to be representative of gay or bisexual populations or using unsatisfactory definitions of homosexuality. Many studies also fail to differentiate between findings among gay and bisexual men, making comparisons between these men difficult. Given these caveats, what is known about the mental health of gay men?

PREVALENCE OF MENTAL DISORDERS

Depressive and Anxiety Disorders

Multiple studies in the 1980s and early 1990s reported equivocal findings regarding higher rates of depressive and anxiety disorders in gay men. Tross et al. (1987) reported a slightly elevated prevalence for current major depressive disorder. Williams et al. (1991) reported a higher lifetime prevalence of affective disorders in gay men compared with national estimates in the North American Epidemiologic Catchment Area study but no elevated prevalence of current disorders. Throughout the 1980s, many small studies, aimed mainly at elucidating the effects of human immunodeficiency virus (HIV), reported raised rates of mental health problems even in healthy gay men (e.g., Atkinson et al. 1988). These findings were later confirmed in more rigorous studies in the United States, Australia, Holland, and the United Kingdom. In these studies, elevated rates of major depression and panic disorder (Cochran and Mays 2000), bipolar disorder (Pillard 1998), and anxiety and depression (Gilman et al. 2001; Herek et al. 1999; Jorm et al. 2002; King et al. 2003; Mills et al. 2004; Sandfort et al. 2001) were reported. Odds ratios, which express the level of risk relative to heterosexual men, are 2.9 (confidence interval [CI] = 1.54–5.57) for mood disorders, 2.61 (CI = 1.44–4.74) for anxiety disorders (Sandfort et al. 2001), and 1.48 (CI = 1.09–2.01) for any psychiatric disorder (King et al. 2003). Bisexual men appear to be at greater risk than gay men (Jorm et al. 2002; Warner et al. 2004). African American gay men may be at even greater risk of psychiatric morbidity than their white counterparts, although some of this research is confounded by use of populations at risk for or infected with HIV (e.g., see Cochran and Mays 1994). Ethnic minority gay men live as minorities within minorities and may experience multiple levels of discrimination. They also have to cope with affirming two types of cultural and personal identity (Greene 1994).

Studies employing probabilistic sampling of the general population are hampered by the low prevalence of gay men among those men who are recruited and consequent problems of low power (Gilman et al. 2001; Jorm et al. 2002). Furthermore, definition of sexuality is often based on simple measures of same-sex activity. Prevalence rates of gay men in the range of 2.8% (Sandfort et al. 2001) and 1%–1.6% (Jorm et al. 2002) strongly suggest that many gay men evade the surveys or avoid declaring their sexuality when participating. In contrast, epidemiological studies with very large samples of gay men may recruit participants in ways that threaten external validity (generalizability; Herek et al. 1999; King et al. 2003). Occasionally researchers resort to combining gay men and lesbians in their analyses in order to achieve sufficient power (e.g., Fergusson et al. 1999; Jorm et al. 2002). Given that the origins of homosexuality in men and women and the life experiences of gay men and lesbians are likely to be different, this procedure risks conflating both estimates and confounders of observed associations between sexual orientation and mental health. Even studies that randomly recruit gay men living in gay neighborhoods (Mills et al. 2004) may include participants not typical of all gay men in the community. For example, men who have sex with other men—but who do not live in gay neighborhoods—are less likely to report having only male sexual partners, to identify themselves as gay, and to have sought HIV antibody testing (Mills et al. 2001).

Although prospective studies are uncommon, two have been performed in New Zealand. Both were conducted in birth cohorts and found increased rates of mental disorder in people who reported some degree of same-sex attraction or behavior (Fergusson et al. 1999; Skegg et al. 2003). Advantages of these studies include the longer time span of the research, more wide-ranging assessments, and use of composite measures of sexual orientation that examined sexual attraction, sexual identity, and same-sex contacts. The main disadvantage is the low numbers of gay men surveyed, a problem that forced Fergusson et al. (1999) to combine gay men and lesbians in at least some of their analyses.

A comprehensive literature review evaluated the mental health of gay and bisexual people as reported in studies published between 1970 and 2001. A meta-analysis of data from 10 studies indicated that gay men were approximately twice as likely as heterosexual men to experience a mental disorder at some point in their lives (odds ratios are 2.66 [95% CI=2.07–3.64] for mood disorders, 2.43 [CI=1.78–3.30] for anxiety disorders, and 1.45 [CI=1.10–1.91] for substance use disorders) (Meyer 2003). Although the search strategy for papers was not clearly defined in the meta-analysis, the degree of risk approximates other published findings for gay men, in which the odds ratio for any current psychiatric disorder after adjustment for likely confounders was 1.48 (CI=1.09–2.01) (King et al. 2003).

Eating Disorders

Evidence has been accumulating since the early 1980s that gay men may be at particular risk for eating disorders, with prevalence rates approximately three times those of heterosexual men, at least in clinical populations. This finding has been linked to pressures to be slim and physically attractive that are assumed to be greater in gay than heterosexual men (Herzog et al. 1991; Yager et al. 1988). Thus the concern is seen as mirroring women's concerns about weight and shape (Bailey 1999). There is a tendency here to associate "feminine" characteristics with gay men, a concern discussed later in the chapter. Although it seems that gay men have greater concerns about body image than their heterosexual counterparts (Strong et al. 2000), body dissatisfaction and the pursuit of a muscular physique are significant issues for many men (Olivardia et al. 2004; Pope et al. 2000).

The psychopathology of full- and partial-syndrome eating disorders is strikingly similar in men and women (Woodside et al. 2001), but men with anorexia nervosa generally focus more on exercise and muscularity than do women with the disorder. In fact, the body image disturbance characteristic of muscle dysmorphia, seen in men who are compulsive weight trainers, may be associated with anorexia nervosa in men (see Chapter 13, "Body Image and Muscularity"). Recent evidence suggests that the increased prevalence of eating disorders in gay men may have been exaggerated (Hausmann et al. 2004). Unfortunately, the largest study to date of men with eating disorders in nonclinical populations did not inquire about sexual orientation because the topic was considered "too sensitive" (Woodside et al. 2001). Because sexual confusion and fear are common in women with anorexia nervosa, a more parsimonious explanation might be that men or women who are confused and anxious about sexual maturity may be prone to these disorders (Herzog et al. 1984). Given the social ambivalence about homosexuality, this explanation may be particularly applicable to the etiology of eating disorders in gay men.

Mental Health of Older Gay Men

Many early studies of gay men (and lesbians) focused on the concerns of older people. Although some data suggest that older gay men have better psychological well-being than do their younger counterparts (Bennett and Thompson 1980; King et al. 2003; Warner et al. 2003), few studies have directly compared older gay men with similarly aged heterosexual people (Carlson and Steuer 1985; King et al. 2003). Many mental health and social issues impact older gay populations (Van de Ven et al. 1997). Besides concerns that affect all people as they age, such as failing health, death of a partner, and increasing personal care needs, other potential problems that may affect older gay men include the effects of social and legal hostility that they may have experienced in early life. Gay men of retirement age have lived at least part of their lives when male homosexual behavior was illegal in Britain and the United States and "coming out" was far more difficult than it is today. An emphasis in the gay community on youthful attractiveness may also lead to isolation and loneliness. Gay people are less likely to marry and have children and are less likely to live within a mutually supportive long-term relationship (Berger 1980). As a way of compensating for these factors, they may invest more time and effort in work. At retirement, this raison d'être is lost, and gay men may face greater existential anxiety and mental illness than do heterosexual men. This situation may be compounded by lack of support from children and grandchildren.

Deliberate Self-Harm and Suicide

Evidence of sexual orientation as a risk factor for deliberate self-harm and suicide has steadily accumulated since the 1970s. In a study of 1,023 men, of whom 67% were homosexual, Bell and Weinberg (1978) reported an odds ratio of 7.4 (CI=4.1–13.1) for lifetime prevalence of attempted suicide among the homosexual men. In 1989, the *Report of the Secretary's Task Force on Youth Suicide* in the United States noted that gay youth are two to three times more likely to attempt suicide than other young people and that gay youth comprise up to 30% of completed youth suicides annually (Gibson 1989. This report led to considerable public and scientific debate, and subsequent studies have provided mixed evidence in support of the findings.

Much clinical research can be categorized in four main groups: cross-sectional (usually retrospective), prospective, postmortem, and twin-based. Retrospective studies of gay and bisexual men in the United States and United Kingdom indicate that they have higher lifetime rates of deliberate self-harm than do heterosexual men (Cochran and Mays 2000; Gilman et al. 2001; Hershberger and D'Augelli 1995; King et al. 2003; Lock et al. 1999; Mills et al. 2004). Although suicide rates in ethnic minority populations in Western countries have traditionally been stable and lower than in whites, recent evidence indicates that this trend is changing and that sexuality is a factor (O'Donnell et al. 2004). However, cross-sectional studies of people attending emergency departments have not always confirmed that gay men are overrepresented (Buhrich and Loke 1988).

Prospective studies are arguably the most powerful sources of evidence for etiological factors in mental disorders, deliberate self-harm, and suicide, but such studies are expensive, uncommon, and hampered by insufficient numbers of gay and bisexual participants. Three prospective studies of youths have found increased rates of suicidal ideation and attempts in those who reported same-sex attraction or behavior (Fergusson et al. 1999; Skegg et al. 2003; Wichstrom and Hegna 2003). In Skegg et al. (2003), 25% of men had a risk for deliberate self-harm that was attributable to same-sex attraction. In a cohort study in Norway (Wichstrom and Hegna 2003) that lasted more than 7 years, approximately 3,000 adolescents who identified themselves as gay, lesbian, or bisexual reported increased prevalence rates of deliberate self-harm as compared with heterosexual adolescents and had increased precipitating factors of depression, eating disorders, conduct disorders, a greater number of sexual partners, younger age at first same-sex contact, alcohol use, and drug use.

Psychological postmortem studies in which the circumstances of a suicide victim's life are reconstructed through interviews with friends and family rarely consider homosexuality as a risk factor (Cavanagh et al. 2003). In the three that have considered homosexuality, gay men were not overrepresented among those who had committed suicide (Rich et al. 1986; Robins 1981; Shaffer et al. 1995), and risk factors associated with suicide such as drugs and alcohol were found equally in gay and heterosexual suicides (Rich et al. 1986). Coroners' studies, which similarly gather data after the event, also do not find a raised prevalence of gay men among individuals completing suicide, although most studies have been conducted in the context of acquired immunodeficiency syndrome (AIDS) (Ndimbie et al. 1994).

Twin-study methodologies limit likely confounders of differences in mental health status and suicidal thoughts between gay and straight men. Herrell et al. (1999) studied 103 male twin pairs on a twin registry who were born between 1937 and 1959 and who were discordant for sexual orientation. Being homosexual was defined as ever having had a male sexual partner. All had served in the U.S. military. The homosexual twins were 4.1 times (CI=2.1–8.2) more likely to report ideas of suicide and 6.5 times (CI=1.5–28.8) more likely to have attempted to kill themselves. However, the age and military status of these men mean that they would have experienced greater opposition to their homosexuality than is generally seen today, a factor that may have increased the estimates of risk found.

Misuse of Drugs and Alcohol

Adolescent and young adult gay men appear particularly prone to substance abuse and dependence, and such substance use has important consequences for their long-term health. Given the association between substance use disorders and a variety of serious health consequences of which young gay men are at increased risk, including HIV infection and suicide, there is a need for improved prevention and treatment of substance abuse and dependence. Several epidemiological studies report that gay men are more likely than heterosexual men to use recreational drugs (King et al. 2003) and abuse them (e.g., Gilman et al. 2001). Many findings, however, are equivocal (Sandfort et al. 2001). Among gay and bisexual people, lesbian women appear to be at greatest risk (Meyer 2003; Sandfort et al. 2001). Although substance abuse is 1.47 times more common in gay than heterosexual men (Meyer 2003), it is less clear whether gay men are at increased risk for alcohol abuse or dependence. Some large, controlled studies have reported few differences in alcohol use between gay and straight men (Gilman et al. 2001; King et al. 2003; Sandfort et al. 2001), although others have observed increased rates of drinking and dependence (Meyer 2003). Lifetime prevalence of DSM-III-R (American Psychiatric Association 1987) alcohol abuse was higher in heterosexual than in gay men in one Dutch study based on probability sampling (Sandfort et al. 2001).

Rates of tobacco use among gay men exceed those of the general population, ultimately leading to increased rates of tobacco-related disease. Using a household-based sample, Stall et al. (1999) found that two-fifths of gay men smoked tobacco, a higher rate than the 29% reported for men at a national level. Adolescent gay males are more likely to smoke tobacco than are their heterosexual peers, and higher numbers of male sexual partners correlate with higher rates of tobacco use (as well as drug use, victimization, and the use of violence) (DuRant et al. 1998).

REASONS FOR VULNERABILITY TO MENTAL ILLNESS

Stress and Social Exclusion

Homosexuality has been considered shameful and depraved throughout most of human history. Although there were brief times when it was tolerated or regarded as acceptable in certain parts of the world, such as ancient Greece and imperial Rome, these were exceptions. Hostility toward same-sex attraction and behavior became extensive in Europe by the latter half of the twelfth century, reaching a peak in the thirteenth and fourteenth centuries. This situation reflected increasing intolerance in ecclesiastical and secular institutions toward Christian heretics, sorcerers, and Jews, and these sentiments gradually extended to include any divergence from the standards of the majority. This intolerance was incorporated into theological, moral, and legal compilations of the late Middle Ages and influenced European culture for centuries (Boswell 1980). Gay men were subjected to institutionalized prejudice, social exclusion (even within families), and antihomosexual hatred and violence, and they often internalized a sense of shame about their sexuality (King et al. 2003; Meyer 2003).

Risk factors for emotional distress that have been identified are lack of a partner (Mills et al. 2004); social isolation (Diaz et al. 2001; Wichstrom and Hegna 2003); hesitation to identify oneself as gay or bisexual (Mills et al. 2004); verbal or physical violence (Mills et al. 2004); bullying, particularly at school or college (Warner et al. 2004); day-to-day experiences of discrimination (Mays and Cochran 2001); conflict between religious beliefs and sexual orientation (Warner et al. 2004); and chronic stress and low self-esteem arising from membership in a minority sexual group (Diaz et al. 2001; Meyer 2003). Parental rejection of a son because of his sexual orientation generally has a severe emotional impact on a gay man. Internalized homophobia has been identified as a risk factor for substance dependence (Kus 1989), and Davies and Neal (1996) have suggested that substance abuse and dependence among gay men and lesbians may represent a manifestation of internalized homophobia. Homophobic legislation around the world may be an important factor in generating distress, but widespread social prejudice appears to be a greater influence (Bagley and D'Augelli 2000; Mathy 2002). The terms that have evolved to describe people who seek out same-sex love, partnership, and sexual practice embodied historical and social values (Bourdieu 1991), and most, such as "queer" and "dyke," were used to denigrate and devalue. Such terms have recently been reclaimed by a confident gay and lesbian community as its members are more often seen in the public as agents who interact effectively with society, thereby neutralizing such attitudes. However, there is a risk that effective coping can come to be expected of most who are in stressful or adverse social conditions and failure to cope will be regarded as a personal rather than a societal failing (Meyer 2003).

Deviation From Normal Development

Even before Magnus Hirschfeld's celebrated speculations that homosexuality was a form of psychological hermaphroditism, there were claims that it was a deviation from normal development (Hirschfeld 1920). It would seem likely that genetic and environmental influences determine sexual orientation, although there is no consensus on the heritability of male homosexuality (Kirk et al. 2000). Evidence continues to be published claiming physical anomalies in gay men (and lesbians as well) that distinguish homosexual men from heterosexual men (Lindesay 1987; Martin and Nguyen 2004; McCormick et al. 1990). Similar reasoning is used to suggest that if physiological and physical anomalies exist in gay men, developmental defects may also herald neuropsychiatric vulnerability. A related idea on developmental differences is that atypical levels of prenatal androgens lead to homosexuality and that, consequently, gay men have more sex-atypical traits and are less aggressive than are heterosexual men (Bailey 1999). That gay men's levels of neuroticism are similar to those of women is seen as further corroborative evidence. Such theories are often based on uncritical acceptance of sexist stereotypes of personality and behavioral differences between men and women. Although space precludes a full discussion of the evidence for and against biological differences between gay and heterosexual men, considerably more scientific investigation of this topic is needed before such claims can be validated.

Lifestyles

A third explanation for the elevated rates of psychiatric disorders in gay men is that the disorders are a consequence of the men's lifestyles, particularly as related to substance use disorders (Bailey 1999). Commercial venues such as clubs and bars in which gay and bisexual people meet might make it likely for gay men to consume more alcohol than their heterosexual counterparts. However, epidemiological studies often do not support this notion. Consistent with the elevated risk for drug use, abuse, and dependence in gay men, prolonged drug use, whether as a sexual or general stimulant, may make gay men particularly vulnerable to physical (such as sexual infection) and psychological disorders. This vulnerability may diminish in societies that become more accepting of gay men as valued and respected members of society who might meet prospective partners at places of work and in other such settings that are usual for heterosexual men.

HELP SEEKING AND USE OF SERVICES

Despite the gloomy history of gay men's experiences of psychiatry, it appears that they seek help for emotional difficulties more often than do heterosexual men. My research in the United Kingdom (King et al. 2003) has shown that gay men are more likely than heterosexual men to attend their family physicians or psychiatry services for help with emotional problems. The finding that gay men are more likely to have emotional disorders than heterosexual men contributes to this finding, but the evidence also suggests that gay men are prepared to seek help. What sort of help they receive when they seek treatment is another matter.

Disclosure of Sexual Orientation to Health Care Providers

Most of the data regarding gay men's relationships with health care providers have centered on HIV and sexual health. Much less research has examined gay men's consulting behavior for general health and emotional issues. Research in the 1990s suggested that there was often a poor relationship between gay men and their general practitioners (Fitzpatrick et al. 1994), and more recent evidence suggests that the situation has not improved much. Many gay men are reluctant to discuss their sexual orientation with their family doctors and find discussing sexual issues particularly difficult (Elford et al. 2000). Likely contributors to this uneasiness include the history of HIV infection in gay men and the assumptions that are presumed to arise from this history in many doctors' minds. A substantial minority of physicians feel uncomfortable treating gay and bisexual men, and a majority do not ask their patients routinely about sexual orientation (Owen 1996). Disclosure of sexual orientation is essential for the provision of sensitive and effective mental health care. However, research suggests that gay men's experience of antihomosexual bias is potentially as common in making contact with health care services as it is in wider society (Pharr 1988; Wilton 1997, 2000). The elusive but more pervasive heterosexism, or "heteronormativity," can have a substantial impact on the treatment experiences of gay men (Wilton 2000). Many try to hide their gay identity while in contact with mental health services.

Health Care Experiences

The London-based Project for Advice, Counselling and Education and the U.K. charity Mind have both published evidence on difficulties gay men (and lesbians) experience in mental health care (Golding 1997; Project for Advice, Counselling and Education 1998). The difficulties include depreciation of their domestic circumstances, refusal to accept partners as next of kin, excessive curiosity on the part of health staff about gay lives, concern about confidentiality, and fear that gay people's sexuality will be regarded as a pathology requiring attention. In response, a gay and bisexual–affirmative strand of mental health services provision is slowly developing (Davies and Neal 1996). Mental health professionals are increasingly interested in the varying strategies used by gay people to cope with social hostility and in ways to increase the self-esteem and well-being of gay people. These mental health professionals are much less likely to regard homosexuality as a condition requiring attention. However, this process is developing slowly, and gay people continue to hesitate about being open with health professionals (Klitzman and Greenberg 2002; Potter 2002) and recount upsetting and disturbing encounters with mental health professionals who have poor training and conservative mindsets (King and McKeown 2004). There is an urgent need for improved training of doctors in the care of gay and bisexual people (Tesar and Rovi 1998). Data indicate that improvements in students' knowledge and attitudes occur after appropriate small-group training (Dixon-Woods et al. 2002; Wald et al. 2002).

A small number of community and hospital-based services are developing in Western countries specifically for gay and bisexual people with major mental illness. One recent study compared gay and bisexual people accessing such services with heterosexual patients with similar disorders (Hellman et al. 2004). Few differences were found between the two groups in the nature of the disorders or their presentations. However, little was said about disparities in the need for or nature of the care given, and methodological difficulties inherent in such studies limited the conclusions.

Gay Health Care Providers

Sometimes prejudice occurs in the opposite direction, with gay health professionals becoming the targets of discriminatory reactions from patients or from training institutions. Many gay health care providers are unable to be open about the gender of their partners or discuss even the most rudimentary aspects of their private lives for fear of discrimination ("Being a Gay Doctor" 1995; "Being a Gay Medical Student" 1998). The origin of these reactions appears to be emotional rather than arising from fears of infection. People taking part in a Canadian survey reported that they would be "uncomfortable" consulting a doctor whom they knew to be gay but often could not elaborate on what they meant (Druzin et al. 1998). There is also prejudice against acceptance of gay men as trainees in psychoanalysis. Traditional training institutes for psychoanalysis discriminate against openly gay applicants on the grounds that homosexuality is a mental pathology (Bartlett et al. 2001; Friedman and Lilling 1996), although this situation has changed for the better in recent years, particularly in the United States (Isay 1997).

Reparative Therapy

The particular history of homosexuality being viewed as a mental illness continues to influence some aspects of mental health care provision. Reparative therapy, which claims that homosexual people may be made heterosexual, continues to be promoted by psychoanalysts and religiously oriented professionals who hold entrenched views that homosexuality can be cured (Drescher 1998; Haldeman 1994). The word "reparative" reveals the assumption behind such treatments and recalls early psychoanalytic concepts of heterosexuality as the basic template that will arise when the homosexual "perversion" is addressed. Despite one renowned claim for limited efficacy (Spitzer 2003) and the storm of correspondence that followed it ("Peer Commentaries on Spitzer" 2003), there is no evidence that reparative treatments enable men to change their sexual orientation, and it is likely that they promote prejudice against homosexuality and increase suffering for gay men and their families.

PUBLIC HEALTH AND PREVENTION OF MENTAL DISORDERS

Despite the many ethnic, cultural, and age-related differences among them, gay men share experiences of stigma, discrimination, rejection, and violence (Meyer 2001). Thus, public mental health interventions may help address these men's needs and prevent psychological disorders. Many public health initiatives have come from voluntary organizations that have originated in Western countries to provide gay-friendly service to men and their families. Unfortunately, because of the potential for gay men to hide their status, it is challenging to collect the types of routine data that are important for health planning. Government documents, such as *Healthy People 2010* (U.S. Department of Health and Human Services 2000) in the United States and the *National Suicide Prevention Strategy* in England (Department of Health 2004), say little about gay issues, likely because of lack of data. Few countries in the world collect details of sexual orientation during their censuses, usually out of concerns to not invade privacy and to ensure full participation. This situation needs to change if gay people are ever to become fully visible as citizens. It is important to remember, however, that increased interest in the public health of gay men arose out of a concern to protect homosexual men from unsafe sexual practices in the era of AIDS. Thus there is a danger that placing sexual orientation in the public mental health domain might lead to further movements to "normalize" homosexuality and lead consequently to its further medicalization and the entrenchment of negative attitudes (Meyer 2001; Miller 2001).

CONCLUSION

The process by which gay men have achieved a coherent sense of identity over the past century has been hindered by deeply held views in society that homosexuality is a criminal, moral, or mental problem. Furthermore, when parents who find they have a gay son are disappointed or hostile, discrimination strikes the heart of the nuclear family, something rarely seen in other settings. When mental health problems occur in gay men, therefore, feelings of shame and despair from childhood and adolescence may be reawakened and pose a threat to gay men's sense of identity or even their lives. Recent debates about the links between human rights and health highlight the need for the nonjudgmental recognition of sexual orientation (Miller 2001). More data on gay men (and lesbians and bisexual people) are needed to enable effective prevention and treatment of mental disorders and suicide. Methodological approaches should be used to help ensure anonymity when health and general population statistics are collected.

Education and continuing professional development of health and social care providers should cover 1) the relationship between sexuality and mental well-being; 2) how sexuality fits into the wider context of a person's life experiences and mental health; 3) the increased risk of self-harm, suicide, and abuse of recreational drugs by gay men; and 4) how to respond appropriately to gay men in a mental health setting. This training should aim to ensure that gay men receive help from professionals who are sensitive to their lives and needs. In particular, professionals should avoid extremes of regarding same-sex attraction as the underlying cause of psychological difficulties; ignoring sexuality altogether; or displaying excessive curiosity about gay men's lives and domestic circumstances. Health and social care agencies should monitor the particular experiences and satisfaction levels of gay men as consumers of services. Mechanisms for responding appropriately to feedback should be enacted, and successful methods (those achieving high levels of satisfaction) should be communicated to the larger network of health care providers.

KEY POINTS

- Until the late twentieth century, homosexuality was regarded at best as a vice and at worst as a mental illness.

- The historical record of institutionalized discrimination against gay men has had negative consequences on gay men's mental health.

- Gay and bisexual men appear to be at greater risk than heterosexual men for all forms of nonpsychotic mental disorders.

- Gay and bisexual men are at greater risk of self-harm.

- Gay and bisexual men may be reluctant to reveal their sexuality to health care providers for fear of negative reactions or inappropriate care.

- Health service professionals are improving in their attitudes toward and practice with gay men, but many still need greater awareness of the gay lifestyle and its associations with health.

- So-called reparative therapy to change homosexuals to heterosexuals has very little evidence of efficacy and has the potential to cause considerable psychological harm.

PRACTICE GUIDELINES

1. Take account of the relationship between sexual orientation and mental health.

2. Be aware of the increased risk of self-harm and abuse of recreational drugs by gay men.

3. Avoid concluding that same-sex attraction is the underlying cause of psychological difficulties.

4. Do not ignore sexual orientation altogether or be excessively curious about gay men's lives and domestic circumstances.

5. Monitor gay men's experience and satisfaction with mental health care services.

REFERENCES

American Psychiatric Association: Diagnostic and Statistical Manual of Mental Disorders, 2nd Edition. Washington, DC, American Psychiatric Association, 1968

American Psychiatric Association: Diagnostic and Statistical Manual of Mental Disorders, 3rd Edition. Washington, DC, American Psychiatric Association, 1980

American Psychiatric Association: Diagnostic and Statistical Manual of Mental Disorders, 3rd Edition, Revised. Washington, DC, American Psychiatric Association, 1987

Atkinson JH, Grant I, Kennedy CJ, et al: Prevalence of psychiatric disorders among men infected with human immunodeficiency virus. Arch Gen Psychiatry 45:859–864, 1988

Bagley C, D'Augelli AR: Suicidal behaviour in gay, lesbian and bisexual youth. BMJ 320:1617–1618, 2000

Bailey JM: Homosexuality and mental illness. Arch Gen Psychiatry 56:883–884, 1999

Bartlett A, King M, Phillips P: Straight talking: an investigation of the attitudes and practice of psychoanalysts and psychotherapists in relation to gays and lesbians. Br J Psychiatry 179:545–549, 2001

Bayer R: Homosexuality and American Psychiatry: The Politics of Diagnosis. New York, Basic Books, 1981

Being a gay doctor. Student BMJ 3:385–386, 1995

Being a gay medical student. Student BMJ 6:431–432, 1998

Bell A, Weinberg MS: Homosexualities: A Study of Diversity Among Men and Women. New York, Simon & Shuster, 1978

Bennett KC, Thompson NL: Social and psychological functioning of the ageing male homosexual. Br J Psychiatry 137:361–370, 1980

Berger RM: Psychological adaptation of the older homosexual male. J Homosex 5:161–175, 1980

Boswell J: Christianity, Social Tolerance and Homosexuality. Chicago, IL, University of Chicago Press, 1980

Bourdieu P: Language and Symbolic Power. Cambridge, England, Polity Press, 1991

Buhrich N, Loke C: Homosexuality, suicide, and parasuicide in Australia. J Homosex 15:113–129, 1988

Bullough VL: Caelius Aurelianus: on acute diseases and on chronic disease, in Sexual Variance in Society and History. Edited by Bullough VL. New York, Wiley, 1976, pp 143–144

Carlson HM, Steuer J: Age, sex-role categorization, and psychological health in American homosexual and heterosexual men and women. J Soc Psychol 125:203–211, 1985

Cavanagh JTO, Carson AJ, Sharpe M, et al: Psychological post-mortem studies of suicide: a systematic review. Psychol Med 33:395–405, 2003

Cochran SD, Mays VM: Depressive distress among homosexually active African American men and women. Am J Psychiatry 151:524–529, 1994

Cochran SD, Mays V: Lifetime prevalence of suicide symptoms and affective disorders among men reporting same-sex sexual partners: results from NHANES III. Am J Public Health 90:573–578, 2000

Davenport-Hines R: Sex, Death and Punishment: Attitudes to Sex and Sexuality in Britain Since the Renaissance. London, England, Collins, 1990

Davies D, Neal C (eds): Pink Therapy: A Guide for Counsellors and Therapists Working With Lesbian, Gay and Bisexual Clients. Buckingham, England, Open University Press, 1996

Dean L, Meyer IH, Robinson K, et al: Lesbian, gay, bisexual and transgender health: findings and concerns. J Gay Lesbian Med Assoc 4:101–151, 2000

Department of Health: National Suicide Prevention Strategy. London, England, Department of Health, 2004

Diaz RM, Ayala G, Bein E, et al: The impact of homophobia, poverty and racism on the mental health or gay and bisexual Latino men: findings from 3 US cities. Am J Public Health 91:927–932, 2001

Dixon-Woods M, Regan J, Roberston N, et al: Teaching and learning about human sexuality in undergraduate medical education. Med Educ 36:432–440, 2002

Drescher J: I'm your handyman: a history of reparative therapies. J Homosex 36:19–42, 1998

Druzin P, Shrier I, Yacowar M, et al: Discrimination against gay, lesbian and bisexual family physicians by patients. CMAJ 158:593–597, 1998

DuRant R, Krowchuk D, Sinal S: Victimization, use of violence, and drug use at school among male adolescents who engage in same-sex sexual behavior. J Pediatr 133:113–118, 1998

Elford J, Bolding G, Maguire M, et al: Do many men discuss HIV risk reduction with their GP? AIDS Care 12:287–290, 2000

Faulkner AH, Cranston K: Correlates of same-sex sexual behavior in a random sample of Massachusetts high school students. Am J Public Health 88:262–266, 1998

Felski R: The Gender of Modernity. Cambridge, MA, Harvard University Press, 1995

Fergusson DM, Horwood LJ, Beautrais AL: Is sexual orientation related to mental health problems and suicidality in young people? Arch Gen Psychiatry 56:876–880, 1999

Fitzpatrick R, Dawson J, Boulton M, et al: Perceptions of general practice among homosexual men. Br J Gen Pract 44:80–82, 1994

Friedman RC, Lilling AA: An empirical study of the beliefs of psychoanalysts about scientific and clinical dimensions of male homosexuality. J Homosex 32:79–89, 1996

Garofalo R, Wolf RC, Kessel S, et al: The association between health risk behaviors and sexual orientation among a school-based sample of adolescents. Pediatrics 101:895–902, 1998

Gibson P: Gay Male and Lesbian Youth Suicide. U.S. Department of Health and Human Services: Report of the Secretary's Task Force on Youth Suicide. Washington, DC, Government Printing Office, 1989

Gilbert N: Researching Social Life. London, England, Sage, 1993

Gilman SE, Cochran SD, Mays VM, et al: Risk of psychiatric disorders among individuals reporting same-sex sexual partners in the National Comorbidity Survey. Am J Public Health 91:933–939, 2001

Golding J: Without Prejudice: Mind Lesbian, Gay and Bisexual Health Awareness Research. London, England, Mind, 1997

Greene B: Ethnic-minority lesbians and gay men: mental health and treatment issues. J Consult Clin Psychol 62:243–251, 1994

Haldeman DC: The practice and ethics of sexual orientation conversion therapy. J Consult Clin Psychol 62:221–227, 1994

Hausmann A, Mangweth B, Walch T, et al: Body-image dissatisfaction in gay versus heterosexual men: is there really a difference? J Clin Psychiatry 65:1555–1558, 2004

Hellman RE, Sudderth L, Avery AM: Major mental illness in a sexual minority psychiatric sample. J Gay Lesbian Med Assoc 6:97–106, 2004

Herek GM, Gillis JR, Cogan JC: Psychological sequelae of hate-crime victimization among lesbian, gay, and bisexual adults. J Consult Clin Psychol 67: 945–951, 1999

Herrell R, Goldberg J, True WR, et al: Sexual orientation and suicidality: a co-twin control study in adult men. Arch Gen Psychiatry 56:867–874, 1999

Hershberger SL, D'Augelli AR: The impact of victimization on the mental health and suicidality of lesbian, gay, and bisexual youths. Dev Psychol 67:65–74, 1995

Herzog DB, Norman DK, Gordon C, et al: Sexual conflict and eating disorders in 27 males. Am J Psychiatry 141:989–990, 1984

Herzog DB, Norman KL, Warsaw M: Body image dissatisfaction in homosexual males. J Nerv Ment Dis 179:335–347, 1991

Hirschfeld M: Die Homosexualität des Mannes und des Weibes. Berlin, Germany, Louis Marcus Books, 1920

Hooker E: The adjustment of the male overt homosexual. Journal of Prospective Techniques 21:18–31, 1957

Isay R: Becoming Gay: The Journey to Self-Acceptance. New York, Henry Holt, 1997

Johnson AM, Mercer CH, Erens B, et al: Sexual behaviour in Britain: partnerships, practices and HIV risk behaviours. Lancet 358:1835–1842, 2001

Jorm AF, Korten AE, Rodgers B, et al: Sexual orientation and mental health: results from a community survey of young and middle-aged adults. Br J Psychiatry 180:423–427, 2002

Kennedy H: Karl Heinrich Ulrichs: first theorist of homosexuality, in Science and Homosexualities. Edited by Rosario VA. New York, Routledge, 1997, pp 27–45

King M, Bartlett A: British psychiatry and homosexuality. Br J Psychiatry 174: 106–113, 1999

King M, McKeown E: Gay and lesbian identities and mental health, in Identity and Health. Edited by Kelleher D, Leavey G. New York, Routledge, 2004, pp 149–169

King M, McKeown E, Warner J, et al: Mental health and quality of life of gay men and lesbians in England and Wales: a controlled, cross-sectional study. Br J Psychiatry 183:552–558, 2003

King M, Smith G, Bartlett A: Treatments of homosexuality in Britain since the 1950s, an oral history: the experience of professionals. BMJ 328:429–432, 2004

Kinsey AC, Pomeroy WB, Martin CE: Sexual Behavior in the Human Male. Philadelphia, PA, WB Saunders, 1948

Kirby M: The 1973 deletion of homosexuality as a psychiatric disorder: 30 years on. Aust N Z J Psychiatry 37:674–677, 2003

Kirk KM, Bailey JM, Dunne MP, et al: Measurement models for sexual orientation in a community twin study. Behav Genet 30:345–356, 2000

Klitzman RL, Greenberg JD: Patterns of communication between gay and lesbian patients and their health care providers. J Homosex 42:65–75, 2002

Kus RJ: Alcoholism and non-acceptance of gay self: the critical link. J Homosex 15:25–41, 1989

Lemert EM: Social Pathology. New York, McGraw-Hill, 1951

Lindesay J: Laterality shift in homosexual men. Neuropsychologia 25:965–969, 1987

Lock J, Steiner H: Gay, lesbian, and bisexual youth risks for emotional, physical, and social problems: results from a community-based survey. J Am Acad Child Adolesc Psychiatry 38:297–304, 1999

Martin JT, Nguyen DH: Anthropometric analysis of homosexuals and hetero-sexuals: implications for early hormone exposure. Horm Behav 45:31–39, 2004

Mathy RM: Homosexual legislation does not reduce suicidal intent in sexual minority groups (letter). BMJ 325:1176, 2002

Mays VM, Cochran SD: Mental health correlates of perceived discrimination among lesbian, gay and bisexual adults in the United States. Am J Public Health 91:1869–1876, 2001

McConaghy N, Blaszczynski A: Initial stages of validation by penile volume as-sessment that sexual orientation is distributed dimensionally. Compr Psy-chiatry 32:52–58, 1991

McCormick CM, Witelson SF, Kingstone E: Left-handedness in homosexual men and women: neuroendocrine implications. Psychoneuroendocrinol-ogy 15:69–76, 1990

McWhirter DP, Sanders SA, Reinisch JM: Homosexuality/Heterosexuality. New York, Oxford University Press, 1990

Mendelson G: Homosexuality and psychiatric nosology. Aust N Z J Psychiatry 37:678–683, 2003

Meyer IH: Why lesbian, gay, bisexual, and transgender public health? Am J Public Health 91:856–859, 2001

Meyer IH: Prejudice, social stress and mental health in lesbian, gay and bisexual populations: conceptual issues and research evidence. Psychol Bull 129: 674–697, 2003

Michaels S: The prevalence of homosexuality in the United States, in Textbook of Homosexuality and Mental Health. Edited by Cabaj RP, Stein TS. Wash-ington, DC, American Psychiatric Press, 1996, pp 43–63

Miller AM: Uneasy promises: sexuality, health and human rights. Am J Public Health 91:861–864, 2001

Mills TC, Stall R, Pollack L, et al: Health-related characteristics of men who have sex with men: a comparison of those living in "gay ghettos" with those liv-ing elsewhere. Am J Public Health 91:980–983, 2001

Mills TC, Paul J, Stall R, et al: Distress and depression in men who have sex with men: the Urban Men's Health Study. Am J Psychiatry 161:278–285, 2004

Ndimbie OK, Perper JA, Kingsley L, et al: Sudden unexpected death in a male homosexual cohort. Am J Forensic Med Pathol 15:247–250, 1994

O'Donnell L, O'Donnell C, Wardlaw DM, et al: Risk and resiliency factors influ-encing suicidality among urban African American and Latino youth. Am J Community Psychol 33:37–49, 2004

Olivardia R, Pope HG Jr, Borowiecki JJ, et al: Biceps and body image: the rela-tionship between muscularity and self-esteem, depression and eating dis-order symptoms. Psychology of Men and Masculinity 5:112–120, 2004

Owen WF Jr: Gay and bisexual men and medical care, in Textbook of Homosex-uality and Mental Health. Edited by Cabaj RP, Stein TS. Washington, DC, American Psychiatric Press, 1996, pp 673–685

Peer commentaries on Spitzer. Arch Sex Behav 32:419–468, 2003

Pharr S: Homophobia: A Weapon of Sexism. Inverness, CA, Chardon Press, 1988

Pillard RC: Sexual orientation and mental disorder. Psychiatr Ann 18:52–56, 1998

Pope HG Jr, Phillips KA, Olivardia R: The Adonis Complex: The Secret Crisis of Male Body Obsession. New York, Free Press, 2000

Potter J: Do ask, do tell. Ann Intern Med 137:341–343, 2002

Project for Advice, Counselling and Education: Diagnosis: Homophobic. The Experiences of Lesbians, Gay Men and Bisexuals in Mental Health Services. London, England, Project for Advice, Counselling and Education, 1998

Rich CL, Fowler RC, Young D, et al: San Diego Suicide Study: comparison of gay to straight males. Suicide Life Threat Behav 16:448–457, 1986

Robins E: The Final Months: A Study of the Lives of 134 Persons Who Committed Suicide. New York, Oxford University Press, 1981

Sandfort TGM, de Graaf R, Bijl R, et al: Same-sex sexual behavior and psychiatric disorders: findings from the Netherlands Mental Health Survey and Incidence Study (NEMESIS). Arch Gen Psychiatry 58:85–91, 2001

Sell RL, Wells JA, Wypij D: The prevalence of homosexual behavior and attraction in the United States, the United Kingdom and France: results of national population-based samples. Arch Sex Behav 24:235–248, 1995

Shaffer D, Fisher P, Hicks MP, et al: Sexual orientation in adolescents who commit suicide. Suicide Life Threat Behav 25:64–71, 1995

Sharp D: Telling the truth about sex. Lancet 359:1084, 2002

Skegg K, Nada-Raja S, Dickson N, et al: Sexual orientation and self-harm in men and women. Am J Psychiatry 160:541–546, 2003

Smith G, Bartlett A, King M: Treatments of homosexuality in Britain since the 1950s, an oral history: the experience of patients. BMJ 328:427–429, 2004

Spitzer RL: Can some gay men and lesbians change their sexual orientation? 200 participants reporting a change from homosexual to heterosexual orientation. Arch Sex Behav 32:403–417, 2003

Stall RD, Greenwood GL, Acree M, et al: Cigarette smoking among gay and bisexual men. Am J Public Health 89:1875–1878, 1999

Strong SM, Williamson DA, Netemeyer RG, et al: Eating disorder symptoms and concerns about body differ as a function of gender and sexual orientation. J Soc Clin Psychol 19:240–255, 2000

Tesar CM, Rovi SL: Survey of curriculum on homosexuality/bisexuality in departments of family medicine. Fam Med 30:283–287, 1998

Tross S, Hirsch D, Rabkin B, et al: Determinants of current psychiatric disorders in AIDS spectrum patients, in Programs and Abstracts of the Third International Conference on AIDS, Washington, DC, June 1987

U.S. Department of Health and Human Services: Healthy People 2010, Vols 1 and 2, 2nd Edition. Washington, DC, U.S. Department of Health and Human Services, 2000

Van de Ven P, Rodden P, Crawford J, et al: A comparative demographic and sexual profile of older homosexually active men. J Sex Res 34:349–360, 1997

Wald KD, Rienzo BA, Button JW: Sexual orientation and education politics: gay and lesbian representation in American schools. J Homosex 42:145–168, 2002

Warner JP, Wright L, Blanchard M, et al: The psychological health and quality of life of older lesbians and gay men: a snowball sampling pilot survey. Int J Geriatr Psychiatry 18:754–755, 2003

Warner J, McKeown E, Griffin M, et al: Rates and predictors of mental illness in gay men: results from a survey based in England and Wales. Br J Psychiatry 185:479–485, 2004

Weeks J: Sex, Politics and Society: The Regulation of Sexuality Since 1800. London, England, Longman, 1989

Weeks J: Coming Out: Homosexual Politics in Britain From the Nineteenth Century to the Present. London, England, Quartet Books, 1990

Wichstrom L, Hegna K: Sexual orientation and suicide attempt: a longitudinal study of the general Norwegian adolescent population. J Abnorm Psychol 112:144–151, 2003

Williams J, Rabkin J, Remien R, et al: Multidisciplinary baseline assessment of homosexual men with or without human immunodeficiency virus infection, II: standardized clinical assessment of current and lifetime psychopathology. Arch Gen Psychiatry 48:124–130, 1991

Wilton T: Good for You: A Handbook to Lesbian Health and Wellbeing. New York, Continuum International Publishing Group, 1997

Wilton T: Sexualities in Health and Social Care: A Textbook. Buckingham, England, Open University Press, 2000

Woodside DB, Garfinkel PE, Lin E, et al: Comparisons of men with full or partial eating disorders, men without eating disorders, and women with eating disorders in the community. Am J Psychiatry 158:570–574, 2001

World Health Organization: The ICD-10 Classification of Mental and Behavioural Disorders. Geneva, Switzerland, World Health Organization, 1992

World Health Organization: Pocket Guide to the ICD-10 Classification of Mental and Behavioural Disorders. Geneva, Switzerland, World Health Organization, 1994

Yager J, Kurtzman F, Landsverk J, et al: Behaviors and attitudes related to eating disorders in homosexual male college students. Am J Psychiatry 145:495–497, 1988

OVERCOMING STIGMA AND BARRIERS TO MENTAL HEALTH TREATMENT

DEBORAH A. PERLICK, PH.D.
LAUREN N. MANNING, B.A.

Case Vignette

Theodore, a successful investment banker, husband, and father, began experiencing pronounced insomnia in his mid-40s. Unaware of any psychological stressors or emotional difficulties that might help explain this problem, he sought help from his primary care physician for what he viewed as a medical problem. When his physical examination failed to reveal an organic basis for his problem, he accepted a referral to a female psychiatric social worker for treatment of psychogenic insomnia.

From the outset, Theodore had difficulty allowing the therapist to set basic treatment parameters, such as the frequency of sessions and billing procedures; he demanded to be seen four times a week and insisted on paying in cash. In sessions, he related his daily activities without disclosing any emotions, even when discussing arguments with his wife. If problems arose in the marriage, he questioned his commitment

We would like to thank Robert A. Rosenheck, M.D., and Brett Silverstein, Ph.D., for their conceptual and editorial comments and contributions to this chapter.

to the relationship with his wife. He seemed unable either to examine his own feelings or to empathize with those of his wife.

As therapy progressed and Theodore became invested in treatment, he engaged in games of one-upmanship. For example, he would spend several hours reading Freud before sessions and then interpret his own behavior to the therapist. He began remembering and reporting dreams, which he found unsettling. After the therapist returned from a trip with a suntan, he reported a dream of naked girls windsurfing in Hawaii and discontinued treatment shortly thereafter.

Large, population-based surveys and more intensive studies of specific groups such as college students have almost universally demonstrated that men are less likely than women to seek professional help with mental health providers for their emotional problems. Men are therefore at risk not only for continued experience of symptoms of psychological distress but also for physical health problems associated with continued stress and specific, treatable mental disorders such as depression (Cochran 2001; Cochran and Rabinowitz 2000).

This chapter reviews mental health treatment–seeking behaviors of men versus women and discusses potential explanations for underutilization of mental health services by men experiencing psychological distress. Our approach is guided by current theories of stigma toward mental illness and the role of mental illness stigma as a barrier to treatment seeking (e.g., Corrigan 2004; Perlick 2001) and by theoretical perspectives on masculine gender-role socialization and help seeking (e.g., Addis and Mahalik 2003). Integrating these two perspectives within the general framework of stress and coping theory (Lazarus 1991; Lazarus and Folkman 1991), we hypothesize a model to describe men's coping with symptoms of psychological distress through their seeking of professional mental health treatment. After reviewing gender differences in mental health help–seeking, we describe our overall model and review the literature on the major constructs and relationships within the model that are needed to understand male behavior regarding help seeking as well as the consequences of this behavior. Next, we discuss how issues serving as barriers to initiating treatment also appear to influence men's experience of the treatment process and willingness to continue in treatment. Finally, we discuss potential solutions to overcoming barriers to male treatment participation.

EVIDENCE FOR MALE UNDERUTILIZATION OF MENTAL HEALTH SERVICES

Large epidemiological investigations such as the Epidemiologic Catchment Area study and the National Comorbidity Survey show that fewer than half of those individuals with mental disorders receive professional help for their symptoms (Kessler et al. 1994; Millman 2001; Regier et al. 1993). Although underutilization thus represents a problem for both men and women, gender-focused analyses of these studies have consistently demonstrated that men are less likely than women to seek help for mental health problems (Kessler et al. 1981; Leaf and Bruce 1987; Leaf et al. 1988; Lin et al. 1996; Rhodes et al. 2002). For example, Lin et al. (1996) found that 9.7% of women interviewed in the Ontario Health Survey sought help with mental health practitioners for psychiatric problems during the past year, as compared with only 5.8% of men who sought such help. The gender difference in this sample remained significant after controlling for type of mental disorder and socioeconomic factors (Rhodes et al. 2002). Similarly, Kessler et al. (1981) examined gender differences in psychiatric help–seeking from four epidemiological surveys and concluded that women consistently sought professional help at a higher rate than men with comparable emotional problems.

Smaller, nonepidemiological studies of college or medical students (Leong and Zachar 1999; O'Neil et al. 1995), university employees (Carpenter and Addis 2000), and adolescents (Boldero and Fallon 1995) have also found that men are less likely to seek psychiatric help for emotional problems. Additional studies conducted in more ethnically and socioeconomically diverse samples found that male Latino students and American Indians were less likely than their female counterparts to seek mental health treatment (Robin et al. 1997; Stanton-Salazar et al. 2001) and that Italian American and Greek American men and male Taiwanese college students had less positive attitudes toward psychological treatment than their female counterparts (Ponterotto et al. 2001; Yeh 2002). Although there is some evidence that men may be equally or more likely than women to be referred to more restrictive or specialized forms of treatment such as inpatient mental health or substance abuse programs (e.g., Schober and Annis 1996) or may use mental health services more than women in economically disadvantaged settings (e.g., Albizu-Garcia et al. 2001), the evidence overall indicates that men are far less disposed to seek mental health treatment for emotional problems than women. Despite the consistency of the findings, there has been relatively little empirical examination of reasons for male underutilization of mental health services. Although a coherent body of research examining gender differences in psychiatric help–seeking attitudes has emerged, there is a lack of studies examining reasons for gender differences in actual use of services.

MODEL OF MASCULINE APPRAISAL AND COPING WITH PERSONAL PSYCHOLOGICAL PROBLEMS

Figure 17–1 presents our hypothesized model of male mental health help–seeking behavior. Our model is based on the stress and coping approach outlined by Lazarus (1991), which posits that coping is a process that is influenced both by the individual's assessment of the severity of the threat or stressor (primary appraisal) and by the individual's own evaluation of his or her ability to manage the threat (secondary appraisal). In our model, a *threat* is defined as a life stress or personal problem (e.g., job loss, divorce) sufficiently serious to cause psychological distress using objective standards (e.g., life stress ratings). *Primary appraisal* is defined as the individual's recognition of the problem as a threat to his well-being beyond those posed by his daily routine. *Secondary appraisal* is defined as the individual's acknowledgment that he does not possess sufficient or appropriate resources to enable self-resolution of the problem. As a corollary, secondary appraisal also includes acknowledgment that seeking outside help is desirable or necessary. In our model, *coping* is dichotomized into seeking (or not seeking) help from a mental health professional or making an initial visit but discontinuing treatment after just one or two sessions. The *treatment process* is viewed as influenced by client characteristics and interpersonal (i.e., transference-countertransference) issues relating to male gender-role socialization and includes strategies for optimizing the value of treatment. Outcome is either positive (i.e., improved symptom management) or negative (i.e., continued stress as well as psychological distress or depression due to conflict over help seeking related to gender-role concerns).

It is hypothesized that two sets of culturally embedded beliefs and values—*masculine ideology* and *mental illness stigma*—influence men's stress and coping processes by affecting their primary and secondary appraisal. Drawing on both the clinical theoretical literature and empirical studies of help-seeking attitudes, we later describe the potential influences of these beliefs on male mental health service use. Although our model views male gender-role socialization and mental illness stigma as separate constructs influencing appraisal of need for treatment, our model is consistent with the contention of Mahalik et al. (2003) that men experience a gender-specific stigma against help seeking.

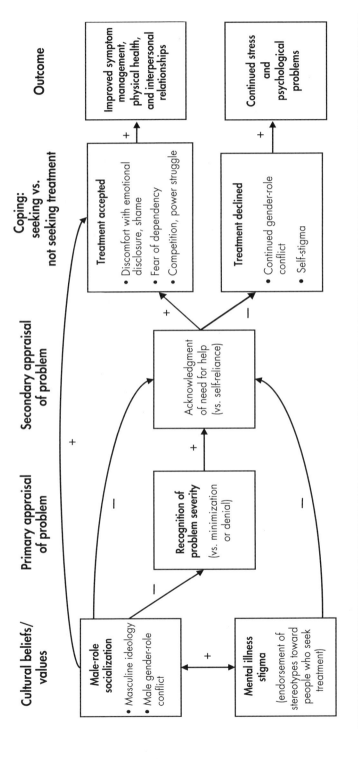

FIGURE 17–1. Hypothesized model of the influence of mental illness stigma and male-role socialization on men's appraisal of serious personal stress/problems and treatment-seeking behavior.

MALE-ROLE SOCIALIZATION, PROBLEM RECOGNITION, AND ACKNOWLEDGMENT OF NEED FOR HELP

Research and theory on help seeking have identified male-role social-ization and socially proscribed male gender roles as barriers to help seeking among men (Addis and Mahalik 2003; Blazina and Marks 2001; Blazina and Watkins 1996; Bursley 1996; Good and Wood 1995; Good et al. 1989, 1995; Leong and Zachar 1999; Mahalik 1999; Mahalik et al. 2003; O'Neil 1982; O'Neil et al. 1995; Robertson and Fitzgerald 1992; Timlin-Scalera et al. 2003; Wisch et al. 1995). Men identifying with tra-ditional views of masculinity are generally reluctant to ask for help of any kind. According to Good et al. (1990),

> Men are prohibited from "giving voice" to that which is perceived as "unmasculine," such as fears, vulnerabilities, and insecurities. Thus, for many men, normal life reactions are denied expression and perhaps eventually even blocked from self-awareness. Hence, at the very thought of seeking counseling, conceptions of gender may have a notable impact. (p. 379)

Gender roles represent socially constructed values, norms, and cog-nitive schemata for role-appropriate behavior of men versus women that are internalized through social reinforcement from early childhood (Bem 1981; Chodorow 1978; Gilligan 1982; Silverstein and Perlick 1995). Our model of male treatment-seeking behavior hypothesizes that tradi-tional male-role socialization and male gender roles serve as barriers to help seeking for men in distress, by affecting both primary and second-ary appraisal (see Figure 17–1). Support for our model of the effects of gender-role socialization on treatment seeking comes from three schools of research and theory: psychoanalytic theory, feminist theory, and so-cial-psychological research on gender roles and help seeking.

Psychoanalytic and Feminist Views

The classic psychoanalytic perspective posits that as part of the healthy resolution of the Oedipus conflict, the young boy must separate or "dis-identify" from his mother in order to move closer to the father and to cre-ate a more secure male gender identity (Greenson 1968) that condones aggression but decries other forms of emotional expression as weak and "feminine." A more relational psychoanalytic perspective (e.g., Pollack 2001, 2003) views such early societally prescribed separations as a "trau-matic disruption of the early holding environment" rather than as part of the sequence of normal development. In either case, the impact of this normative shift and concomitant loss of emotional connection often leads in late adolescence and adulthood to what Pollack (2001) terms a "normative false self-development" characterized by

> (1) partial affective-intellectual split; (2) anger prominence, rage, or repression personality; (3) walling off of vulnerable core self: "mask of masculinity"; (4) phobic avoidance or denial of interdependent object relations: sexualized self-object yearnings; (5) shame sensitive or shame phobic; (6) action blunting of empathic recognition; (7) incapacity to translate feelings into language: alexithymia; (8) harsh unconscious self-criticism, sometimes projected onto others; (9) perfectionistic need to master; (10) inability to grieve or mourn; and (11) vulnerability to substance abuse and depression (male type). (p. 530)

Like the psychoanalytic view, the feminist perspective emphasizes gender differences in early childhood development. Based on clinical experience, Chodorow (1978) concluded that whereas girls were experienced by the mother as like her and tended to remain in this primary relationship, sons were experienced as different and were pushed out (or pushed themselves out), with a resulting loss of empathy with the mother, identification with a distant father, and internalization of the masculine societal values of independence and emotional detachment. In a similar vein, based on her research on moral development, Gilligan (1982) argued that women see themselves and the world in terms of connectedness and are threatened by isolation, whereas men see the world in terms of autonomy and are threatened by intimacy.

Whereas psychoanalytic theories of male-role socialization suggest that men are less likely both 1) to recognize their emotional problems as a result of being socialized to mask their emotions (primary appraisal) and 2) to acknowledge their need for help as a result of their need to control or master their shame and sensitivity (secondary appraisal), feminist theories relate more exclusively to problems in acknowledging the need for help as a result of the need for independence (secondary appraisal).

Social Psychological Theory and Research

Social psychological research on gender roles and help seeking has emphasized the self-evaluative aspects of gender-role socialization and the adverse effects of trying to live up to socially prescribed masculine gender ideals. O'Neil (1981, 1982) coined the term *masculine mystique* to summarize the societal expectations of the male gender role: 1) the expression of emotions or feelings is a sign of vulnerability and weakness in men; 2) seeking help indicates weakness, vulnerability, and/or incompetence in men; and 3) any interpersonal relationships that elicit or cultivate emotions, feelings, or physical contact are inherently feminine and best avoided by men.

Pleck and colleagues (Pleck et al. 1993; Thompson and Pleck 1986) developed the construct of masculine ideology to operationalize and measure the degree to which a person has internalized the societal expectations of the male gender role. According to Pleck, internalization of masculine ideology results in gender-role strain or conflict because stereotyped societal norms around gender ideals are often contradictory, inconsistent, and unattainable. Symptoms of gender-role conflict include depression and anxiety (Cournoyer and Mahalik 1995; Good and Mintz 1990; Sharpe and Heppner 1991). Paradoxically, men who have high degrees of male gender-role conflict may face a "double jeopardy"—they are more likely to be depressed but less likely to seek help (Good and Wood 1995).

MASCULINE IDEOLOGY

Primary Appraisal: Recognition of Problem Severity

Masculine ideology and male gender-role conflict influence treatment seeking through primary appraisal because this process relies on the individual's ability to assess the severity of the stressful situation or problem, which requires making affective and cognitive judgments (Lazarus 1991, pp. 144–145). Because male ideology labels the expression of feelings as a sign of vulnerability, men have been socialized to avoid experiencing feelings and may have genuine difficulty in identifying their affective response to a stressor in order to estimate its severity (Good et al. 1990; Heppner and Gonzalez 1987).

Such a lack of emotional awareness is thought to be so pervasive among men that some theorists have adopted the term *normative alexithymia* to describe it. *Alexithymia* is defined as the inability to recognize and verbally express feelings (Levant 2001). Levant (2001), who described normative alexithymia as a common occurrence of emotional rigidity among men that develops as a result of male-role socialization, argued that this emotional incapacity prevents men from recognizing their problems. In support of this theory, empirical studies have demonstrated that normative alexithymia—or emotional restrictedness—is positively associated with measures of male gender-role conflict and masculine ideology (A.R. Fischer and Good 1997; Levant et al. 2003). Measures of gender-role conflict have been negatively and significantly associated with an attitudinal measure of recognition of personal need for professional help (Good and Wood 1995). Consistent with findings from correlational studies based on self-report measures, Timlin-Scalera et al. (2003) concluded based on interviews with high school males that "many appeared to lack insight into their own problems and need for services" (p. 347).

Results of a study correlating college students' reports of depressive and physical symptoms with subsequent use of mental health services suggest that men are particularly prone to overlook physical manifestations of emotional distress (O'Neil et al. 1995). Although this study found no gender differences in the prevalence of depressive symptoms or in the association between depressive symptoms and service use, there was a differential association by gender for physical symptoms of distress: two physical symptoms of distress (difficulty in breathing and chest pain) were positively related to service use among females but not among males. Finally, Kessler et al. (1981) analyzed data from four large-scale epidemiological surveys, demonstrating that although higher levels of depressive symptoms were significantly related to perceptions of having a problem for both genders, the link between morbidity and recognition was weaker for men than for women. For example, within the top decile of the Center for Epidemiologic Studies Depression Scale scores in one study, 46% of men versus 65% of females translated their distress into problem recognition. Thus, convergent sources of information—data from social-psychological, interview, and epidemiological studies—are consistent with psychoanalytic and feminist theoretical perspectives that men have greater difficulty in recognizing signs of emotional distress than women.

Secondary Appraisal: Acknowledgment of Need for Help

Male-role socialization influences treatment seeking through secondary appraisal, conceptualized as the acknowledgment of need for help, because male ideology places a premium on self-reliance, and the inability to solve one's own problems is viewed as a sign of weakness (Mahalik 1999; O'Neil 1981, 1982; Pollack 2001, 2003). This view is consistent with observations that although some men make independent decisions to seek therapy, many more are "urged, coaxed, or mandated" into treatment by their family, employers, physicians, or legal authorities (Brooks and Good 2001) and that those males who do request therapy are often in more serious difficulty than comparable females (Kirschner 1978; Rice 1969).

Empirical support for the hypothesis that male-role socialization serves as a barrier to acknowledgment of need for help comes from studies evaluating the association between negative attitudes toward help seeking and traditional masculine values, using the Attitudes Toward Seeking Professional Psychological Help Scale (E.H. Fischer and Turner 1970). This scale is composed of four factors: 1) recognition of personal need for professional psychological help, 2) tolerance of stigma associated with psychological help, 3) interpersonal openness regarding one's problems, and 4) confidence in the mental health profession. Studies using this scale have consistently found that men who experience high gender-role conflict or who strongly identify with masculine ideology exhibit significantly more negative attitudes toward help seeking than do women (Johnson 1988; Komiya et al. 2000; Leong and Zachar 1999; Robertson and Fitzgerald 1992) and other men who have lower male gender-role conflict (Blazina and Marks 2001; Blazina and Watkins 1996; Good and Wood 1995; Good et al. 1989; Wisch et al. 1995).

MENTAL ILLNESS STIGMA

A variety of negative characteristics, including violence, childishness, and incompetence, have been ascribed to people who are mentally ill (Corrigan 2004; Corrigan and Watson 2002; Farina 1998; Gabbard and Gabbard 1992; Hyler et al. 1991; Link and Phelan 1999; Mayer and Barry 1992; Monahan 1992; Wahl 1995). Studies have found that employers (Bordieri and Drehmer 1986; Farina and Felner 1973; Link 1987; Olshansky et al. 1960), families of patients (Lefley 1992; Wahl and Harman 1989), mental health workers (Keane 1990; Lyons and Ziviani 1995; Mirabi et al. 1985; Page 1980; Scott and Philip 1985), and prospective landlords (Page 1977, 1983, 1995) all endorsed devaluing statements about or discriminated against mentally ill individuals. Link et al. (1987, 1989) argued that because people with mental illness internalize the devaluing or discriminatory attitudes of society at large, they anticipate discrimination or rejection by others and develop coping strategies, such as secrecy about their illness, to avoid the rejection they anticipate.

Seeking treatment for an emotional problem identifies the seeker as a member of the group of the mentally ill and thereby exposes the individual to potential social rejection and feelings of low self-esteem associated with acknowledging an inability to manage the problem on his or her own (Deane and Chamberlain 1994; Komiya et al. 2000; Scher 1979). In support of concerns about social rejection, one study demonstrated that college students who believed their conversational partners were seeking psychological therapy formed more negative impressions than those students who did not hold such beliefs about their partners

(Sibicky and Dovidio 1986). Therefore, we hypothesize that to avoid the experience of low self-esteem or anticipated social rejection, men are less likely to acknowledge their own need for help if they themselves endorse negative stereotypes toward people who have emotional problems or seek treatment for these problems (see Figure 17–1). Supporting this hypothesis, Cooper et al. (2003) found that members of the general public were less likely to seek care themselves if they blamed mentally ill individuals for their conditions and withheld help to them. These investigators also reported that scores on a dimension of stigma assessing social avoidance of people with mental illness were negatively associated with help seeking on the Attitudes Toward Seeking Professional Psychological Help scale. Conversely, Good and Wood (1995) found that tolerance for stigma was significantly and positively associated with acknowledgment of the need for help assessed on the same scale, and Sirey et al. (2001) found an inverse relationship between stigmatizing attitudes and adherence with antidepressant medication. These findings are consistent with results from the Epidemiologic Catchment Area study that endorsement of negative attitudes about mental illness predicted low service utilization among respondents at risk for psychiatric disorder (Leaf et al. 1988).

PROBLEM APPRAISAL AND THE DECISION TO SEEK HELP

As discussed earlier, masculine ideology, gender-role conflict, and mental illness stigma influence the male appraisal of the severity of emotional problems and acknowledgment of the importance of seeking professional help. In making a decision whether to make an appointment with a mental health professional, an individual balances the degree of distress against the proscriptions for help seeking. Kushner and Sher (1991) discussed the decision to seek help as determined by the resolution of an approach-or-avoidance conflict, in which the approach aspects include the degree of mental distress and pressure or encouragement from others and the avoidance aspects include fear of stigma and degree of endorsement of male ideologies around self-reliance. Researchers have noted that due to male-role proscriptions that devalue help seeking, men who elect to enter treatment for emotional problems are generally more distressed (e.g., Kirschner 1978; Rice 1969).

Another aspect of the decision-making process is the degree of perceived benefits. Although this aspect of help-seeking behavior in men has received relatively little attention to date, Blazina and Marks (2001) reported that among male patients with highly conflicted gender roles, those patients who had had a previous mental health treatment experience had fewer negative attitudes toward therapy than did their counterparts without such experience, possibly because these patients had experienced a previous reduction in symptoms and therefore had a higher expectation of positive results. Additional variables, including personality and situation, might also help determine how the conflict is resolved between masculine ideologies regarding help seeking and need for relief from personal distress. Addis and Mahalik (2003) suggested that the decision for men to seek help in specific help-seeking contexts is moderated by several basic social-psychological processes, including perceptions of the normativeness and ego-centrality of the problem, the characteristics of potential helpers and of the men's social groups, and perceived loss of control.

THE TREATMENT PROCESS

General Treatment Issues

Even after deciding to seek treatment, the male patient—and therefore the treatment process—continues to be influenced by the same gender-role proscriptions and stigma concerns about help seeking. As Scher et al. (1987) pointed out,

> Men are restrained and constrained because of the male role. The expectations of that role cause men to be emotionally flat or repressed, imbued with a competitive spirit, fearful of intimacy, untutored in emotional responsiveness....Therapists working with men must be aware of these qualities and understand their effect on therapy, be patient, and respect the integrity of their clients. (p. 29)

In fact, feelings of weakness for relying on others and fear of dependency may be exacerbated by adopting the patient role (Parsons 1951), which inherently places the therapist in the superior position as the one who is more knowledgeable regarding the areas or problems for which the patient is seeking help. Because the decision to enter treatment is frequently conflicted for men, shortly after entering treatment the male patient may experience a period of what social cognitive scientists refer to as *postdecision dissonance* or *postdecisional regret* (Brehm 1956; Festinger 1957, 1964), a time in which the male patient's initial concerns and reservations are acutely reexperienced. Such concerns can be conceptualized as treatment resistances and need to be addressed by the therapist. Addressing treatment resistances is an initial task in psychotherapy (e.g., Freud 1916/1959) because unacknowledged treatment resistances can either lead to premature termination or diminish the patient's ability to benefit from treatment. A growing group of clinical researchers studying masculine ideology and treatment have recommended various treatment strategies to address these resistances, described in "Solutions to Treatment Barriers" later in this chapter.

Treatment Resistances

Researchers and clinicians addressing the impact of masculine ideology and gender-role conflict on the process of psychotherapy have identified three interrelated barriers or resistances to therapy relating to male-role socialization and expectations: 1) discomfort with emotional expression or self-disclosure, 2) fear of dependency or vulnerability, and 3) need to maintain control and power (see Figure 17–1). The behavior of men entering treatment may not reflect "resistance" or "evidence that the client…does not want to address his problems" so much as a "mismatch between the relational style of the client and the norms of the counseling setting" (p. 45), leading the traditional male to feel uncomfortable (Kiselica 2001). Although we appreciate this cautionary note, the term *resistance* need not imply a lack of cooperation on the part of the patient, and we use it here to refer to a diverse group of issues that pose potential threats to the integrity and potential gains from treatment. Both patient and therapist should address any treatment resistances for successful achievement of therapeutic goals.

Although some theorists (i.e., Mahalik 1999; Mahalik et al. 2003) have delineated several different masculine "scripts" to encompass the stereotypical gender-role behaviors that men enact in and out of treatment, the three types of resistance described earlier are often closely interrelated in practice. To the extent that men are socialized to value strength, self-sufficiency, and control of their interpersonal and emotional lives, both 1) the situational "demands" of traditional psychotherapy of openness to internal experience and expression of emotions and 2) the normative feelings of respect, positive regard, and even dependency that develop toward the therapist over time (i.e., the positive transference) constitute a threat to the maintenance of the masculine ideal.

Along these lines, Pollack (2001, 2003) has articulated a syndrome of *defensive autonomy* to describe the valued yet intrinsically false sense of self-sufficiency that men bring to the treatment setting. According to his relational perspective, defensive autonomy is an effort to block the overt expression of all strong, positive feelings in order to protect against the buried grief and mourning experienced in relation to the socially mandated disidentification with the mother (Chodorow 1978; Greenson 1968) that occurs in early childhood. Pollack (2003) viewed this disidentification as a premature push for separation that results in a loss of emotional connection and an evocation of feelings of shame when the masked feelings of loss and vulnerability begin to surface in the course of therapy, either in connection with a relationship in the individual's life or in relation to the transference. As Pollack (2003) noted,

> In psychotherapy we see many male adolescents who are frightened about some aspect of their developing life they cannot master. These boys are most afraid of the very fact that they are afraid. They have been brought up to believe that a man must not seek help at a time when he needs it most, and so they deny being dependent upon the therapy or the therapist. (p. 1207)

Other writers have also emphasized as barriers or resistances to effective psychotherapy both the difficulties male patients experience in identifying and expressing their affective reactions and the feelings of shame and embarrassment that emerge when they do (e.g., Heppner and Gonzales 1987; Mahalik et al. 2003; Sher 1979). Heppner and Gonzales (1987) noted that it can be "doubly embarrassing" for the male patient to reveal his perceived inadequacies to another man. One 55-year-old Hispanic man who was referred by his urologist to a female psychologist for treatment of psychogenic erectile dysfunction stated that he would never be able to discuss this difficulty with a male therapist, especially with a male psychiatrist. Despite the presence of depressive features that suggested the utility of a psychopharmacology consultation, he resisted this recommendation for close to 2 years because it represented to him further painful acknowledgment of the severity of his difficulties. Only after sufficient remission of his self-blame and low self-esteem through cognitive and supportive interventions was he able to tolerate the narcissistic injury attendant with exposing his perceived deficiencies; he was referred to a psychiatrist and in fact chose a male psychiatrist when presented with referrals to practitioners of both genders.

In an effort to tolerate or manage the ego-dystonic experience of feelings, vulnerability, and shame that may be evoked on entering treatment, men may attempt to save face by controlling the therapeutic process or devaluing the treatment or therapist (Carlson 1987; Heppner and Gonzales 1987; Pollack 2003). Carlson (1987) noted that the need for a male patient to assert his power and control in the therapeutic relationship may be particularly prominent with a female therapist: "These power dynamics in the relationship of the male client with a female counselor appear early....For a male to enter therapy and abdicate power to a woman, with whom he is usually expected to be dominant, is very stressful" (p. 44).

Carlson (1987) noted that the male client may also expect the female therapist to defer to his perceptions of the situation rather than question them or consider alternative views.

TREATMENT STRATEGIES

There are two main viewpoints on how to best address the treatment barriers and resistances described earlier within the context of ongoing treatment: 1) modification of existing treatment methods and 2) development of new techniques.

Modification of Existing Methods

One school of thought is to maintain the traditional format of psychotherapy but to modify it by emphasizing the therapist's need to be sensitive to gender-role socialization treatment resistances, to empathize with and respect the need for these defensive operations, to promote a collaborative working alliance, and to venture into examining feelings and vulnerabilities with caution. As Heppner and Gonzales (1987) stated, "The counselor needs to be cognizant of the male client's anxiety, especially early in therapy, being careful not to push too much too fast" (p. 32). Mahalik et al. (2003) emphasized that from the outset of treatment, clinicians should work to identify the expectations that male patients have about therapy and correct those that are erroneous—for example, by reassuring the patient that he will not be coerced to reveal what he does not want or is not ready to disclose. The therapist should regularly check with the patient regarding his experience of the therapy process in order to elicit any unrealistic fears or concerns that, if left uncorrected, might threaten the treatment (Heppner and Gonzales 1987). Pollack (2003) observed that if the patient's defensive autonomy is challenged prematurely, he may either terminate treatment or devalue the therapy or the therapist. Pollack advocated a relational psychoanalytic approach in which the therapist empathizes with the patient's fears and resistance and recreates an "early holding environment" by remaining calm and noncritical in the face of devaluation:

> With many young men…I have found it necessary to modify psychoanalytic psychotherapy not so much in its frequency, duration, or self-reflective model but rather in the arena of supporting the patient's need to believe, for long periods of time and without challenge to his denial, that both the therapy and therapist are almost unimportant to him. (p. 1208)

Carlson (1987) discussed techniques for addressing the power dynamics in the therapeutic relationship, dynamics that she believed are particularly prominent in treatments with a female therapist. She recommended explaining that the patient is in charge of defining the direction of the therapy and of educating the therapist about who he (the patient) is. However, she cautioned that, as mentioned earlier, the patient may expect the female therapist to defer to his perceptions of the situation rather than to question them or consider an alternative view, and that supporting this expectation and reinforcing sex role stereotypes within the context of the therapeutic relationship compromises the treatment. One man in psychoanalysis with a female therapist talked to the preclusion of analyst input. The therapist's comments or interpretations, when introduced, were generally discarded, and her questions and clarifications generally went unheeded. This man had a domineering wife, and in the treatment setting he appeared determined to get the upper hand. Only after the therapist called attention to this process in the treatment repeatedly and queried why the patient would bother coming to treatment if he was not interested in hearing the therapist's point of view did the patient begin to consider and evaluate the therapist's comments.

Development of New Techniques

A second, more radical viewpoint is that the fundamental parameters of psychotherapy should be altered to better match male gender-role expectations. Because male-role socialization places a premium on rational, logical thought and behavior, interventions developed for men have emphasized principles of cognitive therapy. An example is the "Choice, Change, and Confusion Reduction" treatment described by Good and May (1987). This treatment model is task oriented in that it conceptualizes the treatment goal as initially defining the choice or problem to be addressed. Over the course of treatment, the therapist assists the patient in learning and employing decision-making or problem-solving skills to achieve this goal. Therapeutic skills might include collecting relevant information and working with the patient to accurately evaluate the data collected.

Mahalik (1999) used Bem's (1981) cognitive theory of the development of gender-role schemata to describe a cognitively based intervention for men that relies on identifying the specific gender role–related "shoulds" and "musts" to which men learn to strive to adhere. Mahalik argued that these "shoulds" are best conceptualized as cognitive distortions, as defined by Beck (1963, 1964), in that they prescribe unattainable goals or unrealistic expectations for men that lead to gender-role strain and symptoms such as anxiety, depression, and substance abuse. Mahalik (1999) proposed eight areas of specific gender-related cognitive distortions in men that are associated with gender-role strain: success, power, emotional control, fearlessness, self-reliance, primacy of work, men as playboys, and disdain of homosexuals. Distortions within these domains can be monitored, identified, and challenged using techniques of cognitive therapy such as searching for disconfirming evidence and substituting more rational responses.

Mahalik's application of cognitive therapy principles to gender-role development and strain theory provides practitioners with clear, well-developed guidelines for addressing gender-role behavior that produces strain and symptoms. However, as Scher et al. (1987) noted, although men are most likely to experience symptom relief through cognitive interventions, such interventions may also reinforce the trait of

> excessive detachment from self and other.…Because self-awareness and self-exploration are narrowly defined in the cognitive-behavioral perspective, difficulties with therapy ensue. There is collusion with the restricting traditional male gender role. That is, the relationship component in therapy is ignored, and men are prematurely hooked into therapy for less valid reasons, for example, cognitive control versus the development of relationship awareness. (p. 389)

Scher et al. (1987) advocated a model of therapy called *masculist therapy* that emphasizes relationships and relies on a cooperative relationship between patient and therapist as a model for nontherapeutic relationships. Masculist therapy focuses on issues specifically related to male gender roles—emotional constriction, dominance, low self-disclosure, and competition—and helps the patient to "integrate these issues in a more humane way than is typical" (p. 390).

Gender aware therapy, which is grounded in feminist theory (Good et al. 1990), similarly regards conceptions of gender as integral aspects of the therapeutic process and helps patients to evaluate the impact of gender scripts on their lives in order to facilitate their freedom to choose whether to subscribe to these scripts or not. Like other therapies based on feminist theory, gender aware therapy de-emphasizes the expert role of the therapist in favor of a more collaborative, egalitarian role that short-circuits the competitive urge or drive in men.

A nontraditional type of therapy for school-age boys that emphasizes relationship aspects of the treatment has been described by Kiselica (2001). In order to correct for what he views as a mismatch between the parameters of traditional psychotherapy and the relational styles of adolescent boys, he advocates altering both the parameters of treatment (e.g., use of settings outside the office such as a gym, park, or restaurant; holding "office hours" for drop-in sessions instead of scheduled appointments) and the contents of sessions, including use of humor, self-disclosure, and issue-specific discussions.

TREATMENT PREFERENCES

Despite the different theoretical perspectives on appropriate treatment strategies for men, little research has been conducted to determine which kinds of treatments men find more acceptable or effective. Studies of college men describe different treatment approaches using a variety of formats such as pamphlets and videotapes in an effort to determine the most appealing form of treatment for men. Robertson and Fitzgerald (1992) found that college men with more masculine attitudes reacted more positively to brochures advertising alternative services such as classes, workshops, seminars, and circulating videotapes than they did to brochures advertising traditional mental health services offered by the university. Similarly, Wisch et al. (1995) found that highly gender-role-conflicted college men who viewed a videotape depicting emotion-focused therapy were significantly less willing to seek help than were 1) highly gender-role-conflicted men who viewed a videotape depicting cognition-focused therapy and 2) low gender-role-conflicted men in both the emotion-focused and cognition-focused conditions. Blazina and Marks (2001) adapted the brochure design employed by Robertson and Fitzgerald (1992) to advertise individual therapy, psychoeducational services, or a men's support group as treatment options to college men. Their results showed that highly gender-role-conflicted men had negative reactions to all three types of treatment but were significantly less accepting of the men's group and significantly more accepting of individual therapy. Attending a men's group might cause anxiety over the possibility of having to express emotions in the presence of other men—an action prohibited by male-role socialization. Men who experience high gender-role conflict may in fact be psychologically maladjusted, therefore recognizing on some level that if they were to seek treatment for their problems it would be in an individual setting.

OVERCOMING TREATMENT BARRIERS

We suggest four potential avenues for overcoming the barriers to mental health treatment–seeking described earlier in this chapter: 1) facilitating changing norms for male social role–appropriate behavior at both the societal and individual level, 2) modifying or developing treatments that better fit with the social-role constraints under which men currently operate, 3) expanding current research paradigms on male mental health treatment–seeking, and 4) incorporating material on masculine ideology and treatment resistances into standard training for physical as well as mental health practitioners.

Facilitating Changing Norms for Male Social Role–Appropriate Behavior

Men are particularly susceptible to negative attitudes toward treatment seeking because of the male social-role expectations of strength and self-reliance. Corrigan and Penn (1999) identified three strategies to reduce these negative attitudes: *protest* (e.g., challenging inaccurate representations of mental illness), *education*, and *contact* (recruitment or engagement of people with mental illness). Evidence on the value of protest is mixed, whereas results of education programs to reduce mental illness stigma have suggested positive, although somewhat transient, effects for participants (Corrigan 2004). Because men's negative attitudes toward treatment seeking are likely the result of gender-role socialization initiated during preschool years, real change in societally transmitted values needs to start with parenting groups, religious institutions, and literature handed out during visits to the obstetrician or Lamaze classes. To promote better ways of helping to resolve common problems experienced by adolescents and preadolescents, school health classes and programs that address other important health topics might also incorporate material that advocates students' seeking guidance from mental health professionals instead of resorting to substance use. In line with research on the value of contact, high school students at upper grade levels who have benefited from such assistance could contribute testimonials in such settings to their younger peers.

Modifying or Developing Modified Treatments to Match Male Social-Role Biases

We described examples of such treatment approaches earlier in this chapter, in the section "Treatment Strategies." Here we note that the development of gender-matched treatments is a double-edged sword: although such approaches may make needed help more available to some men, the creation of such treatments also represents an inherent if subtle collusion and reinforcement of current male gender stereotypes that have been shown to have adverse effects for some men (Cournoyer and Mahalik 1995; Good et al. 1995; Hayes and Mahalik 2000; Sharpe and Heppner 1991). The field of differential therapeutics (Beutler and Clarkin 1990) investigates methods for determining which types of treatments are most appropriate for which individuals, and screening methods might be developed to help predict which men might benefit most from modified traditional treatment versus gender-specific types of treatment (e.g., gender aware therapy). Methods such as *motivational interviewing* (Miller and Rollnick 1991), which is a patient-centered, low-reactance (i.e., less confrontational) approach with demonstrated efficacy in engaging patients in substance abuse treatment programs, might be adapted to help guide highly ambivalent yet highly distressed males into treatment.

Expanding Current Research Paradigms

As we noted earlier, most of the empirical research done on male treatment-seeking to date has focused on attitudes toward help seeking rather than on measuring predictors of actual service use. Although epidemiological surveys report data on actual service use, the ability to include mediating variables in such studies to help explain gender differences is inherently limited. Studies of actual mental health service use across a variety of settings are needed that incorporate measures of stigma, masculine ideology, and masculine gender-role conflict as well as measures of symptom distress and salient individual differences. Also needed are studies of what types of treatment men find most acceptable and from which they believe they will most benefit. Corrigan (2004) noted that it is important that future research distinguish between people who are deterred from seeking treatment to avoid the public discrimination that comes from labels (public stigma) and those who avoid seeking treatment with its attendant label of mental illness in order to protect themselves from a loss of self-esteem (self-stigma).

Our model and review of the literature suggest that future studies also need to distinguish between primary appraisal (problem recognition) and secondary appraisal (acknowledgment of need for help). Campaigns to normalize mental health treatment–seeking are unlikely to help motivate men or boys who may not recognize or may greatly minimize the degree of the stressors confronting them. Identifying differential predictors of primary and secondary appraisal may help to develop more finely targeted interventions.

Incorporating Material on Masculine Ideology Into Standard Training Programs

As discussed in the section "Treatment Strategies," therapists should be sensitive to the unvoiced needs of their male patients and tolerant of resistances that emerge as men begin to engage in emotional disclosure and other behaviors that counter socially prescribed male gender roles. Training for mental and physical health practitioners and educators should foster an understanding of the difficulties men may experience in expressing their emotional needs verbally and teach these practitioners to identify emotional distress or related problems such as substance abuse and somatization. Training for psychotherapists should also examine the therapist's countertransference to male patients, with a focus on his or her own orientation toward gender norms. For example, as Wester and Vogel (2002) noted, the traditional male's preoccupation with success and competition also has the potential to interfere with the appropriate conduct of psychotherapy because some male therapists may feel the need to outperform their clients (Hayes 1984). Other studies have shown that male therapists high in restricted emotionality and restricted affectionate behavior between men (two indices of gender-role conflict) report less empathy for, and more interpersonal difficulties with, both gay and highly emotional clients. Through appropriate training and supervision, therapists may learn their own strengths and limitations as providers and optimize their therapeutic approaches.

CAVEATS

Several caveats warrant mention regarding the discussion in this chapter. The stress and coping framework of primary and secondary appraisal that we have utilized here is most applicable to males seeking treatment for stress-induced symptoms of psychological distress or males seeking treatment for stress-induced exacerbations of a preexisting mental disorder. Additional parameters may help explain barriers to men's use of mental health services when they have chronic conditions unrelated to situational stress. Although we expect that male-role socialization and stigma would continue to serve as barriers to service use for men with serious mental illness, the effects of these factors may be reduced and other factors not examined here may be more salient. Because most studies to date have focused on treatment seeking of men with less severe disorders, little is known about the barriers to mental health treatment of men with more serious mental illnesses.

Although we have focused attention on barriers to effective mental health treatment for men and potential ways to reduce these barriers, we do not mean to imply that these barriers and treatment resistances apply uniquely to men. Women who assume traditionally "masculine" roles or jobs such as corporate executives or police officers may share some of the attitudes and concerns that lead to treatment barriers or resistances for men. Additionally, although the data from epidemiological studies suggest there are fewer barriers to mental health treatment for women than for men, women also experience conflict or ambivalence in relation to traditional gender-role expectations (Silverstein and Perlick 1995), and such conflict may be expected to pose challenges to, or dilute the effectiveness of, mental health treatment for women, although in different ways from those we have described for men (e.g., Flordh 1992; Kolod 2002; Lutwak 1998). Increasing awareness about how traditional gender-role stereotypes serve as barriers to mental health treatment may help to lessen men's need to rigidly adhere to such stereotypes, ones that limit the capacity for personal growth both inside and outside of treatment.

CONCLUSION

We have posited that men in psychological distress are faced with appreciable barriers to seeking mental health treatment and are less likely to seek help than are equally distressed female counterparts. We have argued that these barriers stem from discrimination and devaluation of persons with mental illness on the one hand and from the anticipated risks of violating male gender-role behavioral proscriptions on the other. We adopted a stress and coping framework of primary and secondary appraisal to suggest that these barriers are manifested in multiple steps of the treatment-seeking process. Male-role prohibitions against expressing emotion may prevent men from accurately appraising the severity of their problems and acknowledging a need for help. Men who overcome these treatment-entry barriers and initiate treatment, we argue, still must contend with the same adverse societal influences, in the forms of self-stigma, decrements in self-esteem, feelings of discomfort and anxiety evoked by the emotional demands of psychotherapy, and potential social ostracism from peers or family espousing traditional masculine ideals or mental illness stigma. As a response to these problems, we identified four potential solutions to help reduce the adverse effects of mental illness stigma and male-role socialization on the treatment-seeking process and to increase men's ability to seek help for their emotional problems free from disapprobation from themselves or others:

1. Facilitate changing norms for male social role–appropriate behavior.
2. Modify or develop modified treatments to match male social-role biases.
3. Expand current research paradigms.
4. Incorporate material on masculine ideology into standard training programs.

KEY POINTS

- Barriers to men's seeking mental health treatment stem from discriminatory and devaluing attitudes toward people with mental illness and from anticipated risks of violating male gender-role behavioral proscriptions.

- These factors also influence men's ability to identify emotional problems and to recognize the need to seek help from a mental health professional.

PRACTICE GUIDELINES

1. Therapists should be sensitive to the unvoiced needs of their male patients and be tolerant of resistances that emerge as men begin to engage in emotional disclosure and other behaviors that counter socially proscribed male gender roles.

2. Male patients with female therapists may experience different important treatment resistances than male patients with male therapists, and therapists of both genders should be cognizant of these potential resistances.

REFERENCES

Addis ME, Mahalik JR: Men, masculinity, and the contexts of help seeking. Am Psychol 58:5–14, 2003

Albizu-Garcia CE, Alegria M, Freeman D, et al: Gender and health services use for a mental health problem. Soc Sci Med 53:865–878, 2001

Beck AT: Thinking and depression, I: idiosyncratic content and cognitive distortions. Arch Gen Psychiatry 9:324–333, 1963

Beck AT: Thinking and depression, II: theory and therapy. Arch Gen Psychiatry 10:561–571, 1964

Bem S: Gender schema theory: a cognitive account of sex typing. Psychol Rev 88:354–364, 1981

Beutler LE, Clarkin JF: Systematic Treatment Selection: Toward Targeted Therapeutic Interventions. New York, Brunner/Mazel, 1990

Blazina C, Marks L: College men's affective reactions to individual therapy, psychoeducational workshops, and men's support group brochures: the influence of gender-role conflict and power dynamics upon help-seeking attitudes. Psychotherapy 38:297–305, 2001

Blazina C, Watkins CE Jr: Masculine gender role conflict: effects on college men's psychological well-being, chemical substance usage, and attitudes toward help seeking. J Couns Psychol 43:461–465, 1996

Boldero J, Fallon B: Adolescent help-seeking: what do they get help for and from whom? J Adolesc 18:193–209, 1995

Bordieri J, Drehmer D: Hiring decisions for disabled workers: looking at the cause. J Appl Soc Psychol 16:197–208, 1986

Brehm JW: Postdecision changes in the desirability of alternatives. J Abnorm Soc Psychol 52:384–389, 1956

Brooks GR, Good GE (eds): The New Handbook of Psychotherapy and Counseling With Men, Vols 1 and 2. San Francisco, CA, Jossey-Bass, 2001

Bursley KH: Gender role strain and help-seeking attitudes and behavior in college men. Diss Abstr Int 56:3884a, 1996

Carlson NL: Woman therapist: male client, in Handbook of Counseling and Psychotherapy With Men. Edited by Scher M, Stevens M, Good G, et al. Newbury Park, CA, Sage, 1987, pp 39–50

Carpenter KM, Addis ME: Alexithymia, gender and responses to depressive symptoms. Sex Roles 43:629–644, 2000

Chodorow N: The Reproduction of Mothering. Berkeley, University of California Press, 1978

Cochran SV: Assessing and treating depression in men, in The New Handbook of Psychotherapy and Counseling With Men. Edited by Brooks GR, Good GE. San Francisco, CA, Jossey-Bass, 2001, pp 229–245

Cochran SV, Rabinowitz FE: Men and depression: clinical and empirical perspectives. San Diego, CA, Academic Press, 2000

Cooper AE, Corrigan PW, Watson AC: Mental illness stigma and care seeking. J Nerv Ment Dis 191:339–341, 2003

Corrigan P: How stigma interferes with mental health care. Am Psychol 59:614–625, 2004

Corrigan PW, Penn DL: Lessons from social psychology on discrediting psychiatric stigma. Am Psychol 54:765–776, 1999

Corrigan PW, Watson AC: The paradox of self-stigma and mental illness. Clinical Psychology: Science and Practice 9:35–53, 2002

Cournoyer RJ, Mahalik JR: Cross-sectional study of gender role conflict examining college-aged and middle-aged men. J Couns Psychol 42:11–19, 1995

Deane FR, Chamberlain K: Treatment fearfulness and distress as predictors of professional psychological help–seeking. Br J Guid Counc 22:207–217, 1994

Farina A: Stigma, in Handbook of Social Functioning in Schizophrenia. Edited by Mueser KT, Tarrier, N. Boston, MA, Allyn & Bacon, 1998, pp 247–279

Farina A, Felner RD: Employment interviewer reactions to former mental patients. J Abnorm Psychol 82:268–272, 1973

Festinger L: A Theory of Cognitive Dissonance. Stanford, CA, Stanford University Press, 1957

Festinger L: Conflict, Decision, and Dissonance. Stanford, CA, Stanford University Press, 1964

Fischer AR, Good GE: Men and psychotherapy: an investigation of alexithymia, intimacy, and masculine gender roles. Psychotherapy: Theory, Research, Practice, Training 34:160–170, 1997

Fischer EH, Turner JL: Orientation to seeking professional psychological help: development and research utility of an attitude scale. J Consult Clin Psychol 35:79–90, 1970

Flordh C: Longings for fusion and autonomy in the relation between the female analyst and the female patient. International Forum of Psychoanalysis 1:175–179, 1992

Freud S: Some character-types met with in psycho-analytic work (1916), in The Collected Papers of Sigmund Freud, Vol 4. Translated by Riviere J. Edited by Jones E. New York, NY, Basic Books, 1959

Gabbard GO, Gabbard K: Cinematic stereotypes contributing to the stigmatization of psychiatrists, in Stigma and Mental Illness. Edited by Fink PJ, Tasman A. Washington, DC, American Psychiatric Press, 1992, pp 113–126

Gilligan C: In a Different Voice. Cambridge, MA, Harvard University Press, 1982

Good G, May R: Developmental issues, environmental influences, and the nature of therapy with college men, in Handbook of Counseling and Psychotherapy With Men. Edited by Scher M, Stevens M, Good G, et al. Newbury Park, CA, Sage, pp 150–164, 1987

Good GE, Mintz LB: Gender role conflict and depression in college men: evidence for compounded risk. J Couns Dev 69:17–21, 1990

Good GE, Wood PK: Male gender role conflict, depression, and help seeking: do college men face double jeopardy? J Couns Dev 74:69–75, 1995

Good GE, Dell DM, Mintz LB: Male role and gender role conflict: relations to help seeking in men. J Couns Psychol 36:295–300, 1989

Good GE, Gilbert LA, Scher M: Gender aware therapy: a synthesis of feminist therapy and knowledge about gender. J Couns Dev 68:376–380, 1990

Good GE, Robertson JM, O'Neil JM, et al: Male gender role conflict: psychometric properties and relations to distress. J Couns Psychol 42:3–10, 1995

Greenson R: Disidentifying from mother. Int J Psychoanal 49:370–374, 1968

Hayes JA, Mahalik JR: Gender role conflict and psychological distress in male counseling center clients. Psychology of Men and Masculinity 1:116–125, 2000

Hayes MM: Counselor sex-role values and effects on attitudes toward and treatment of nontraditional male clients. Unpublished doctoral dissertation, Ohio State University, Columbus, OH, 1984 [Diss Abstr Int 45:3072, 1984]

Heppner PP, Gonzales DS: Men counseling men, in Handbook of Counseling and Psychotherapy With Men. Edited by Scher M, Stevens M, Good G, et al. Newbury Park, CA, Sage, 1987, pp 30–50

Hyler SE, Gabbard GO, Schneider I: Homicidal maniacs and narcissistic parasites: stigmatization of mentally ill persons in the movies. Hosp Community Psychiatry 42:1044–1048, 1991

Johnson ME: Influences of gender and sex role orientation on help-seeking attitudes. J Psychol 122:237–241, 1988

Keane M: Contemporary beliefs about mental illness among medical students: implications for education and practice. Acad Psychiatry 14:172–177, 1990

Kessler RC, Brown RL, Broman CL: Sex differences in psychiatric help–seeking: evidence from four large-scale surveys. J Health Soc Behav 22:49–64, 1981

Kessler RC, McGonagle KA, Zhao S, et al: Lifetime and 12-month prevalence of DSM-III psychiatric disorders in the United States: results from the National Comorbidity Survey. Arch Gen Psychiatry 51:8–19, 1994

Kirschner LA: Effects of gender on psychotherapy. Compr Psychiatry 19:79–82, 1978

Kiselica MS: A male-friendly therapeutic process with school-age boys, in The New Handbook of Psychotherapy and Counseling With Men. Edited by Brooks GR, Good GE. San Francisco, CA, Jossey-Bass, 2001, pp 43–58

Kolod S: Between women: love and combat. Contemp Psychoanal 38:315–328, 2002

Komiya N, Good GE, Sherrod NB: Emotional openness as a predictor of college students' attitudes toward seeking psychological help. J Couns Psychol 47: 138–143, 2000

Kushner MG, Sher KJ: The relation of treatment fearfulness and psychological service utilization: an overview. Prof Psychol Res Pr 22:196–203, 1991

Lazarus RS: Emotion and Adaptation. New York, Oxford University Press, 1991

Lazarus RS, Folkman S: The concept of coping, in Stress and Coping: An Anthology. Edited by Monat A, Lazarus RS. New York, Columbia University Press, 1991, pp 189–206

Leaf PJ, Bruce ML: Gender differences in the use of mental health–related services: a re-examination. J Health Soc Behav 28:171–183, 1987

Leaf PJ, Bruce ML, Tischler GL, et al: Factors affecting the utilization of specialty and general medical mental health services. Med Care 26:9–26, 1988

Lefley HP: The stigmatized family, in Stigma and Mental Illness. Edited by Fink PJ, Tasman A. Washington, DC, American Psychiatric Press, 1992, pp 127–138

Leong FTL, Zachar P: Gender and opinions about mental illness as predictors of attitudes toward seeking professional psychological help. Br J Guid Counc 27:123–132, 1999

Levant RF: Desperately seeking language: understanding, assessing, and treating normative male alexithymia, in The New Handbook of Psychotherapy and Counseling With Men. Edited by Brooks GR, Good GE. San Francisco, CA, Jossey-Bass, 2001, pp 424–443

Levant RF, Richmond K, Majors RG, et al: A multicultural investigation of masculinity ideology and alexithymia. Psychology of Men and Masculinity 4: 91–99, 2003

Lin E, Goering P, Offord DR, et al: The use of mental health services in Ontario: epidemiologic findings. Can J Psychiatry 41:572–577, 1996

Link BG: Understanding labeling effects in the area of mental disorders and assessment of the effects of expectations of rejection. Am Sociol Rev 52:96–112, 1987

Link BG, Phelan JC: Labeling and stigma, in Handbook of the Sociology of Mental Health. Edited by Aneshensel CS, Phelan JC. New York, Kluwer Academic/Plenum, 1999, pp 481–494

Link BG, Cullen FT, Frank J, et al: The social rejection of former mental patients: understanding why labels matter. Am J Sociol 92:1461–1500, 1987

Link BG, Cullen FT, Struening EL, et al: A modified labeling theory approach to mental disorders: an empirical assessment. Am Sociol Rev 54:400–423, 1989

Lutwak N: Shame, women, and group psychotherapy. Group 22:129–143, 1998

Lyons M, Ziviani J: Stereotypes, stigma and mental illness: learning from fieldwork experiences. Am J Occup Ther 49:1002–1008, 1995

Mahalik JR: Incorporating a gender role strain perspective in assessing and treating men's cognitive distortions. Prof Psychol Res Pr 30:333–340, 1999

Mahalik JR, Good GE, Englar-Carlson M: Masculinity scripts, presenting concerns, and help seeking: implications for practice and training. Prof Psychol Res Pr 34:123–131, 2003

Mayer A, Barry DD: Working with the media to destigmatize mental illness. Hosp Community Psychiatry 43:77–78, 1992

Miller WR, Rollnick S: Motivational Interviewing: Preparing People to Change Addictive Behavior. New York, Guilford, 1991

Millman EJ: The mental health and biosocial context of help seeking in longitudinal perspective: the Midtown Longitudinal Study, 1954 to 1974. Am J Orthopsychiatry 71:450–456, 2001

Mirabi M, Weinman ML, Magnetti SM, et al: Professional attitudes toward the chronic mentally ill. Hosp Community Psychiatry 36:404–405, 1985

Monahan J: Mental disorder and violent behavior: perceptions and evidence. Am Psychol 47:511–521, 1992

O'Neil JM: Patterns of gender role conflict and strain: sexism and fear of femininity in men's lives. Pers Guid J 60:203–210, 1981

O'Neil JM: Gender role conflict and strain in men's lives: implications for psychiatrists, psychologists, and other human service providers, in Men in Transition. Edited by Solomon K, Levy NB. New York, Plenum, 1982, pp 5–40

O'Neil JM, Good GE, Holmes S: Fifteen years of theory and research on men's gender role conflict: new paradigms for empirical research, in A New Psychology of Men. Edited by Levant RF, Pollack WS. New York, Basic Books, 1995, pp 164–206

Olshansky S, Grob S, Ekdahl M: Survey of employment experience of patients discharged from three mental hospitals during the period 1951–1953. Ment Hyg 44:510–521, 1960

Page S: Effects of the mental illness label in attempts to obtain accommodation. Can J Behav Sci 9:85–90, 1977

Page S: Social responsiveness toward mental patients: the general public and others. Can J Psychiatry 25:242–246, 1980

Page S: Psychiatric stigma: two studies of behavior when the chips are down. Can J Commun Ment Health 2:13–19, 1983

Page S: Effects of the mental illness label in 1993: acceptance and rejection in the community. J Health Soc Policy 7:61–68, 1995

Parsons T: The Social System. New York, Free Press, 1951

Perlick DA: Special section on stigma as a barrier to recovery: introduction. Psychiatr Serv 52:1613–1614, 2001

Pleck JH, Sonenstein FL, Ku LC: Masculinity ideology and its correlates, in Gender Issues in Social Psychology. Edited by Oskamp S, Costanzo M. Newbury Park, CA, Sage, 1993, pp 85–110

Pollack WS: "Masked men": new psychoanalytically oriented treatment models for adult and young adult men, in The New Handbook of Psychotherapy and Counseling With Men. Edited by Brooks GR, Good GE. San Francisco, CA, Jossey-Bass, 2001, pp 527–543

Pollack WS: Relational psychoanalytic treatment for young adult males. J Clin Psychol 59:1205–1213, 2003

Ponterotto JG, Rao V, Zwieg J, et al: The relationship of acculturation and gender to attitudes toward counseling in Italian and Greek American college students. Cultur Divers Ethnic Minor Psychol 7:362–375, 2001

Regier DA, Narrow WE, Rae DS, et al: The de facto U.S. mental and addictive disorders service system: Epidemiologic Catchment Area prospective 1-year prevalence rates of disorders and services. Arch Gen Psychiatry 50: 85–94, 1993

Rhodes AE, Goering PN, To T, et al: Gender and outpatient mental health service use. Soc Sci Med 54:1–10, 2002

Rice DG: Patient sex differences and selection for individual therapy. J Nerv Ment Dis 148:124–133, 1969

Robertson JM, Fitzgerald LF: Overcoming the masculine mystique: preferences for alternative forms of assistance among men who avoid counseling. J Couns Psychol 39:240–246, 1992

Robin RW, Chester B, Rasmussen JK, et al: Factors influencing utilization of mental health and substance abuse services by American Indian men and women. Psychiatr Serv 48:826–832, 1997

Scher M: On counseling men. Pers Guid J 58:252–254, 1979

Scher M, Stevens M, Good G, et al (eds): Handbook of Counseling and Psychotherapy With Men. Newbury Park, CA, Sage, 1987

Schober R, Annis HM: Barriers to help seeking for change in drinking: a gender-focused review of the literature. Addict Behav 21:81–92, 1996

Scott DJ, Philip AE: Attitudes of psychiatric nurses to treatment and patients. Br J Med Psychol 58:169–173, 1985

Sharpe MJ, Heppner PP: Gender role, gender-role conflict, and psychological well-being in men. J Couns Psychol 39:240–246, 1991

Sibicky M, Dovidio JF: Stigma of psychological therapy: stereotypes, interpersonal reactions, and the self-fulfilling prophecy. J Couns Psychol 33:148–154, 1986

Silverstein B, Perlick D: The Cost of Competence. New York, Oxford University Press, 1995

Sirey JA, Bruce ML, Alexopoulos GS, et al: Stigma as a barrier to recovery: perceived stigma and patient-rated severity of illness as predictors of antidepressant drug adherence. Psychiatr Serv 52:1615–1620, 2001

Stanton-Salazar RD, Chavez LF, Tai RH: The help-seeking orientations of Latino and non-Latino urban high school students: a critical-sociological investigation. Social Psychology of Education 5:49–82, 2001

Thompson EH Jr, Pleck JH: The structure of male role norms. Am Behav Sci 29:531–544, 1986

Timlin-Scalera RM, Ponterotto JG, Blumberg FC, et al: A grounded theory study of help-seeking behaviors among white male high school students. J Couns Psychol 50:339–350, 2003

Wahl O: Media Madness: Public Images of Mental Illness. New Brunswick, NJ, Rutgers University Press, 1995

Wahl O, Harman C: Family views of stigma. Schizophr Bull 15:131–139, 1989

Wester SR, Vogel DL: Working with the masculine mystique: male gender role conflict, counseling self-efficacy, and the training of male psychologists. Prof Psychol Res Pr 33:370–376, 2002

Wisch AF, Mahalik JR, Hayes JA, et al: The impact of gender role conflict and counseling technique on psychological help seeking in men. Sex Roles 33:77–89, 1995

Yeh CJ: Taiwanese students' gender, age, interdependent and independent self-construal, and collective self-esteem as predictors of professional psychological help–seeking attitudes. Cultur Divers Ethnic Minor Psychol 8:19–29, 2002

INDEX

*Page numbers printed in **boldface** type refer to tables or figures.*